LAPAROSCOPIC SURGERY
IN GYNAECOLOGICAL ONCOLOGY

Laparoscopic Surgery in Gynaecological Oncology

EDITED BY

Denis Querleu
Hôpital Jeanne de Flandre,
59000 Lille, France

Joel M. Childers
Arizona Oncology Associates,
Tucson, Arizona 85712, USA

Daniel Dargent
Hôpital Edouard Herriot,
69374 Lyon, France

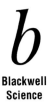

**Blackwell
Science**

© 1999 by
Blackwell Science Ltd
Editorial Offices:
Osney Mead, Oxford OX2 OEL
25 John Street, London WC1N 2BL
23 Ainslie Place, Edinburgh EH3 6AJ
350 Main Street, Malden
   MA 02148 5018, USA
54 University Street, Carlton
   Victoria 3053, Australia
10, rue Casimir Delavigne
   75006 Paris, France

Other Editorial Offices:
Blackwell Wissenschafts-Verlag GmbH
Kurfürstendamm 57
10707 Berlin, Germany

Blackwell Science KK
MG Kodenmacho Building
7–10 Kodenmacho Nihombashi
Chuo-ku, Tokyo 104, Japan

First published 1999

Set by Excel Typesetters Co., Hong Kong
Printed and bound in Italy by
Rotolito Lombarda S.p.A., Milan

The Blackwell Science logo is a
trade mark of Blackwell Science Ltd,
registered at the United Kingdom
Trade Marks Registry

A catalogue record for this title
is available from the British Library

ISBN 0-86542-692-9

Library of Congress
cataloging-in-publication data

Laparoscopic surgery in gynaecological
   oncology/edited by Denis Querleu,
   Joel M. Childers, Daniel Dargent.
         p.   cm.
      Includes bibliographical references.
      ISBN 0-86542-692-9
      1. Generative organs, Female—
   Cancer—Endoscopic surgery.
   2. Laparoscopic surgery. I. Querleu,
   Denis. II. Childers, Joel M.   III.
   Dargent, D.
      [DNLM: 1. Genital Neoplasms,
   Female—surgery.   2. Surgical
   Procedures, Laparoscopic.   3. Genital
   Neoplasms, Female—diagnosis.
   WP   145 L592   1999]
   RG104.7.L36   1999
   616.99′465059—dc21
   DNLM/DLC
   for Library of Congress   98-36147
                                    CIP

DISTRIBUTORS

Marston Book Services Ltd
PO Box 269
Abingdon, Oxon OX14 4YN
(Orders: Tel: 01235 465500
              Fax: 01235 465555)
USA
Blackwell Science, Inc.
Commerce Place
350 Main Street
Malden, MA 02148 5018
(Orders: Tel: 800 759 6102
                    781 388 8250
              Fax: 781 388 8255)
Canada
Login Brothers Book Company
324 Saulteaux Crescent
Winnipeg, Manitoba. R3J 3T2
(Orders: Tel: 204 837-2987)

Australia
Blackwell Science Pty Ltd
54 University Street
Carlton, Victoria 3053
(Orders: Tel: 3 9347 0300
              Fax: 3 9347 5001)

For further information on
Blackwell Science, visit our website:
www.blackwell-science.com

Contents

List of contributors

Mark D. Adelson *730 South Crouse Avenue, Suite 203, Syracuse, New York, NY 13210-1746, USA*

Maurice-Antoine Bruhat *Department of Obstetrics, Gynecology and Reproductive Medicine, Polyclinique de L'Hôtel Dieu, 13 Boulevard Charles de Gaulle, 63033 Clermont Ferrand Cedex 1, France*

Matthew O. Burrell *Institute for Gynecologic Oncology, 980 Johnson Ferry Road, Suite 900, Atlanta, GA 30342, USA*

Michel Canis *Department of Obstetrics, Gynecology and Reproductive Medicine, Polyclinique de L'Hôtel Dieu, 13 Boulevard Charles de Gaulle, 63033 Clermont Ferrand Cedex 1, France*

Charles Chapron *Maternité Cochin-Baudelocque, 123 Boulevard de Port Royal, 75079 Paris Cedex 14, France*

Joel M. Childers *Arizona Oncology Associates, 2625 North Craycroft Road, Suite 201, Tucson, AZ 85712, USA*

Daniel Dargent *Hôpital Edouard Herriot, Pavillon K, Place d'Arsonval, 69374 Lyon Cedex, France*

François Dubecq *35 rue de Turenne, 33000 Bordeaux, France*

Abdou Elhage *Department of Obstetrics and Gynecology, Hotel-Dieu, Beirut, Lebanon*

Keith M. Harrigill *The University Physicians, 1501 North Campbell, Tucson, AZ 85712, USA*

Nicholas Kadar *The New Margaret Hague Women's Health Institute, Jode Professional Plaza, 193 Route 9 South, Suite 2A, Manalapan, NJ 07726, USA*

Dominique Lanvin *Department of Gynecology Oncology, Hôpital Jeanne de Flandre, CHRU, 5900 Lille, France*

Eric Le Goupils *Faculté de Médecine de Lille, Chirurgie Gynécologique Cancerologie, Pavillon Paul Gellé, 91 Avenue Julien Lagache, 59100 Roubaix, France*

Eric Leblanc *Centre Oscar Lambret, Rue Frédéric Combemale, 59000 Lille, France*

Fabrice Lecuru *Department of Maternity, Hôpital Boucicaut, 75015 Paris, France*

Gérard Mage *Department of Obstetrics, Gynecology and Reproductive Medicine, Polyclinique de L'Hôtel Dieu, 13 Boulevard Charles de Gaulle, 63033 Clermont Ferrand Cedex 1, France*

Mitchell Maiman *Department of Obstetrics and Gynecology, Staten Island University Hospital, 475 Seaview Avenue, Staten Island, NY 10305, USA*

Hubert Manhes *Department of Obstetrics, Gynecology and Reproductive Medicine, Polyclinique de L'Hôtel Dieu, 13 Boulevard Charles de Gaulle, 63033 Clermont Ferrand Cedex 1, France*

Patrice Mathevet *Hôpital Edouard Herriot, Pavillon K, Place d'Arsonval, 69437 Lyon Cedex 03, France*

Patrice Mille *Department of Obstetrics, Gynecology and Reproductive Medicine, Polyclinique de L'Hôtel Dieu, 13 Boulevard Charles de Gaulle, 63033 Clermont Ferrand Cedex 1, France*

Hania Moal *Department of Obstetrics, Gynecology and Reproductive Medicine, Polyclinique de L'Hôtel Dieu, 13 Boulevard Charles de Gaulle, 63033 Clermont Ferrand Cedex 1, France*

John Monaghan *Gynaecological Oncology Centre, Queen Elizabeth Hospital, Sheriff Hill, Gateshead, Tyne and Wear NE9 6SX, USA*

Fredrick J. Montz *Department of Gynecology and Obstetrics, Johns Hopkins Hospital, 600 North Wolfe Street, Houck 248, Baltimore, MD 21287-1248, USA*

Fariba Nasserbakht *Department of Surgery, Stanford University School of Medicine, Stanford, CA 94304, USA*

Camran Nezhat *Department of Surgery, Obstetrics and Gynecology, Stanford University School of Medicine, Stanford, CA 94304, USA*

Ceana H. Nezhat *Department of Surgery, Obstetrics and Gynecology, Stanford University School of Medicine, Stanford, CA 94304, USA*

Farr Nezhat *Department of Obstetrics and Gynecology, Stanford University School of Medicine, Stanford, CA 94304 , USA*

Magdy W. Nour *The University Physicians, 1501 North Campbell, Tucson, AZ 85712, USA*

Marie Plante *Department of Obstetrics and Gynecology, Laval University, Chuq-Pavillon, L'Hôtel Dieu de Quebec, 11 Côte du Palais, Quebec G1R 2J6, Canada*

Christophe Pomel *Department of Obstetrics, Gynecology and Reproductive Medicine, Polyclinique de L'Hôtel Dieu, 13 Boulevard Charles de Gaulle, 63033 Clermont Ferrand Cedex 1, France*

Jean-Luc Pouly *Department of Obstetrics, Gynecology and Reproductive Medicine, Polyclinique de L'Hôtel Dieu, 13 Boulevard Charles de Gaulle, 63033 Clermont Ferrand Cedex 1, France*

Denis Querleu *Department of Gynecology Oncology, Hôpital Jeanne de Flandre, CHRU, 59000 Lille, France*

Jacques Raiga *Department of Obstetrics, Gynecology and Reproductive Medicine, Polyclinique de L'Hôtel Dieu, 13 Boulevard Charles de Gaulle, 63033 Clermont Ferrand Cedex 1, France*

Michel Roy *Department of Obstetrics and Gynecology, Laval University, Chuq-Pavillon, L'Hôtel Dieu de Quebec, 11 Côte du Palais, Quebec G1R 2J6, Canada*

Daniel S. Seidman *Department of Obstetrics and Gynecology, Stanford University School of Medicine, Stanford, CA 94304, USA*

Earl A. Surwit *Department of Obstetrics and Gynecology, Division of Gynecologic Oncology, University of Arizona College of Medicine, Tucson, AZ 85724, USA*

Arnaud Wattiez *Department of Obstetrics, Gynecology and Reproductive Medicine, Polyclinique de L'Hôtel Dieu, 13 Boulevard Charles de Gaulle, 63033 Clermont Ferrand Cedex 1, France*

Preface

The introduction of endoscopic surgery to gynaecological oncology is now over 10 years old. The movement started in France and then in the United States, and we consider ourselves fortunate to have been some of the early investigators in the field. We are also blessed in that virtually all the early pioneers in this pursuit have been willing to contribute to this text. We appreciate their willingness to participate in such an enterprise.

As with any oncology text, there is great variation in each author's philosophies on management. Laparoscopy aside, there is not a universal consensus on the management of any gynaecological malignancy. The introduction of laparoscopy in gynaecological oncology only compounds an already complex area, and of course makes a controversial topic even more so. We respect these individual and regional philosophical differences and encourage the reader of this text to read between the lines.

It is not our intent to change your personal beliefs. It *is* our intent to introduce you to alternative surgical techniques that we believe can readily be incorporated into most oncological practices and can improve the quality of life for our patients. We appreciate the infancy of laparoscopy in oncology, and fully recognize that, above all, the survival of our patients is of the utmost importance and cannot be compromised.

We delayed the publication of this first book on laparoscopy in oncology until we genuinely believed that the propagation of this technique was ethically acceptable. We have developed our techniques independently but for many years have worked in a friendly and fecund collaboration, constantly learning from and working with one another to spread and encourage the growth of this technique worldwide. This book is a token of our unified belief in the validity of operative laparoscopy. While our philosophies on oncological management may differ in many respects, spiritually we believe in the philosophy of laparoscopic surgery. Through individualization of patient management and improvement of quality of life, operative laparoscopy may be one of the greatest advances in gynaecological oncology we will see in our lifetimes.

Laparoscopic surgery of cancer is not a technique, it is a philosophy.

Denis Querleu
Joel Childers
Daniel Dargent

1 History of laparoscopic surgery in gynaecological oncology

Fredrick J. Montz

Introduction

Jacobaeus, in 1910, was the first to visualize the peritoneal cavity in the human using an optical instrument [1]. He performed this procedure using a modification of a technique described earlier in the century by Kelling [2]. Kelling had performed his procedure in canines, creating an air pneumoperitoneum with a needle and then inserting a luminated cystoscope that had been developed by Nitze in the 1870s [3]. By contrast, Jacobaeus created the pneumoperitoneum using a trocar, prior to inserting the Nitze cystoscope.

Peritoneoscopy remained generally unused in the USA until the late 1930s. At this time, methods for the coagulation of fallopian tubes using laparoscopy were developed, and the initial clinical reports were published in the early 1940s [4]. In the ensuing four decades there were improvements and variations in laparoscopic sterilization techniques, but little application of this technology in the performance of more 'advanced' procedures.

Following the reports of the use of laparoscopy for the management of tubal gestations in the early 1980s [5,6], the 'flag was literally dropped', and there was a race to apply the laparoscopic approach to almost all intraperitoneal gynaecological procedures that were traditionally performed via laparotomy. Associated with this, certain endoscopic surgeons felt a sense of urgency not only to be the 'first' to perform a given procedure laparoscopically, but also to explore how much use could be made of laparoscopic surgery. This led to the development of innumerable new tools which could be used to facilitate the performance of progressively more complex and intricate operations laparoscopically. It is within this milieu that laparoscopy came to be employed for the management of various gynaecological malignances.

Endometrial cancer

For decades it had been proposed that vaginal hysterectomy was a potential and, at times, preferable route in select women with endometrial cancer. Unfortunately, the vaginal approach did not guarantee adequate adnexal management or thorough exploration of the peritoneal cavity and its contents. Similarly, lymph-node sampling, which became an essential part of the appropriate staging of endometrial cancer following the 1988 recommendation by the Cancer Committee of the International Federation of Gynecology and Obstetrics (FIGO) [7], could not be readily performed via the vagina. Theoretically, the addition of a laparoscopic procedure to the vaginal hysterectomy could potentially correct these deficiencies. Reich proposed, and others proved [8–10], that this was the case in the management of the uterus and the adnexa, whereas in laparoscopic lymph-node dissection or sampling developments were slow.

The first reports on laparoscopic pelvic node sampling/dissection were from cases of cervical and prostate cancer [11,12], with Dargent, in 1989, publishing his now famous report of laparoscopic pelvic node dissection in patients with cervical malignancies. Subsequent investigations confirmed that these techniques were effective for removing the pelvic nodes in patients with prostate cancer, while at the same time having a lower morbidity and being less expensive than the traditional open techniques [13–15]. Despite these advances, the technique of laparoscopic node sampling in the late 1980s was inadequate for surgical staging of endometrial cancer and, for that matter, the majority of malignances that arise from the internal genital organs. This inadequacy was because the sentinel para-aortic lymph nodes were not being sampled. In the early 1990s, multiple centres (Montz and associates [16] using an animal model; Childers and Surwit as well as Querleu and his fellow researchers, humans [17,18]) independently developed various techniques for adequate para-aortic lymph-node sampling. Since the publication of these initial reports, various authors have presented their preliminary experiences at scientific meetings, but only selected reports have been published. To date, the largest and most credible collection is that of the investigators at the University of Arizona in Tucson. In their most recent published series [19], Childers and associates reported on 59 patients who underwent laparoscopically assisted surgical staging as the management of early endometrial cancer. Only 29 patients were considered to be suitable for laparoscopic lymphadenectomy. Childers *et al.* were able to successfully perform a laparoscopic lymphadenectomy in 94% of patients, although they did not complete bilateral para-aortic lymph-node sampling that would meet Gynecologic Oncology Group (GOG) standards in all of the patients. Despite the Arizona Group's impressive results, and also data from Spirtos and colleagues at the Women's Cancer Center in Palo Alto [20], numerous important questions have not been answered. In an attempt to answer some of these questions, the Gynecologic Oncology Group has undertaken a limited-access prospective multicentre trial (GOG 9206) of laparoscopically assisted vaginal hysterectomy with pelvic and para-aortic lymph-node sampling, intraperitoneal exploration and washings in the management of early staged endometrial cancer. Based on the preliminary data from GOG 9206, a phase III randomized clinical trial has been proposed and funded by the National Cancer Institute (NCI). This trial will compare laparoscopic pelvic and para-aortic node sampling with vaginal hysterectomy and bilateral salpingo-oophorectomy to open laparotomy with similar sampling and abdominal hysterectomy/bilateral salpingo-oophorectomy in clinical stage I and IIA, grade 1–3 endometrial adenocarcinoma. This study could become a landmark, as it will be the first time that the rigid standards of a phase III cooperative group trial have been applied to questions regarding laparoscopic surgery.

A continuing treatment dilemma has been how best to manage patients with endometrial cancer who have undergone a hysterectomy without the associated appropriate staging. Childers and Spirtos, combining data from their two separate organizations, were the first to apply laparoscopic surgical staging in the management of these problematical patients. In 1994, these authors reported on 13 patients who were at high risk of extrauterine spread of endometrial cancer [21]. At laparoscopy, previously unappreciated intraperitoneal or retroperitoneal disease was identified in three patients (23%). The Gynecologic Oncology Group has recognized the need to determine the applicability of laparoscopy in these cases, and has instituted a multicentre prospective clinical trial to evaluate laparoscopic staging in incompletely staged endometrial adenocarcinomas (GOG 9403).

Ovarian malignancies

Laparoscopy and early-stage ovarian cancer

From the 1980s, many of the adnexal masses diagnosed in large urban centres in the USA were managed via laparoscopy. It could be expected that a well-characterized series of early ovarian malignancies that had been adequately and properly managed laparoscopically would result. Unfortunately, although there are multiple reports of laparoscopic 'management' of early ovarian cancer, only a handful of reviews in the published literature report adequate and thorough operative staging, including laparoscopic lymph-node sampling, as part of the management of early ovarian malignancies. Querleu, in his 1994 report [22], summarized his experience with 10 patients, eight of whom had presumed early-stage ovarian cancer. Subsequently, Childers *et al.* reported on their experience surgically staging 14 patients with presumed early ovarian cancer [23]. Eight (57%) of the patients in Childers' series had metastatic disease identified; three of these patients had the metastatic disease in their para-aortic lymph nodes. Based on this data, as well as anecdotal experiences from various institutions in the USA, the Gynecologic Oncology Group has instituted a study to evaluate the merit of laparoscopic staging in patients with incompletely staged cancers of the ovary (GOG 9302).

Laparoscopy and advanced-stage ovarian cancer

In the 1970s Bagley and associates were the first to propose that laparoscopy could be used to confirm the presence of an advanced ovarian primary when the diagnosis or spread of disease was uncertain [24]. Based on the knowledge obtained at laparoscopy, the decision could be made whether to proceed to coeliotomy, with an attempt at aggressive cytoreductive surgery, or to institute a cytotoxic drug regimen or other less invasive treatments [25]. The use of laparoscopy for this indication was initially embraced by various centres in the USA. However, at that time there was a general belief in the gynaecologicol oncology community that aggressive pre-chemotherapy cytoreductive surgery, which reduces residual disease to an 'optimal' level, offers a survival advantage. Therefore, diagnostic laparoscopy for the indications described above fell out of favour, and it is now generally felt to be superfluous, if not harmful, to the patient as it may lead to a delay in starting the definitive treatment as well as potentiating spread of the disease.

Laparoscopy and surgical reassessment of ovarian cancer

The hypothesis that laparoscopy could be used to document disease status following initial therapy in women with advanced ovarian malignancies was proposed over 20 years ago. In 1975, Rosenoff *et al.*, in the first report of the use of laparoscopy in surgical reassessment, noted that 39% of patients who were in clinical remission had tumour documented at second-look laparoscopy [26]. Subsequent reviews confirmed this finding, noting that even the availability of tumour-related antigens (CA-125, etc.) did not remarkably improve the clinical diagnostic accuracy. Unfortunately, surgical success rates (i.e. being able to visualize the entire peritoneal cavity without a significant complication) in the early investigations from the late 1970s and 1980s were in the range of 60–75% [27]. Similarly, when compared to second-look laparotomy, false-negative rates were as high as 55% [28]. With the improvements in available instrumentation and operator skill that occurred in the late 1980s and early 1990s, surgical success rates now exceed 90% [29,30], with Krafft and associates reporting an accuracy at predicting pathological disease that rivals second-look laparotomy [31]. In the USA, two single-institution studies have investigated laparoscopic second-look procedures. Childers and associates identified persistent disease in 56% (24/44) of their subjects who were clinically free of disease after initial optimal cytoreductive surgery and platinum-based chemotherapy [23]. Twenty per cent of these patients (five of 24) had only microscopic disease. These five included two patients in whom the para-aortic nodes were the only site of residuum. From our sister institution, Casey and colleagues presented data comparing laparoscopy and laparotomy as reassessment surgery in 154 patients with adnexal malignancies. There was no significant difference noted between the two groups in the ability to detect persistent disease. However, laparoscopy did appear to have the advantages of decreases in blood loss, hospital stay, operation time and cost, although the cost assessment was not performed using current accounting methodologies [32]. Despite these encouraging reports, significant concerns and unanswered questions regarding second-look laparoscopy have persisted, and opinions about its potential usefulness are remarkably divergent. Attempts to undertake a multicentre cooperative investigation to definitively answer these questions have been unsuccessful to date.

Cervical malignancies

Early-stage cervical cancer

Based on the above-described multicentre success at safely and thoroughly performing laparoscopic pelvic lymphadenectomies, there was a resurgence of interest in the performance of radical vaginal (Schauta–Amreich) hysterectomies combined with either trans- or retroperitoneal laparoscopic node dissection. The first two significant reports on this technique came from France

(Querleu in 1991 [33] and Dargent and Mathevet in 1992 [34]). The largest series in the English language literature was published in 1993, and reviews Querleu's experience in performing eight radical vaginal hysterectomies with associated laparoscopic pelvic node dissections [35]. Definitive studies evaluating this technique have been proposed and are now taking place as single-centre investigations by Dargent in France, Roy in Canada and Smith in the USA. A multicentre clinical trial has yet to be initiated.

The first case of an alleged laparoscopic radical abdominal hysterectomy was published in 1992 [36]. Unfortunately there were numerous significant deficiencies in the technique reported. Subsequently, the laparoscopic radical hysterectomy, with the degree of radicality being consistent with the traditional M.D. Anderson classification [37], has been championed by Sedlacek [38] and Spirtos and colleagues [39] at the Women's Cancer Center in Palo Alto. Although the data from Spirtos and associates is encouraging, with complication rates that are on a par with those for a similar case performed in an open manner, Sedlacek's initial experience does indicate that caution is needed. Sedlacek had a urinary tract injury rate approaching 50% in his initial report of 14 patients.

Evidently, we await more encouraging positive reports to tell us which of the laparoscopically associated radical hysterectomy techniques will prove to be of most merit and whether or not, when paired with a laparoscopic node dissection, any will become an acceptable new standard.

Probably the most avant-garde application of laparoscopic surgery in the management of cervical cancer has been that proposed by Dargent. He combined laparoscopic pelvic node dissection with a radical vaginal trachelectomy in women with early stage IB and IIA malignancies who wanted to preserve their fertility [40]. Dargent's published data is remarkably limited and simply reports on early evaluations of feasibility, but no doubt other studies will be published in an attempt to rationally evaluate this technique.

Locally advanced cervical cancer

It has been proposed that preradiation surgical staging with para-aortic lymph-node sampling should be performed in women with locally advanced cervical malignancies. This provides a more accurate definition of the disease spread, to assist in decisions on the resection of bulky nodes and the removal of diseased adnexa or whether to perform an oophoropexy in an attempt to maintain gonadal function. Unfortunately, there are significant disadvantages of operative and postoperative morbidity in patients receiving radiation therapy. In 1991 Querleu was the first to report the value of laparoscopic pelvic lymph-node dissection in patients with cervical cancer who went on to receive radiotherapy [41]. However, Childers published data in 1992 claiming that laparoscopic para-aortic lymphadenectomy could obtain the same information as that obtained via extraperitoneal lymph-node sampling, while being performed on a day-case basis with a lower associated morbidity and a shortened recovery time [42]. Unfortunately, the data from Querleu and Childers, as well as that from Fowler et al. [43], are limited, with a predominance of early stage cases, and include few, if any, patients who underwent para-aortic node sampling with or without subsequent radiotherapy. Despite these weaknesses, both Childers' and Fowler's articles shed light on the issue of adequacy of a laparoscopic dissection. When compared with coeliotomy, between 75% and 100% of nodes were removed, with only a single patient (out of a combined total of 30) having a positive (microscopic) node that was not removed at laparoscopy and subsequently identified at laparotomy.

Dargent employed an extraperitoneal laparoscopic approach [44]. This approach was first proposed by urological surgeons completing preradiation pelvic node sampling in patients with prostate cancer, and has the theoretical advantages of being able to keep intraperitoneal adhesion formation to a minimum while limiting the potential for herniation through a sleeve site. However, there is no data to support this theory. In the first investigation attempting to clarify these uncertainties, Fowler et al. compared pelvic adhesion formation following transperitoneal laparoscopic pelvic lymphadenectomy to the same procedure performed via an extraperitoneal approach using a porcine model [45]. Their data, from 10 animals treated with laparoscopy and nine treated with an extraperitoneal approach, did not demonstrate a statistically significant difference in adhesion scores. Fowler has proposed that transperitoneal laparoscopic pelvic lymphadenectomy may not induce the degree of adhesion formation that is associated with transperitoneal laparotomy. To date, there have been no published human trials comparing extraperitoneal laparoscopic lymph-node sampling to either intraperitoneal laparoscopic sampling or the more traditional approaches.

The Gynecologic Oncology Group had proposed to complete a trial to obtain data on not only transperitoneal laparoscopic para-aortic lymph-node sampling in patients with locally advanced cervical cancer but also information on the safety and thoroughness of laparoscopic pelvic lymphadenectomies in women for whom a radical abdominal hysterectomy had been proposed (GOG 9207). However, this protocol was amended to investigate only the latter group of patients. Therefore it is unlikely that all of the questions regarding the safety of preradiation laparoscopic para-aortic node sampling will be answered in the foreseeable future.

Conclusion

The use of laparoscopy in the management of gynaecological malignancies is a relatively new field, and reported research is still adding to the knowledge-base. The advances made so far, although far behind those the readers of the third edition of this text will probably be conversant with, are substantial. The pioneers in this field have been successful because of the remarkable technical advances in instrumentation coupled with their own vision and determination.

References

1 Jacobaeus HC (1910). Uber die Moglichkeit die Zystoskopie bei Untersuchung seroser Hohlungen anzuwenden. *Munich med Wschr* **57**:2090–2092.

2 Kelling G (1902). Uber Oesophagoskopie, Gastroskopie und Colioskopie. *Munich med Wschr* **49**:21–24.

3 Nitze M (1879). *Uber eine neue Beleuchtungsmethode der Hoblen des menschlichen Korpers*, Vol 20. Wein: Med Presse, 851–858.

4 Power FH, Barnes AC (1941). Sterilization by means of peritoneoscopic fulguration: a preliminary report. *Am J Obstet Gynecol* **41**:1093–1097.

5 Bruhat MA, Manhes H, Mage G, Pouly J-L (1980). Treatment of ectopic pregnancy by means of laparoscopy. *Fertil Steril* **33**:411–414.

6 DeCherney AH, Diamond MP (1987). Laparoscopic salpingostomy for ectopic pregnancy. *Obstet Gynecol* **70**:948–950.

7 International Federation of Gynecology and Obstetrics (1989). Annual report on the results of treatment in gynecologic cancer. *Int J Gynecol Obstet* **28**:189–190.

8 Reich HJ, DeCaprio J, McGlynn F (1989). Laparoscopic hysterectomy. *J Gynecol Surg* **5**:213–216.

9 Summit R, Stovall T, Lipscomb G, Ling F (1992). Randomized comparison of laparoscopically assisted vaginal hysterectomy with standard vaginal hysterectomy in an outpatient setting. *Obstet Gynecol* **80**:894–898.

10 Boike GM (1993). Laparoscopic assisted vaginal hysterectomy in a university hospital: a report of 82 cases in comparison with abdominal and vaginal hysterectomy. *Am J Obstet Gynecol* **168**:1690–1701.

11 Dargent D, Salvat J (1989). *L'Envahissement Ganglionnaire Pelvien*. Paris: McGraw-Hill.

12 Gershman A, Daykhovsky L, Chandra M, Danoff D, Grundfest WS (1990). Laparoscopic pelvic lymphadenectomy. *J Laparoscop Endoscop Surg* **1**:63–68.

13 Schuessler WW, Vancaillie TG, Reich H, Griffin DP (1991). Transperitoneal endosurgical lymphadenectomy in patients with localized prostate cancer. *J Urol* **145**:988–991.

14 Parra RO, Anduus C, Boullier J (1992). Staging laparoscopic pelvic lymph node dissection: comparison of results with open pelvic lymphadenectomy. *J Urol* **147**:875–878.

15 Bowsher WG, Clarke A, Clarke DG, Costello AJ (1992). Laparoscopic pelvic lymph node dissection. *Br J Urol* **70**:776–779.

16 Herd J, Fowler JM, Shenson D, Lacey S, Montz FJ (1992). Para-aortic lymph node sampling: development of a technique. *Gynecol Oncol* **44**:271–276.

17 Childers JM, Surwit EA (1992). Case report: combined laparoscopic and vaginal surgery for the management of two cases of stage 1 endometrial cancer. *Gynecol Oncol* **45**:46–48.

18 Querleu D (1993). Laparoscopic para-aortic node sampling in gynecologic oncology: a preliminary experience. *Gynecol Oncol* **49**:24–29.

19 Childers JM, Brzechffa PR, Hatch KD, Surwit EA (1993). Laparoscopically Assisted Surgical Staging (LASS) of endometrial cancer. *Gynecol Oncol* **51**:33–38.

20 Spirtos NM, Schlaerth JB, Spirtos T, Schlaerth A, Indaman P, Kimball R (1995). Laparoscopic bilateral pelvic and para-aortic lymph node sampling: an evolving technique. *Am J Obstet Gynecol* **173**:105–111.

21 Childers JM, Spirtos NM, Brainard P, Surwit EA (1994). Laparoscopic staging of the patient with incompletely staged early adenocarcinoma of the endometrium. *Obstet Gynecol* **83**:597–600.

22 Querleu D, LeBlanc E (1994). Laparoscopic infrarenal paraaortic lymph node dissection for restaging of carcinoma of the ovary or fallopian tube. *Cancer* **73**:1467–1472.

23 Childers J, Lang J, Surwit E, Hatch K (1995). Laparoscopic surgical staging of ovarian cancer. *Gynecol Oncol* **59**:25–33.

24 Bagley CM, Young RC, Schien PS *et al* (1973). Ovarian cancer metastatic to the diaphragm frequently undiagnosed at laparotomy. A preliminary report. *Am J Obstet Gynecol* **116**:397–404.

25 Ozols RF, Fisher RI, Anderson T *et al* (1981). Peritoneoscopy in the management of ovarian cancer. *Am J Obstet Gynecol* **140**:611–619.

26 Rosenoff SH, DeVita VT, Hubbard S, Young RC (1975). Peritoneoscopy in the staging and follow-up of ovarian cancer. *Semin Oncol* **2**:223–228.

27 Berek JS, Griffiths CT, Leventhal JM (1981). Laparoscopy for second-look evaluation in ovarian cancer. *Obstet Gynecol* **61**:189–193.

28 Piver MS, Lele SB, Barlow JJ *et al* (1980). Second look laparoscopy prior to proposed second look laparotomy. *Obstet Gynecol* **55**:571–577.

29 Lele SB, Piver MS (1986). Interval laparoscopy as predictor of response to chemotherapy in ovarian carcinoma. *Obstet Gynecol* **68**:345–348.

30 Marti Vicente A, Sainz S, Soriano G *et al* (1990). Utilidad de la laparoscopia como metodod do 'second look' en las neoplasias de ovario. *Rev Esp Enferm Dig* **77**:275.

31 Krafft W, Konig EM, Schrimer A *et al* (1990). 'Second-look operation' oder second-look laparoskopie zur Sicherung der kompletten Remission beim Ovarialkarzinom. *Zentralbl Gynakol* **112**:767–772.

32 Casey AC, Farias-Eisner R, Pisani A *et al* (1996). What is the role of reassessment laparoscopy in the management of gynecologic cancers in 1995? *Gynecol Oncol* **60**:454–461.

33 Querleu D (1991). Hysterectomies de Schauta–Amreich et Schauta–Stoeckel assistees per coelioscopie [Letter]. *J Gynecol Obstet Biol Reprod* **20**:747.

34 Dargent D, Mathevet P (1992). Radical laparoscopic vaginal hysterectomy. *J Gynecol Obstet Biol Reprod* **21**:709–710.

35 Querleu D (1993). Case report: laparoscopically assisted radical vaginal hysterectomy. *Gynecol Oncol* **51**:248–250.

36 Nezhat CR, Burrell MO, Nezhat FR, Benigno BB, Welander CE (1992). Laparoscopic radical hysterectomy with paraaortic and pelvic node dissection. *Am J Obstet Gynecol* **166**:864–866.

37 Piver MS, Rutledge F, Smith JP (1974). Five classes of extended hysterectomy for women with cervical cancer. *Obstet Gynecol* **44**:265–272.

38 Sedlacek TV (1995). Laparoscopic radical hysterectomy: the next evolutionary step in the treatment of invasive cervical cancer. *J Gynecol Tech* **1**:223–230.

39 Spirtos NM, Schlaerth JB, Kimball RE, Leiphart VM, Ballon SC (1996). Laparoscopic radical hysterectomy (type III) with aortic and pelvic lymphadenectomy. *Am J Obstet Gynecol* **174**:1763–1768.

40 Dargent D, Brun JL, Remy I (1994). Pregnancies following radical trachelectomy for invasive cervical cancer. *Gynecol Oncol* **52**:105–108.

41 Querleu D, Leblanc E, Castelain B (1991). Laparoscopic pelvic lymphadenectomy in the staging of early carcinoma of the cervix. *Am J Obstet Gynecol* **164**:579–583.

42 Childers JM, Hatch K, Surwit EA (1992). The role of laparoscopic lymphadenectomy in the management of cervical cancer. *Gynecol Oncol* **47**:38–41.

43 Fowler JM, Carter JR, Carlson JW *et al* (1993). Lymph node yield from laparoscopic lymphadenectomy in cervical cancer: a comparative study. *Gynecol Oncol* **51**:187–191.

44 Dargent D (1993). Laparoscopy in gynecologic cancer. *Current Opin Obstet Gynecol* **5**:294–300.

45 Fowler JM, Hartenbach EM, Reynolds HT *et al* (1994) Pelvic adhesion formation after pelvic lymphadenectomy: comparison between transperitoneal laparoscopy and extraperitoneal laparotomy in a porcine model. *Gynecol Oncol* **55**:25–28.

Section 1
Laparoscopic Techniques in Diagnostic and Staging Laparoscopy

2 Laparoscopic diagnosis of adnexal tumours

Michel Canis, Gérard Mage, Christophe Pomel,
Jacques Raiga, Jean-Luc Pouly, Arnaud Wattiez,
Hubert Manhes and Maurice-Antoine Bruhat

Introduction

Laparoscopic surgery is becoming the gold standard for the diagnosis and the treatment of benign adnexal cystic masses [1–3]. However, this approach remains controversial, because large cystic masses must be reduced in size for extraction. As there is the risk of dissemination, careful preoperative selection is still recommended by most authors [4–6]. However, because of the very high rate of false-positive diagnoses of malignancy given by ultrasound, surgical and pathological examination are still required to distinguish benign and malignant adnexal neoplasms. The laparoscopic approach has not been restricted to entirely cystic lesions, and most large studies have included teratomas and mixed masses [1–3]. It is becoming more and more difficult to know where the limits of laparoscopic surgery lie when very experienced teams propose comprehensive laparoscopic staging of selected cases of stage I ovarian cancer [7–9].

From the recent data about tumour dissemination, surgical diagnosis is the key step in the intraoperative management of adnexal cystic masses. Data from the literature can be summarized as follows.

1 At laparotomy, the surgical rupture and/or puncture of a tumour of low malignant potential has no incidence on the prognosis, provided that the tumour is removed immediately (i.e. during the same surgical procedure) [10–15]. Similarly, despite the controversial results of univariate analysis [16–23], multivariate studies have demonstrated that intraoperative rupture of invasive cancer has no incidence on the prognosis [24–28].

2 These conclusions from patients treated by laparotomy should be confirmed after laparoscopic treatment.

3 By contrast, several reports indicate that when the tumour is not removed immediately, laparoscopic puncture or biopsy may worsen the prognosis of a malignant ovarian tumour [29–36]. Abdominal wall implants have been observed after the biopsy of both invasive cancers and tumours of low malignant potential. Therefore the rule proposed by Maiman et al. appears to be the key to safe surgical management: the surgeon should be able to remove the tumour immediately and entirely [29].

4 Obviously the prognosis of a stage IA ovarian cancer cannot be improved by surgical puncture or any other surgical trauma. Inadequate management of ovarian tumours may, however, occur at laparotomy. In 1986, Helawa and colleagues reported 25 cases of staging laparotomy in early epithelial ovarian cancer [37]. The diagnosis of cancer had been suspected during the primary surgical procedure in only 10 cases (40%). Moreover, three patients had been treated by ovarian biopsy or ovarian cystectomy.

Laparoscopic diagnosis: technique

Preoperative evaluation

Surgical diagnosis is the final step in the diagnosis of an adnexal mass. Intraoperative management depends on information from the preoperative data. With increased experience more and more adnexal masses may be evaluated by laparoscopy. However, the preoperative data which no longer select the patient for laparoscopy or for laparotomy are still essential to help the surgeon choose the most appropriate form of laparoscopic management. This data provides invaluable information about the internal structure and the appearance of the mass.

Our preoperative management protocol has remained basically the same since 1980 [38]. Except for patients who present with an acute pelvic syndrome or whose adnexal mass is discovered incidentally at laparoscopy, the preoperative work-up is as described below.

After clinical examination, all patients undergo an abdominal and a vaginal ultrasound examination. Then unilocular completely anechogenic adnexal cysts <8 cm, when diagnosed in premenopausal patients, are treated for 3 months using an oral contraceptive pill containing 50 µg of oestrogen or are managed expectantly for 3 months. During this time, the patient undergoes a monthly clinical and ultrasound examination. Simple cysts are evaluated by laparoscopy if still present at the end of the treatment or if they are found to have increased in diameter at ultrasound examination. Patients whose adnexal mass is >8 cm in diameter and/or appeared septated, complex, mixed or even mainly solid at ultrasound examination undergo laparoscopic evaluation. Also, over the years, large adnexal cysts (>10 cm) and older patients have been increasingly evaluated by laparoscopy. In the early stages of our experience with laparoscopic diagnosis, highly suspicious masses were managed by laparotomy, whereas this is now reserved to obvious stage III or IV ovarian cancer.

A second vaginal ultrasound examination is routinely performed on the day before surgery. This avoids some unnecessary surgical procedures when the cyst has disappeared. Also this final ultrasound study is essential, as it provides more accurate data about the internal structure of the tumour. Since 1993, this last examination has been made in conjunction with a colour Doppler, which is probably helpful when managing mixed tumours [39,40]. A blood sample is drawn on the day before surgery, so that tumour markers are available for follow-up, but are not used for the preoperative selection.

Patients are informed about the laparoscopic procedure, and that an immediate vertical midline laparotomy might be required if the adnexal cystic mass is found to be malignant or suspicious. A bowel preparation is administered to all patients on the day before surgery.

The technique of laparoscopy and the instruments used have been described elsewhere [40,41]. To avoid blind puncture of large masses, the Veress needle is inserted in the left upper quadrant perpendicular to the anterior abdominal wall. Once a satisfactory pneumoperitoneum has been obtained, the umbilical trocar is inserted cautiously. Ancillary trocars are inserted perpendicular to the abdominal wall, to allow a reliable excision of the trocar site when looking for abdominal wall metastasis during restaging procedures.

A strict protocol should be used for the surgical diagnosis; most of the guidelines used in our department were designed in 1980 following the comments addressed to a study conducted in the late 1970s. First, a peritoneal fluid sample and/or peritoneal washings for cytological examination are aspirated from the posterior cul-de-sac, or from the paracolic gutters and the vesicouterine cul-de-sac when the pouch of Douglas is obliterated by adhesions or filled by a large adnexal mass. Thereafter the cystic ovary, pelvic peritoneum, contralateral ovary, paracolic gutters, diaphragm, omentum, liver and bowel are carefully inspected. The value of this inspection has been confirmed by Possover *et al.*, who reported that metastases easily accessible to laparoscopic inspection were always present in patients with metastasis of the small bowel and of the mesentery [42]. Because of the magnification pro-

vided by the laparoscope, the inspection of the upper abdomen, particularly of the diaphragm, is better at laparoscopy than at laparotomy [9]. If signs of malignancy such as ascites, peritoneal metastases or extracystic ovarian vegetations are found, the mass is diagnosed as suspicious or malignant.

In the remaining cases, an intracystic evaluation is required to rule out malignancy. This is begun preoperatively using vaginal ultrasound examination. Depending on the patient's age and on the ultrasound appearance, the intraoperative intracystic evaluation will be performed after a puncture [38], or macroscopically after an adnexectomy and extraction using a bag. Adnexal masses are punctured only when they are assumed to be benign from the initial laparoscopic inspection and from the preoperative work-up. Care is always taken to minimize spillage when puncturing and aspirating a cyst. Briefly, the adnexa is grasped and stabilized using an atraumatic forceps placed on the utero-ovarian ligament, so that the puncture can be performed perpendicularly to the ovarian surface. Small cysts are aspirated with a needle connected to a 20- or 50-ml syringe. Cysts of more than 5 cm are punctured with a 5-mm conical trocar and emptied with a 5-mm aspiration lavage device. The cyst fluid is examined macroscopically and sent for delayed cytological examination. The cyst and the pelvic cavity are then washed many times with small volumes, minimizing the spillage and doing everything to avoid contamination of the upper abdomen. Very large cysts (>10 cm) are aspirated by inserting the second puncture trocar high enough to allow visual control of the puncture site. Once the cyst is emptied and washed, it is opened with scissors and the internal cyst wall is carefully inspected. If signs of malignancy are found, the mass is diagnosed as suspicious or malignant.

In postmenopausal patients, or in highly suspicious masses, the puncture is not performed and the intracystic examination is performed after adnexectomy. However, we do not think that a cystectomy without puncture avoids spillage of an intracystic ovarian cancer. If the tumour is invasive, it invades the cleavage plane and thus an excision without puncture or rupture is virtually impossible. Paraovarian cysts may be an exception. Usually non-suspicious paraovarian cysts appear blue because the cyst wall is thin and is covered only by the peritoneum, so that the cyst fluid can be seen through the cyst wall. If there are abnormal intracystic areas, the cyst wall is thicker and appears white, so that intracystic evaluation can often be done without puncture, thus making surgical excision without rupture more realistic.

From 1992 we have used frozen section to decrease the consequences of the false-positive laparoscopic diagnoses of malignancy. The sample sent to the pathologist was either a biopsy or the adnexa, depending on the conditions *in vivo* and on the patient's age.

Results of the laparoscopic diagnosis

It has been demonstrated in our large study published in 1994 that laparoscopic diagnosis of malignancy is reliable and safe when used cautiously (Table 2.1) [38]. All the malignant masses were diagnosed at laparoscopy, but the positive predictive value was only 41.3%. As signs of malignancy such as external or intracystic growths may be encountered in benign masses (Table 2.2), false positives are necessary to ensure that the laparoscopic approach is safe. From our experience, the puncture of an intracystic invasive ovarian cancer is uncommon. Indeed, among 1098 patients evaluated over 14 years, including 42 malignant tumours and 323 masses which were solid or suspicious at ultrasound, a diagnostic puncture was performed in only four intracystic ovarian cancers and in 11 tumours of low malignant potential. Unfortunately, 18 of the 22 invasive cancers were obvious before puncture.

False positives appear to be the main disadvantage of our very cautious approach. Initially, some unnecessary

Table 2.1 Correlation between the laparoscopic and pathological diagnoses (1980–91).

| Laparoscopic diagnosis | n | Pathological diagnosis | | |
		Benign	LMP	Cancer
Benign	773	773	0	0
Suspicious	38	25	11	2
Cancer	8	2	1	5
Total	819	800	12	7

LMP, low malignant potential.

Table 2.2 Signs of malignancy among true-positive (TP) (*n* = 42) and false-positive (FP) (*n* = 69) diagnoses of malignancy (1980–93). Percentages are given in brackets.

	Cancer and low malignant tumours (TP)	Macroscopically suspicious benign lesions (FP)
Turbid fluid	9 (21.4)	5 (7.3)
Extracystic vegetations	18 (42.8)	24 (34.8)
Intracystic vegetations	17 (40.5)	22 (31.8)
Peritoneal metastases	12 (28.6)	0 (0.0)
Ascites	6 (14.3)	0 (0.0)
Abnormal vessels	1 (2.3)	1 (1.5)
Highly suspicious ultrasound	7 (16.6)	13 (18.8)

laparotomies were performed because of this problem and, as demonstrated below, this may induce some unnecessary adnexectomies in the future. To avoid this problem we have used frozen sections since 1992 and, as reported by others, their accuracy has been satisfactory, above 90%. There are advantages with this method, as in 1992 and 1993 only two of the 42 macroscopically suspicious benign adnexal cystic masses were treated by laparotomy. However, frozen section in the diagnosis of ovarian tumours is difficult, with a false-negative rate of about 5% [43,44]. Most false-negative diagnoses are the consequences of inadequate and/or limited sampling [43,44]. We also had two false negatives induced by inadequate sampling. One sample was carried out by pathologists after an oophorectomy for a 23-cm-diameter tumour of low malignant potential which was diagnosed as benign, and treated by bilateral adnexectomy. This 72-year-old patient is alive with no evidence of disease 3 years later. In the second case, the sample was carried out by a surgeon to decide the treatment of a 15-cm solid adnexal mass in a 21-year-old patient. As the pathologist found calcified tissue in the small biopsy specimen, a mature teratoma was diagnosed, an adnexectomy was performed, the tumour was morcellated and extracted through a 4-cm transverse incision. The final pathological diagnosis was a grade I immature teratoma [45]. A second-look laparoscopy was performed 3 weeks later and a gliomatosis peritonei with mature and immature implants was found [46].

From the experience above the following conclusions about frozen sections and laparoscopy are proposed.
1 Frozen sections should not be used to decide the treatment of the ovary. If the mass is macroscopically suspicious the 'entire adnexa' should be removed. The only exception to this rule is adnexal masses with a small (<5 mm) solitary vegetation, when the local conditions (diameter of the mass, pelvic adhesions, etc.) allow satisfactory macroscopic inspection of the tumour. In such cases, there is only one suspicious area and the incidence of malignancy in this group is less than 20% [47]. Using this approach, out of 18 patients less than 40 years old diagnosed with a laparoscopically suspicious mass, eight (44.4%) were treated conservatively by laparoscopy despite a small intracystic vegetation. However, this approach should be used very carefully, and if there is any doubt an adnexectomy should be performed.
2 Frozen sections are essential to decide on the staging procedure, and also the treatment of the contralateral adnexa and of the uterus, thus avoiding a second surgical procedure.
3 If frozen sections are not available, macroscopically suspicious ovarian masses should be removed completely and immediately.

Current surgical management

The choice between laparoscopy and laparotomy will be discussed later. First the choice between oophorectomy and cystectomy will be discussed, and this depends on: (i) the results of the inspection of the external surface of the ovary and of the peritoneal cavity; (ii) the ultrasound appearance; and (iii) the patient's age.

Extracystic signs of malignancy are found

An adnexectomy is performed except when a solitary vegetation is found and frozen section is used, as described above. In the same way frozen section helps to decide the treatment when a small vegetation is found on the contralateral ovary, or on the peritoneum in a young patient with a non-suspicious cystic mass.

No extracystic signs of malignancy are found

a THE ULTRASOUND APPEARANCE WAS NOT SUSPICIOUS (ENTIRELY CYSTIC, OR ONLY ONE THIN SEPTA)

a–1 In patients <40 years old, conservative treatment can be achieved in most cases [1]. An endocystic inspection confirms the findings of the ultrasound examination. As confirmation of numerous previous ultrasound studies [47–52], in our studies the incidence of cancer among patients less than 50 years old treated for an entirely cystic mass was only 0.3%. The only cancer was diagnosed at laparoscopy from a turbid fluid and endocystic papillary growths of less than 1 mm in diameter. An adnexectomy was performed, frozen-section diagnosis was doubtful and the restaging procedure performed 3 weeks later was negative, although the diagnosis of cancer had been confirmed at permanent sections.

If endocystic signs of malignancy are found, a unilateral adnexectomy should be performed except in the case of a small solitary vegetation as described above.

a–2 In patients aged 40–50 years, the management is the same.

a–3 Postmenopausal patients and patients over 50 years old are treated by bilateral adnexectomy. Both adnexae are removed and extracted with an endopouch to prevent spillage. The adnexectomy is always bilateral, as we have observed malignant recurrences several years after conservative treatment of a benign serous cyst in menopausal patients [1]. Similarly, Randall *et al.* reported malignant recurrences after unilateral adnexectomy in patients of more than 45 years old [53].

We elected not to remove a normal-appearing uterus because of the added operating time and morbidity. However, the uterus is always carefully evaluated with routine Pap smears and hysteroscopy. A total hysterectomy should be performed in patients with a previous history of cervical intraepithelial neoplasia, or who are at risk from endometrial cancer.

b THE ULTRASONOGRAPHIC APPEARANCE WAS SUSPICIOUS (Table 2.3)

b–1 In young patients (<40 years old) the choice has to be made between conservative and radical treatment. Most of these masses are benign and can be treated conservatively, so that a routine adnexectomy seems unacceptable (Table 2.3).

Among these patients the laparoscopic inspection allows a reliable diagnosis of: functional cysts which are identified using previously reported macroscopic signs such as a normal utero-ovarian ligament and scanty coral-like vessels (Table 2.4); endometriomas which are recognized from the ovarian adhesions and the peritoneal

Table 2.3 Pathological diagnosis according to age in patients with lesions which are solid or suspicious at ultrasound.

Pathological diagnosis	Age group*			
	<40 years	40–49 years	≥50 years	Total
Functional	23 (11.7)	7 (10.8)	3 (4.8)	33 (10.2)
Serous	18 (9.2)	6 (9.2)	26 (41.9)	50 (15.5)
Paraovarian	3 (1.5)	2 (3.1)	1 (1.6)	6 (1.9)
Mucinous	9 (4.6)	5 (7.7)	8 (12.9)	22 (6.8)
Dermoid	103 (52.6)	16 (24.6)	9 (14.5)	128 (39.6)
Endometrioma	26 (13.3)	25 (38.5)	1 (1.6)	52 (16.1)
LMP [1]	6 (3.1)	1 (1.5)	5 (8.1)	12 (3.7)
Cancer	8 (4.1)	3 (4.6)	9 (14.5)	20 (6.2)

LMP, low malignant potential.
* n = 196 (<40 years); 65 (40–49 years); 62 (≥50 years); 323 (total).

Table 2.4 Laparoscopic criteria to distinguish a functional cyst from a benign ovarian neoplasm.

	Benign neoplasm	Functional cyst
Uteroovarian ligament	Lengthened	Normal
Cyst wall	Thick	Thin
Cyst vessels	Comb like from the hilum	Scanty, coral like
Fluid	Clear or chocolate, mucinous or sebaceus	Saffron yellow
Internal appearance	Smooth	Retinal-like aspect
Cystectomy	Possible	'Impossible'

implants; and suspicious paraovarian cysts with solid contents which may be seen through the cyst wall. Moreover, teratomas may be diagnosed by an ultrasound examination or a CT scan.

In the remaining cases, which represent less than 10% of the patients aged less then 40 years, the management should be adapted to each case.

1 If only one small intracystic papillary formation is found at ultrasound, the endocystic examination with frozen section may allow conservative treatment.

2 By contrast, if there are numerous papillary formations, if the tumour is mixed or mainly solid, if numerous vessels with a low resistance index [54] are found or if the tumour is very large, an adnexectomy without puncture is the most reasonable treatment.

The unknown consequences of a puncture on the prognosis means that a routine adnexectomy cannot be justified.

b–2 In patients aged 40–50 years, laparoscopy remains an important diagnostic tool given the frequency of functional and paraovarian cysts and endometriomas (Table 2.3), but difficult cases are managed by adnexectomy.

b–3 In postmenopausal patients and patients over 50 years old, the incidence of malignant tumours is high (22.6%), laparoscopic diagnosis is mainly helpful for inspection of the diaphragm and the upper abdomen. All benign masses are treated by bilateral adnexectomy.

Adnexectomy for macroscopically suspicious adnexal masses: laparoscopy or laparotomy?

This question is crucial, for the following reasons: (i) laparoscopic adnexectomy is becoming a standard procedure which could easily be used for many suspicious masses; but (ii) if we accept laparoscopic adnexectomy for macroscopically suspicious masses, we also accept the possibility of a laparoscopic adnexectomy for early ovarian cancer.

However, there are no data available to demonstrate that laparoscopy has no influence on the prognosis of a stage I ovarian cancer when compared with laparotomy. Although the surgical procedures are similar, the prognosis may be different, as there are several essential differences between laparoscopy and laparotomy (see Chapter 14) [55].

At laparoscopy the intra-abdominal pH is lower [56]. This is important, because when carbon dioxide is used, lactated Ringer's solution has been shown to have a protective effect against postoperative adhesions [57]. Moreover, the increased intra-abdominal pressure may be a disadvantage when considering intraoperative disse-

mination of malignant cells. Finally, when performing a laparoscopic adnexectomy the risk of traumatic embolism could be increased as the procedure is slower and carried out with more manipulation and without traction on the pedicles.

The advantages of laparoscopy over laparotomy are well known. Although these advantages are very attractive, they cannot justify a possible dissemination or decrease in the survival rate of patients with early ovarian cancer. Moreover, the cosmetic result is probably similar when comparing a laparotomy tailored to the size of the tumour and a laparoscopic adnexectomy followed by an incision large enough to allow easy extraction without morcellation of the tumour.

This question can be illustrated using the results obtained in our department among 351 patients in 1992 and 1993. Only 42 of the 330 benign masses (12.7%) were found to be macroscopically suspicious at laparoscopy, and of these five (1.5%) were treated by laparotomy, thus avoiding many laparotomies. However, two cases of dissemination occurred after a laparoscopic adnexectomy for ovarian cancer. The first case, induced by the treatment of an immature teratoma, is described above. In the second case a 5-cm solid tumour with external vegetations, but no visible peritoneal metastases, was found in a 33-year-old patient who was operated on for infertility. A laparoscopic adnexectomy was performed and the ovary was extracted using a bag. As the diagnosis of invasive cancer was not confirmed by frozen section, the staging procedure was delayed. At the permanent-section stage an invasive serous cystadenocarcinoma was diagnosed and it was decided to carry out restaging. Three weeks later numerous vegetations of less than 1 mm were found in the posterior cul-de-sac at laparoscopy. A laparotomy and a classic radical treatment were performed. Although the diagnosis of peritoneal metastases had been confirmed by the biopsies performed at laparoscopy, the peritoneal vegetations were almost impossible to see at laparotomy. Several explanations can be proposed to explain this dissemination: the spontaneous evolution of the tumour, the worsening of the prognosis induced by a surgical procedure or a change in the prognosis induced by the laparoscopic approach.

When deciding between laparoscopy and laparotomy, some situations are simple and appear as reasonable and almost definitive limits of laparoscopic surgery. For example, a laparotomy is required: (i) in patients with ascites and peritoneal dissemination; and (ii) to treat friable solid ovarian tumours and large tumours with big solid components which cannot be placed in a bag and whose extraction would require such a large abdominal incision that the advantage of laparoscopy is questionable. By contrast, a laparoscopic adnexectomy is very attractive for the removal of a 5-cm cystic mass with an internal vegetation of less than 1 cm in a postmenopausal patient.

If laparoscopic treatment is decided on, the procedure should be atraumatic for the tumour and an adnexectomy should always be performed. The identification of the ureter is the first step. The adnexa should be placed in a bag as soon as possible. The extraction should be achieved without morcellation. An extensive peritoneal lavage should be carried out at the end of the procedure.

Staging

If the diagnosis of cancer is confirmed by frozen section, the staging procedure should be performed immediately.

If an ovarian cancer has been treated by adnexectomy or by inadequate procedures such as puncture, biopsy or partial resection, a restaging procedure should be performed as soon as possible. The steps for complete staging have been described by other authors [58]. However, if the tumour has been managed and/or removed by laparoscopy, two additional steps can be included.

1 The procedure begins by laparoscopy, because the peritoneal metastases possibly induced by the first surgical procedure may be very small and more easily and reliably seen and biopsied using the magnification provided by the laparoscope, as in a case described above.

2 Excision of the previous trocar entry sites is performed routinely, despite reports that the incidence of abdominal wall metastases at the trocar sites is very low (0.3%), as reported by Childers *et al.* [59].

The decision on treatment of the contralateral adnexa and of the uterus made according to the stage of tumour, the pathological diagnosis, the grade of the lesion, and the patient's age and previous reproductive history. This restaging procedure is performed by laparoscopy whenever possible [8].

Conclusion

Diagnostic laparoscopy is essential in the assessment of masses found to be suspicious at ultrasound. It allows macroscopic diagnosis and laparoscopic treatment of a large number of benign lesions. Many laparotomies are avoided by diagnosing non-ovarian masses, such as extensive pelvic adhesions, which may appear suspicious at ultrasound. Moreover, the initial laparoscopy can be used to assess the upper abdomen better than with laparotomy and to choose the abdominal incision, avoiding the treatment of an ovarian cancer by a low transverse incision.

However, until long-term results of large prospective studies have defined the limits and the contraindications for the endoscopic treatment of macroscopically suspicious lesions, great caution must be used in these cases. Laparotomy should be totally accepted as a surgical treatment and not be considered as only the result of a failure of laparoscopy. One case of tumour dissemination is not worth one thousand laparotomies avoided!

References

1 Canis M, Mage G, Wattiez A *et al* (1992). Kystes de l'annexe: Place de la coelioscopie en 1991. *Contracept Fertil Sex* **20**:345–352.

2 Nezhat F, Nezhat C, Welander CE, Benigno B (1992). Four ovarian cancers diagnosed during laparoscopic management of 1011 women with adnexal masses. *Am J Obstet Gynecol* **167**:790–796.

3 Hauuy JP, Madelenat P, Bouquet de la Jolinière J, Dubuisson JB (1990). Chirurgie per coelioscopique des kystes ovariens indications et limites à propos d'une série de 169 kystes. *J Gynecol Obstet Biol Reprod* **19**:209–216.

4 Parker WH, Levine RL, Howard FM, Sansone B, Berek JS (1994). A multicenter study of laparoscopic management of selected cystic masses in postmenopausal women. *J Am Coll Surg* **179**:733–737.

5 Hulka J, Parker WJ, Surrey M, Phillips J (1992). American association of gynecologist laparoscopist survey of management of ovarian masses in 1990. *J Reprod Med* **7**:599–602.

6 Shalev E, Eliyahu S, Peleg D, Tsabari A (1994). Laparoscopic management of adnexal cystic masses in postmenopausal women. *Obstet Gynecol* **83**:594–596.

7 Querleu D, Leblanc E (1994). Laparoscopic infrarenal paraaortic lymph node dissection for restaging of carcinoma of the ovary and of the tube. *Cancer* **73**:1467–1471.

8 Pomel C, Provencher D, Dauplat J *et al* (1995). Laparoscopic staging of early ovarian cancer. *Gynecol Oncol* **58**:301–306.

9 Childers JM, Lang J, Surwit EA, Hatch KD (1995). Laparoscopic surgical staging of ovarian cancer. *Gynecol Oncol* **59**:25–33.

10 Hart WR, Norris HJ (1973). Borderline and malignant tumors of the ovary. Histologic criteria and clinical behaviour. *Cancer* **31**:1031–1045.

11 Katzenstein ALA, Mazur MT, Morgan TE, Kao MS (1978). Proliferative serous tumors of the ovary. Histologic features and prognosis. *Am J Surg Pathol* **2**:339–355.

12 Colgan TJ, Norris HJ (1983). Ovarian epithelial tumors of low malignant potential: a review. *Int J Gynecol Pathol* **1**:367–382.

13 Tasker M, Langley FA (1985). The outlook for women with borderline epithelial tumors of the ovary. *Br J Obstet Gynaecol* **92**:969–973.

14 Kliman L, Rome RM, Fortune DW (1986). Low malignant potential tumors of the ovary: a study of 76 cases. *Obstet Gynecol* **68**:338–344.

15 Hopkins MP, Kumar NB, Morley GW (1987). An assessment of the pathologic features and treatment modalities in ovarian tumors of low malignant potential. *Obstet Gynecol* **70**:923–929.

16 Williams TJ, Symmonds RE, Litwak O (1973). Management of unilateral and encapsulated ovarian cancer in young women. *Gynecol Oncol* **1**:143–148.

17 Webb MJ, Decker DG, Mussey E, Williams TJ (1973). Factors influencing survival in stage I ovarian cancer. *Am J Obstet Gynecol* **116**:222–228.

18 Malkasian GD, Melton LJ III, O'Brien PC, Greene MH (1984). Prognostic significance of histologic classification and grading of epithelial malignancies of the ovary. *Am J Obstet Gynecol* **149**:274–284.

19 Grogan RH (1967). Accidental rupture of malignant ovarian cysts during surgical removal. *Obstet Gynecol* **30**:716–720.

20 Einhorn N, Nilsson B, Sjovall K (1985). Factors influencing survival in carcinoma of the ovary. Study of a well-defined Swedish population. *Cancer* **55**:2019–2025.

21 Sigurdsson K, Alm P, Gullberg B (1983). Prognostic factors in malignant epithelial ovarian tumors. *Gynecol Oncol* **15**:370–380.

22 Sainz de la Cuesta R, Goff BA, Fuller AF, Nikrui N, Rice W (1994). Prognostic significance of intraoperative rupture of malignant ovarian neoplasm. *Gynecol Oncol* **52**:111 (abstr 34).

23 Petru E, Lahousen M, Tamussino K et al (1994). Lymphadenectomy in stage I ovarian cancer. *Am J Obstet Gynecol* **170**:656–662.

24 Dembo AJ, Davy M, Stenwig AE, Berle EJ, Bush RS, Kjorstad K (1990). Prognostic factors in patients with stage I epithelial ovarian cancer. *Obstet Gynecol* **75**:263–273.

25 Sevelda P, Vavra N, Schemper M, Salzer H (1990). Prognostic factors for survival in stage I epithelial ovarian carcinoma. *Cancer* **65**:2349–2352.

26 Finn CB, Luesley DM, Buxton EJ et al (1992). Is stage I epithelial ovarian cancer overtreated both surgically and systemically? Results of a five-year cancer registry review. *Br J Obstet Gynaecol* **99**:54–58.

27 Vergote IB, Kaern J, Abeler VM, Pettersen EO, De Vos LN, Trpé CG (1993). Analysis of prognostic factors in stage I epithelial ovarian carcinoma: importance of degree of differentiation and deoxyribonucleic acid ploidy in predicting relapse. *Am J Obstet Gynecol* **160**:40–52.

28 Sjovall K, Nilsson B, Einhorn N (1994). Prognostic incidence of intraoperative rupture of malignant ovarian tumor with immediate surgical treatment. In: Bruhat M-A, ed. *Proceedings of the 1st European Congress on Gynecologic Endoscopy*. London: Blackwell Science, 107–108.

29 Maiman M, Seltzer V, Boyce J (1991). Laparoscopic excision of ovarian neoplasms subsequently found to be malignant. *Obstet Gynecol* **77**:563–565.

30 Crouet H, Heron JF (1991). Dissémination du cancer de l'ovaire lors de la chirurgie coelioscopique: un danger réel. *Presse Med* **20**:1738–1739.

31 Benifla JL, Hauuy JP, Guglielmina JN et al (1992). Kystectomie percoelioscopique: découverte histologique fortuite d'un carcinome ovarien. Case report. *J Gynecol Obstet Biol Reprod* **21**:45–49.

32 Canis M, Mage G, Wattiez A et al (1993). Tumor implantation after laparoscopy. In: Hunt RB, ed. *Endoscopy in Gynecology*. American Association of Gynecological Laparoscopists 20th Annual Meeting Proceedings. Santa Fe Springs, CA.

33 Trimbos JB, Haville NF (1993). The case against aspirating ovarian cyst. *Cancer* **72**:828–831.

34 Blanc B, Nicoloso E, d'Ercole C, Cazenave JC, Boubli L (1993). Hazards of systematic laparoscopic treatment of ovarian pathology. 2 cases. *Presse Med* **22**:1732–1734.

35 Hsiu JG, Given FT, Kemp GM (1986). Tumor implantation after diagnostic laparoscopic biopsy of serous ovarian tumors of low malignant potential. *Obstet Gynecol* **68S**:90S–93S.

36 Blanc B, Boubli L, D'ercole C, Nicoloso E (1994). Laparoscopic management of malignant ovarian cysts: a 78-case national survey. Part 1: pre-operative and laparoscopic evaluation. *Eur J Obstet Gynecol Reprod Biol* **56**:177–180.

37 Helawa ME, Krepart GV, Lotocki R (1986). Staging laparotomy in early epithelial ovarian carcinoma. *Am J Obstet Gynecol* **154**:282–286.

38 Canis M, Mage G, Pouly JL, Wattiez A, Manhes H, Bruhat MA (1994). Laparoscopic diagnosis of adnexal cystic masses: a 12 year experience with long term follow up. *Obstet Gynecol* **83**:707–712.

39 Valentin L, Sladkevicius P, Marsal K (1994). Limited contribution of doppler velocimetry to the differential diagnosis of extrauterine pelvic tumors. *Obstet Gynecol* **83**:425–433.

40 Carter JR, Lau M, Fowler JM, Carlson JW, Carson LF, Twiggs LB (1995). Blood flow characteristics of ovarian tumors: implications for ovarian cancer screening. *Am J Obstet Gynecol* **172**:901–907.

41 Bruhat M-A, Mage G, Pouly J-L, Manhes H, Canis M, Wattiez A (1992). *Operative Laparoscopy*. New York: McGraw-Hill.

42 Possover M, Mader M, Zielinski J, Pietrzak K, Hettenbach A (1995). Is laparotomy for staging early ovarian cancer an absolute necessity? *J Am Assoc Gynecol Laparoscopists* **2**:285–287.

43 Obiakor I, Maiman M, Mittal K. et al (1991). The accuracy of frozen sections in the diagnosis of ovarian neoplasms. *Gynecol Oncol* **43**:61–63.

44 Twaalfhoven FCM, Peters AAW, Trimos JB, Hermans J, Fleuren GJ (1990). The accuracy of frozen section diagnosis of ovarian tumors. *Gynecol Oncol* **41**:189–192.

45 Norris HJ, Zirkin HJ, Benson WL (1976). Immature malignant teratoma of the ovary. A clinicopathologic study of 58 cases. *Cancer* **37**:2359–2372.

46 Shefren G, Collin J, Soriero O (1991). Gliomatosis peritonei with malignant transformation: a case report and review of the literature. *Am J Obstet Gynecol* **164**:1617–1621.

47 Granberg S, Wikland M, Jansson I (1989). Macroscopic characterization of ovarian tumors and the relation to the histological diagnosis: criteria to be used for ultrasound evaluation. *Gynecol Oncol* **35**:139–144.

48 Herrmann UJ, Locher GW, Goldhirsch A (1987). Sonographic patterns of ovarian tumors: prediction of malignancy. *Obstet Gynecol* **69**:777–781.

49 Andolf E, Jorgensen C (1989). Cystic lesions in elderly women, diagnosed by ultrasound. *Br J Obstet Gynaecol* **96**:1076–1079.

50 Goldstein SR, Subramanyam B, Snyder JR, Beller U, Raghavendra N, Beckman M (1989). The postmenopausal cystic adnexal mass: the potential role of ultrasound in conservative management. *Obstet Gynecol* **73**:8–10.

51 Granberg S, Norstrom A, Wikland M (1990). Tumors in the lower pelvis as imaged by vaginal sonography. *Gynecol Oncol* **37**:224–229.

52 Luxman D, Bergman A, Sagi J, David MP (1991). The postmenopausal adnexal mass: correlation between ultrasonic and pathologic findings. *Obstet Gynecol* **77**:726–728.

53 Randall CL, Hall DW, Armenia CS (1962). Pathology in the preserved ovary after unilateral oophorectomy. *Am J Obstet Gynecol* **84**:1233–1241.

54 Bourne TH (1991). Transvaginal color Doppler in gynecology. *Ultrasound Obstet Gynecol* **1**:359–373.

55 Canis M, Mage G, Wattiez A et al (1994). The role of laparoscopic surgery in gynecologic oncology. *Curr Opin Obstet Gynecol* **6**:210–214.

56 Perry CP, Tombrello R (1993). Effect of fluid instillation on postlaparoscopy pain. *J Reprod Med* **38**:768–770.

57 Sahakian V, Rogers RG, Halme J, Hulka J (1993). Effects of carbon dioxide-saturated normal saline and Ringer's lactate on postsurgical adhesion formation in the rabbit. *Obstet Gynecol* **82**:851–853.

58 Hoskins WJ (1994). Epithelial ovarian carcinoma: principles of primary surgery. *Gynecol Oncol* **55**:S91–S96.

59 Childers JM, Aqua KA, Surwit EA, Hallum AV, Hatch KD (1994). Abdominal-wall tumor implantation after laparoscopy for malignant conditions. *Obstet Gynecol* **84**:765–769.

3 Transumbilical pelvic lymphadenectomy

Denis Querleu and Eric Leblanc

Introduction

Attempts had been made at node sampling by a limited retroperitoneal approach [1–3], then, in 1987, Dargent and Salvat [4] described a panoramic retroperitoneal approach for removal of the interiliac nodes. Since 1988 [5,6] we have used interiliac pelvic lymphadenectomy by laparoscopy in a significant number of patients. Later progress in laparoscopy enabled extension of the dissection to the common iliac area, and thus a full pelvic lymphadenectomy could be performed. However, not all patients with gynaecological cancer benefit from a radical pelvic lymphadenectomy, and in early (IA2 and IB1) cervical cancers interiliac lymphadenectomy only is recommended.

General principles

The patient gives informed consent to the laparoscopic procedure, but she should be prepared for progression on to a laparotomy in the event of technical difficulties or complications. A general anaesthetic is administered with tracheal intubation.

The patient is placed in the supine position without any flexion of the hips, as flexed legs may limit movements of the instruments in all directions in the abdomen. The legs are placed with a 30° angle, to enable the surgeon to stand between them when exploring the upper quadrants of the abdomen and when performing the common iliac lymphadenectomy. To explore the interiliac area and the true pelvis, it is usual to stand at the left side of the patient, but, when exploring the left lateral part of the abdomen and pelvis, it may be more useful to stand on the right side. Again, the common iliac and the para-aortic areas are best explored by standing between the legs of the patient. Two monitor screens are needed, one at the legs and one at the head of the patient.

As the vast majority of patients have a cervical or endometrial tumour, a cannula is not usually placed in the uterus. Indeed, the cannula is not necessary for the completion of lymphadenectomy, even in the lateropelvic

area, or for exploration of the abdominal cavity. Obviously a cannula is not used if there has been a previous hysterectomy.

A pneumoperitoneum is created and a 10-mm laparoscope is introduced through a minimal umbilical incision. In patients who have undergone previous laparotomy, an open laparoscopy may be preferable. The video camera is attached. After a preliminary observation of the liver surface, the appendix and the internal genitalia, two ancillary 5-mm and one 10-mm incisions are made through which ancillary instruments are introduced. The 10-mm port is used to accommodate specific instruments such as a clip applier and to extract the lymph nodes.

The placement of the ancillary incisions is quite important, and must not be affected by aesthetic considerations, but by the need to make optimal use of the instruments in different areas of the pelvis and abdomen. When the diagnostic procedure is limited to the pelvis, and specially the interiliac area, the 5-mm incisions are made in the right and left inguinal areas, approximately 4 cm above the inguinal fold, usually lateral to the inferior epigastric vessels. If a para-aortic lymphadenectomy is to be performed, the two 5-mm incisions are made approximately 10 cm lateral to the umbilicus. Both the pelvis and the para-aortic area may usually be reached through these last portals. The 10-mm incision is placed in the midline, approximately 4 cm above the symphysis pubis. In some patients with a very short distance between the umbilicus and the pubis, it may be useful to place this 10-mm port slightly lateral to the midline, usually on the right.

The exploratory and operative procedure require 4.5-mm scissors, a grasping forceps, an irrigation-aspiration device and a coagulation forceps. For fine haemostasis close to the ureter, the bowel or large vessels bipolar ferceps are most suitable, but monopolar electrosurgery may be used elsewhere. Removal of the lymph nodes from the abdomen is performed with a three-arm retractable Dargent forceps (Lépine) or within an endoscopic bag or, in most cases, under the protection of a reducer. However, it is essential to avoid even minimal contamination of the abdominal wall with specimens that could be malignant. The nodes will be removed after each step to make a precise pathological diagnosis of each area (i.e. obturator, hypogastric, common iliac, external iliac). The retraction of the bowel may require an additional port, either a 4.5 mm for the use of a probe or a closed forceps, or a 10 mm for the use of an endoretractor (Endoretract).

The entire surface of the parietal peritoneum and the surfaces of the intraperitoneal organs are observed. Material for peritoneal cytological examination must be obtained. Biopsies, when required, are taken by sharp dissection.

A classification of the level of lymphadenectomy has been used (Fig. 3.1) to clarify the description of the technique, and to help in comparisons between published papers. Level 1 is the interiliac dissection. It may be divided into two parts, anterior (1a, including the nodes located in the obturator fossa and the nodes located between the external iliac artery and vein) and posterior (1b, including the nodes located between the external and internal iliac artery and the deep obturator nodes located at the angle between the external iliac vein and the first hypogastric vein). Level 2 is the level required to complete a full pelvic dissection. It may be divided into three parts. Part 2a includes the lateral chain of the external iliac nodes on both sides. Part 2b includes the lateral chain of the common iliac nodes on both sides. Part 2c is located in the middle line; it includes the medial chains of the right and left common iliac nodes and the presacral nodes. Level 3

(lower aortic, below the inferior mesenteric artery) and level 4 (infrarenal, from the inferior mesenteric artery to the left renal vein) are not dealt with in this chapter.

Lymph-node sampling

In some operations intended only for staging, lymph-node sampling is the only procedure. Enlarged nodes may be identified by inspection or palpation of the nodal areas; however, enlargement is not specific for malignancy, and observation through the peritoneum is not necessarily accurate. The peritoneum overlying the suspect node is opened with scissors after identification of the ureter. The first goal of observation of the suspect node is to assess adherence to, or even involvement with, iliac vessels. When the diseased node is strongly adherent to a large vessel, attempts at removal may be hazardous, and needle aspiration for cytological examination is indicated. More frequently, the suspect node is not fixed, and removal is advised for pathological examination. Partial biopsy is inadvisable, as contamination of the peritoneal cavity or the retroperitoneal tissue could follow. Sampling of the entire node is preferable: the node is gently grasped, bluntly separated from the surrounding structures and removed through a large port. Clips may be applied on unresectable nodes for later radiological localization. After simple observation, selective lymph-node sampling or lymph-node dissection, the peritoneum is left opened. Fine-needle aspiration product or removed nodes may be immediately processed and read by the pathologist.

Laparoscopic interiliac dissection

As reported by other authors [4], pelvic dissection is in our practice limited to the interiliac area in all cases of endometrial cancer and in early cervical carcinomas. The rationale is that the sentinel nodes are in this area, and involvement of common iliac or para-aortic nodes is quite rare (less than 2%) when interiliac nodes are not involved. The interiliac area is defined (see Fig. 3.1) as the area between the external and internal iliac arteries. The dissection encompasses the obturator area, the medial and middle chains of the external iliac lymph nodes, and the internal iliac lymph nodes. The lateral chain of the external iliac area is not removed to avoid late lymphoedema. The common iliac vessels are not dissected.

When the procedure is only diagnostic, the infundibulopelvic ligament is left intact, and is retracted cranially along with the ureter when necessary. On the left side, the sigmoid colon usually has to be freed from the pelvic brim for a better view. To achieve this, the paracolic gutter is incised and the sigmoid colon is mobilized. The psoas muscle is identified, then the iliac arteries and the ureter

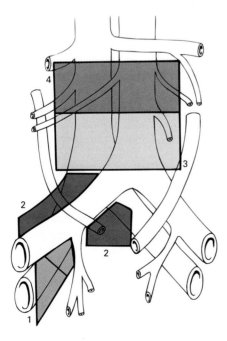

Fig. 3.1 Definition of levels 1–4 for lymph-node dissection. (Redrawn from Querleu [7] with permission.)

crossing the common iliac artery. When oophorectomy is planned, the operation may start with division of the infundibulopelvic ligament. This occasionally makes identification of the common iliac arteries and of the ureters easier. Haemostasis of the ovarian vessels is not in the remit of this chapter; bipolar cautery is safe and is a cheap procedure. However, it is usually preferable to leave the infundibulopelvic ligament intact during interiliac lymphadenectomy, particularly on the right side.

For right interiliac lymphadenectomy without division of the ovarian vessels, the patient is placed in a slight Trendelenburg position. The external iliac vessels, the umbilical artery and the ureter are usually identified under the peritoneal surface. The procedure begins with an incision of the pelvic peritoneum between the round and infundibulopelvic ligaments, parallel to the axis of external iliac vessels. The round ligament is grasped with a forceps to put the peritoneum in tension. The peritoneum is incised from the obliterated umbilical artery medially to the psoas muscle laterally, then it is easily torn or incised further to open the whole area between the round and infundibulopelvic ligaments (Fig. 3.2). The paravesical space is entered. Moderately dense connective tissue is found under the peritoneum, forming the roof of the paravesical space. This tissue must be incised or separated by blunt dissection. A blunt instrument (a closed forceps or the tip of an aspiration–irrigation cannula) is placed in the retroperitoneal space. Further identification of the external iliac vessels is carried out. In obese patients, it may be necessary to identify first the psoas muscle laterally, then the external iliac artery and, finally, the external iliac vein medial to the artery. In thin patients, the external iliac vein and the umbilical

artery are immediately identified. When the umbilical artery is not immediately visible, even after peritoneal opening, its position can be suggested by following its direction from the umbilicus to its crossing with the round ligament.

The paravesical space is then developed by blunt dissection between the umbilical artery medially and the external iliac vessels laterally (Fig. 3.3). The umbilical artery, along with the lateral wall of the bladder, is pushed medially to widen the paravesical space. Opening the paravesical space down to the level of the pelvic floor, well under the level of the obturator pedicle, is recommended. This can usually be achieved without any significant bleeding by following the lateral aspect of the bladder. The bottom of the paravesical space will then be used to store dissected nodes before removal, avoiding potential contamination of the peritoneal cavity by metastatic cells. The small amount of lymph fluid and blood from the dissection area will also collect in this area, leaving the operative field clear.

The obturator nerve is identified directly or by blunt dissection of the areolar tissue under the external iliac vein, parallel to the axis of the vessels. When the nerve is not immediately visible, it may be observed later at the obturator foramen, after identification of the pubic bone. The obturator nerve is easily dissected caudally to the point where it leaves the pelvis, by blunt dissection parallel to its axis. The cellulolymphatic area below the external iliac vein is then clearly visible. An anterior obturator vein is usually present, joining the external iliac vein to the main obturators veins. This vein may be dissected free or cut between clips or after electrodesiccation with bipolar forceps. The fatty tissue between the obturator nerve and the external iliac vein is then grasped with a grasping forceps in one hand, and thoroughly separated from the pelvic wall by blunt dissection with the tip of an instru-

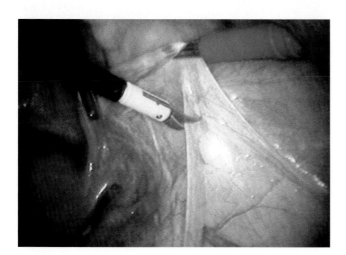

Fig. 3.2 Incision of the lateropelvic peritoneum (right side). The round ligament is elevated and the peritoneal fold artificially created is incised.

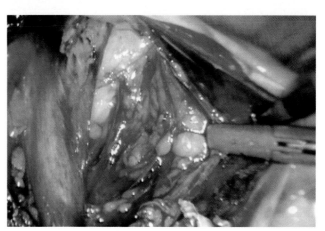

Fig. 3.3 Opening the paravesical space (left side).

ment held by the other hand (Fig. 3.4). The inferior aspect of the external iliac vein is separated by blunt dissection with a closed forceps. At this point, the pelvic bone and the internal obturator muscle are exposed. The caudal part of the connective tissue pedicle is then detached from the area of the obturator foramen and the femoral canal. This is achieved by gentle traction and/or section, with or without haemostasis by electrocautery. The tissue flap is then firmly grasped and moved cranially, then carefully dissected from the external iliac vein and artery laterally and the umbilical artery medially by blunt dissection. The obturator nodes (1a level) are ready for separate removal, as the obturator cellulolymphatic flap is loosely attached to the cephalic part of the dissection, and may be sampled by gentle traction. The removal of the middle chain of the external iliac lymph nodes completes the dissection of the 1a level. This chain is identified between the external iliac artery and vein. The lymphatic flap in this area is grasped and freed by blunt dissection.

The 1b level is then dissected. The nodes located in the hypogastric bifurcation area are gently separated by traction and blunt dissection from the external and internal iliac artery, up to the level of the division of the common iliac artery. Two ways of achieving this goal are possible: the surgeon can either follow the umbilical artery as a guide to the division of the anterior trunk of the hypogastric artery, or follow the external iliac artery. In both cases, the medial aspect of the external iliac vein must be identified and carefully freed. The operation is complete only if the angle between the internal and external iliac artery is dissected. This angle is usually visible only after a retraction of the infundibulopelvic ligament.

The nodes located below the external iliac vein must also be removed, up to the point where the hypogastric

vein (or the most caudal of the hypogastric veins) floods into the external iliac vein. The external iliac vein can either be pushed against the pelvic wall, or it can be dissected free from the pelvic wall. In the first option, the nodes are made visible by the flattening of the external iliac vein; they are grasped with an instrument coming from the opposite side and pulled medially to free them from the pelvic wall and from the external iliac vein. We prefer the second technique (Fig. 3.5), in which the external iliac vein is separated from the pelvic nodes. An instrument coming from the opposite side is used with care to retract the external iliac vein medially; the nodes are then freed from the pelvic wall by blunt dissection with the help of an instrument coming from the ipsilateral side. The retraction of the vein is released, and the nodes can be grasped easily and dissected from the external iliac vein. Care must be taken in this area to avoid injury to the origin of the obturator artery or to the pelvic veins. As there are numerous anatomical variants, the best advice is to fully dissect all the vessels in the area. This full dissection makes possible identification of the lumbosacral trunk and of the ischial spine (Fig. 3.6).

The nodes are extracted from the abdomen. If the reducer is used, it accommodates a grasping forceps. The forceps seizes the nodal chain in one or more parts. The node is placed in the lumen of the reducer, then the reducer is removed from the trocar along with the forceps and nodes. The abdominal part of this step must be followed with the endoscope, to avoid losing nodes in the process. For this purpose, a 10-mm trocar with a transparent sheath is used. Care must be taken to avoid leaving

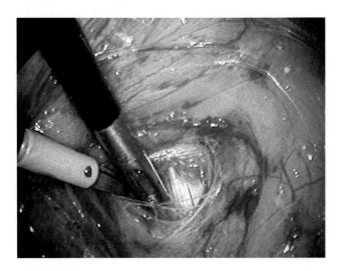

Fig. 3.4 Identification of the Cooper ligament (right side).

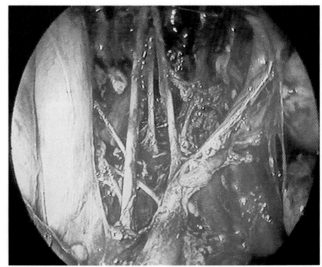

Fig. 3.5 Dissection of the branches of the internal iliac artery (left side). The left external iliac vein and, medial to it, the obturator nerve, are visible on the left.

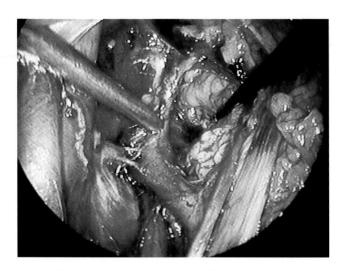

Fig. 3.6 The external iliac vein has been fully separated from the external iliac artery (left side). The vein and the obturator nerve are moved medially (right), making visible the internal iliac vein and its obturator and pudendal affluents, the pelvic bone (bright white surface, bottom left) and the lumbosacral trunk (bottom).

nodes in the dissected area, in the abdomen or in the trocar sheath. Haemostasis is confirmed; a minimal amount of blood may have to be aspirated. At the end of the procedure, the peritoneum is left open to allow drainage of the lymphatic fluid into the abdominal cavity. The same procedure is performed on the opposite side. No drain is left *in situ*.

Laparoscopic full pelvic lymphadenectomy

The removal of nodes lateral to the external iliac artery (level 2a) requires a blunt dissection between the psoas muscle and the external iliac artery, taking care not to injure the psoaic artery. This step may follow or precede the interiliac dissection.

The removal of common iliac nodes may be accomplished without changing position, by extending the incision in the parietal peritoneum above the infundibulopelvic ligament up to the level of the sacral promontory. The ureter must be identified and displaced. The removal of presacral nodes requires an extension of the peritoneal incision and identification of the middle sacral vessels and the left common iliac vein. In practice, this step is usually included in the low para-aortic dissection, and is best performed by standing between the legs of the patient and looking at the screen placed at the head of the patient.

The operating table is placed in a 10° Trendelenburg position and tilted to the left. The bowel is gently retracted towards the left upper quadrant. The aorta is identified under the peritoneum, up to the level of the mesenteric

root. The posterior peritoneum is incised over the lower 3 cm of aorta and the first 2 cm of the right common iliac artery. The left margin of the incision is grasped by the assistant with a forceps and retracted laterally to the left side of the patient, which ensures, in most cases, retraction of the bowel. If this movement is not sufficient to lever the bowel away, an incision in the left upper quadrant is necessary to introduce an additional instrument to retract the bowel loops. The anterior aspect of the lower aorta and vena cava and the aortic bifurcation are identified and freed by blunt dissection.

The retroperitoneal space is then developed laterally under the right and left mesocolons, and the psoas muscles are easily reached. The lumbar ureters and ovarian vessels are identified under the mesocolon and retracted laterally when working on either side. Throughout this step of the operation, there must be careful control of small bleeders. This dissection is much more difficult and hazardous than the easier interiliac dissection. Blunt dissection with the closed end of the atraumatic forceps or with the tip of the aspiration device (used at the same time to clarify the operative field when necessary) can be used. Electrosurgery with monopolar scissors may also be used. As soon as part of a flap is freed from the great vessels, it may be firmly grasped with a forceps and elevated to show its posterior aspect, overlying the vessels or the prevertebral plane. Dissection of the great vessels must proceed with extreme care. All of the small vessels going to or coming from the common iliac veins must be electrodesiccated with bipolar forceps or occluded using clips. A lumbar vein may have to be identified beneath the left common iliac artery. The middle sacral vessels must be identified in front of the prevertebral fascia at the level of the promontory. When moderate bleeding occurs, the surgeon must remain calm and use compression with the tip of a closed atraumatic forceps, the aspiration—irrigation cannula or a sponge. The bleeding stops either spontaneously or after elective haemostasis with clips or electrodesiccation (Figs 3.7 & 3.8).

The goal of this step of the procedure is to identify and to free the nodes lateral to the common iliac arteries (level 2b), the nodes overlying the left common iliac vein and the presacral nodes (level 2c).

The right ureter and ovarian vessels must be reflected laterally to locate and to free the nodes lateral to the right common iliac artery. The nodes are grasped and pulled laterally. The lateral aspect of the right common iliac artery is freed by blunt dissection parallel to its axis. The bifurcation of the right common iliac artery is reached, and the previously performed interiliac dissection is reached.

The nodes lateral to the left common iliac artery are first

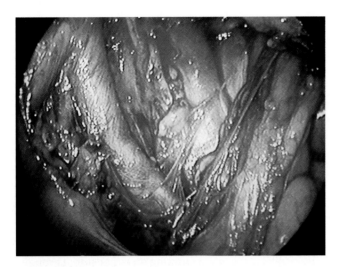

Fig. 3.7 Left common iliac dissection. The posterior parietal peritoneum is opened. The lateral and anterior aspects of the common iliac artery have been dissected, from the aortic bifurcation (top left) to the common iliac bifurcation (bottom). The psoas muscle is visible (middle of the picture).

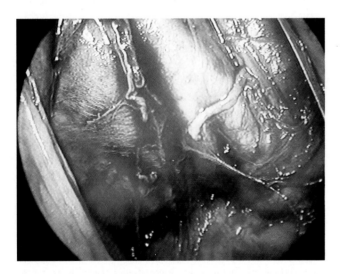

Fig. 3.8 Left common iliac dissection. The medial aspect of the common iliac artery has been dissected. The external and internal artery are identified (right). The bifurcation of the inferior vena cava is visible (left), overlying the promontory (bottom).

freed at the level of the aortic bifurcation. The left ureter is identified under the sigmoid mesocolon and retracted laterally. Care must be taken to avoid injury to the inferior mesenteric artery. When a para-aortic dissection is performed, the inferior mesenteric artery is freed in a caudal direction from its origin. If the origin of the inferior mesenteric is not identified, the left common iliac artery must be followed as close as possible. The inferior mesentery artery is then retracted by reflecting the mesocolon later-

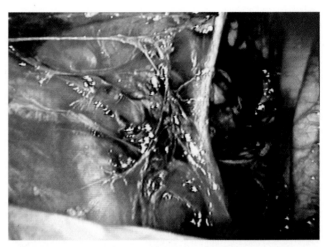

Fig. 3.9 The uterine artery node (right side). The cervical cancer has been injected with dye. The blue dye is visible in the lymphatic channels joining the cervix (top left) to the origin of the uterine artery (centre). The dyes concentrate at the origin of the uterine artery. The ureter is visible (bottom left).

ally. The left lateral common iliac nodes are located under the mesocolon, medial to the ureter, and lateral to the left common iliac artery. They are gradually freed as far as possible under the mesocolon. The sigmoid colon is then retracted medially, and the left lower pelvic dissection is reached to ensure that the entire common iliac artery has been freed down to the level of the hypogastric bifurcation (Fig. 3.9).

The nodes located immediately distal to the bifurcation of the aorta are easily found, overlying the left common iliac vein. They have to be removed with extreme care to avoid even minimal injuries to the vessels. Gradually identify and free the medial aspect of the left common iliac artery, then the anterior face of the common iliac vein, then the medial aspect of the left common iliac vein; this must be performed slowly and carefully, with preventive haemostasis.

The presacral nodes are located in front of the prevertebral fascia, caudal to the origin of the vena cava and medial to the right common iliac artery. The medial aspect of the left common iliac vein must be identified first, as well as the origin of the middle sacral vessels. Exposing the prevertebral fascia is then quite easy. The promontory is exposed, and the presacral space may be partially entered. Finally, the nodes are grasped and freed from the medial aspect of the right common iliac artery.

Haemostasis is checked. The peritoneum is left open.

Paracervical lymphadenectomy (Figs 3.10–3.12)

The removal of the parietal lymph nodes related to the uterus is generally referred to as 'pelvic' lymphaden-

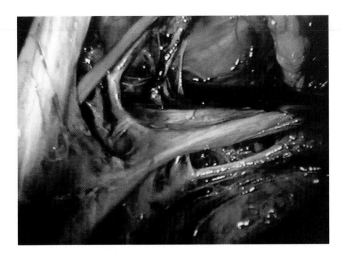

Fig. 3.10 Status of the cardinal ligament (left side) after paracervical lymphadenectomy. The deep uterine veins, the obturator artery, vein and nerve are dissected. No cellulolymphatic tissue is left.

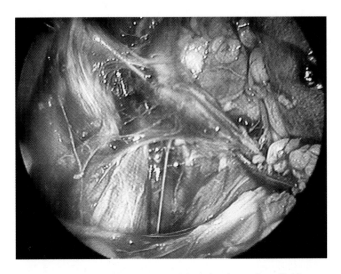

Fig. 3.11 Lumbosacral trunk view of the left pelvic side wall. The vessels are moved medially.

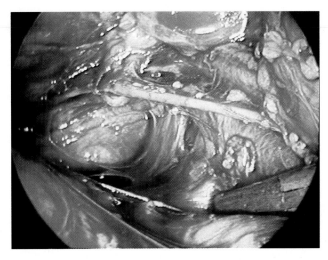

Fig. 3.12 The posterior aspect of the cardinal ligament after paracervical lymphadenectomy (right side). The pararectal space is opened. The faces of the space are the rectum (left), the sacrum (bottom), the cardinal ligament with the middle rectal artery (top), the hypogastric vein and the pelvic wall (right). The space is crossed by the autonomic nerves leaving the sacrum and penetrating the cardinal ligament underneath the middle rectal artery.

ectomy. However, these nodes are not the only ones involved in the natural history of cervical carcinoma. Some lymphatic channels, occasionally interrupted by one or several nodes, may be found running along the uterine artery. They may be selectively removed at laparoscopy by blunt separation from the uterine artery, or their removal may be included in the removal of the entire uterine artery during radical hysterectomy. This step of the operation is quite feasible by laparoscopy, as a part of a full laparoscopic radical hysterectomy or as part of a laparoscopically assisted radical vaginal hysterectomy [8].

Much more frequently, lymph nodes are found in the cardinal ligament (paracervix). They are anatomically spread either in the proximal part of the ligament, close to the uterus or in the distal part of the ligament, closer to the pelvic wall. The proximal part of the ligament cannot be sampled without performing, at the same time, a radical hysterectomy, and it cannot be included in a staging procedure. However, the cellulolymphatic component of the distal part of the ligament may be removed separately from the uterus. This part of the staging procedure has been labelled 'paracervical lymphadenectomy'.

When the cardinal ligament is not macroscopically involved, cancer spreads by lymphatic channel and node involvement. The rationale for the removal of the cardinal ligament is the removal of the lymphatic tissue along with the surrounding fatty tissue of the ligament. Transection of vessels and nerves should be avoided, as this may lead to ischaemic fistula formation and long-term voiding difficulty secondary to bladder denervation. A magnified laparoscopic view, a clean operative field and direct access with the tip of the laparoscope and of the laparoscopic instruments to the deep pelvic structures enable careful dissection of the distal part of the cardinal ligament without unnecessary surgical trauma to the vessels and nerves.

Paracervical lymphadenectomy is the latest achievement of laparoscopic surgery in gynaecological cancer; it involves dissection of the distal part of the cardinal ligament and removal of the parametrial nodes, while sparing the vessels and nerves of the cardinal ligament. In the future this procedure may be used as a complement to a laparoscopic or vaginal modified radical hysterectomy, as it provides the oncological safety of the radical hysterectomy while sparing the patient the high risk of fistula formation and of long-term voiding difficulty associated with classic (distal) radical hysterectomy.

The installation is essentially the same for paracervical as it is for parietal interiliac lymphadenectomy. An instrument is placed in the paravesical space, pushing the bladder medially when the anterolateral side of the cardinal ligament is being worked on, or placed in the pararectal space, pushing the rectum medially for the posteromedial side of the cardinal ligament. As a consequence, the surgeon can work with two hands without any interference from other instruments. When dissecting on the right side, for example, the surgeon stands on the right side of the patient with the instruments placed in the middle line and in the right lower quadrant. The assistant holds the camera in his right hand and a retractor in his left hand, pushing the bladder or rectum towards the left side of the patient.

As the general direction of the cardinal ligament is posterolateral, this ligament has two visible faces—anterolateral and posteromedial. The edge of the ligament is formed by the anterior branch of the internal iliac artery. To start this step of the operation, it is advisable to complete first the parietal lymphadenectomy. As a consequence, the paravesical space is already opened. If necessary, this opening has to be enlarged. Additional blunt dissection is carried out to identify the levator ani. It is usually easy to identify, deeper than the obturator nerve, with its arcus tendineus leaving the ischial spine. In this area, care must be taken to identify, and not to injure, large obturator and parietal veins, as well as the obturator artery which may be quite small. It is then necessary to further develop the medial part of the paravesical space, to move the lateral wall of the bladder, and to free the whole anterolateral aspect of the cardinal ligament as medial as possible. The superior vesical artery is the first landmark. It forms the upper edge of the vesical ligament ('lateral bladder pillar'); its lateral aspect can be entirely freed down to the level of the pelvic floor by blunt dissection.

After this step, the lateral part of the cardinal ligament, between the pelvic wall and the insertion of the vesical ligament, is clearly identified. Its anterolateral aspect is composed of arteries, veins and cellulolymphatic tissue. The vessels include vaginal and inferior vesical arteries, deep uterine veins, vaginal and vesical veins. These veins usually join the deep obturator vein to form the hypogastric vein, but there are numerous possible anatomical variants. The main part of the cellulolymphatic tissue usually lies anterior to the vessels, at the medial part of the common visceral ligament. This part can usually be dissected *en bloc* using blunt dissection, with removal of a rectangular flap measuring approximately 2 cm in width and 1–1.5 cm in height. This flap corresponds to the part of the cardinal ligament removed in type 3 extended hysterectomies after placing a clamp at the root of the cardinal ligament. After the removal of this flap, the deep uterine vein is clearly identified. It is usually joined by vesical and vaginal veins coming from the vesical ligament.

In the distal part of the common visceral ligament, near the pelvic wall, the cellular tissue has to be carefully and gradually removed in small pieces. The vessels are identified, a small amount of fatty tissue is elevated with a grasping forceps, and the vessels are separated from the specimen by gentle blunt dissection. This careful and gradual dissection leads to identification and skeletonization of all the vessels of this part of the pelvic wall, including internal pudendal and deep obturator veins, and some other landmarks, including the ischial spine and, posterior to this, the lumbosacral trunk. It is not necessary to extend the dissection in the greater ischiatic foramen where the fatty tissue becomes more abundant.

The dissection is completed on the posteromedial aspect of the cardinal ligament. The pararectal space is entered, medial to the internal iliac artery. It is further developed by blunt dissection, moving the rectum medially, to identify the promontory and the presacral fascia. In some cases, the first sacral nerve is identified at the level of the first sacral foramen, as well as the parasympathic nerves leaving this nerve and running parallel to the pelvic wall. One aim of this dissection is to spare these nerves. To avoid dividing them, the landmarks are the rectal vessels, which are directed medially, overlying the nervous part of the visceral ligament. The cellulolymphatic tissue of this part of the cardinal ligament is located superficially to the rectal vessels and the nervous part. It is usually less abundant, more dense and more firmly attached to the vessels and to the connective tissue of the ligament than it is on the anterior face of the ligament. Blunt dissection is again advised, but the use of elective bipolar cautery followed by sharp dissection may be necessary.

Management of complications

Potential intraoperative complications are bleeding, injury to the ureter and injury to the obturator nerve. The other complications of laparoscopy and laparoscopic surgery are not specific to the dissection of the lymph nodes and will not be addressed.

Bleeding from small vessels will stop spontaneously or after fine bipolar cautery. Larger bleeders are first managed by compression. While maintaining the compression, clean the area, proceed with the dissection around the origin of bleeding, then slowly remove the instrument used for compression to identify the bleeder. The bleeding may be stopped by the use of clips or bipolar cautery. In some cases, the origin of a bleeder located in the upper interiliac area is impossible to locate. The advice, if significant bleeding does not resume after compression, is to divide the hypogastric artery with a stapler device (EndoGIA). The bleeder can be identified and controlled because of the separation of the two stumps of the artery. In other cases, the bleeding comes from the wall of a large vessel. A hole in a large vein may be controlled with two clips placed in a V fashion. A small bleeder in a large artery may be controlled by a short application of bipolar cautery. Obviously, major-vessel injuries, except injuries to the hypogastric artery, require a laparotomy for repair.

Injuries to the ureter have never occurred in our experience. They must be identified intraoperatively and can be repaired laparoscopically. A lateral opening may be closed with interrupted stitches and intracorporeal sutures. A transsection of the ureter can also be repaired laparoscopically. A ureteral catheter is placed by cystoscopy, pushed to the lower end of the cut ureter, attracted laparoscopically and placed in the upper end of the ureter. It will be used as a stent. The edges of the ureter are approximated with four 4.0 absorbable sutures.

Injury to the obturator nerve may be neglected, considering the minor and sensitive function of this nerve, but a repair may be performed by open surgery.

Postoperative complications are few. The rare symptomatic lymphocyst may be drained under ultrasound guidance.

Results

Laparoscopic pelvic lymphadenectomy appears to yield a satisfactory assessment of pelvic nodes with a minimum of surgical trauma. We have performed 350 interiliac dissections, including 252 interiliac dissections for cervical carcinoma. In 1997, the average yield was 20.1 nodes. The number of nodes removed in the obturator area (average 5–7 [6]) is comparable to the number removed by laparotomy (average 4.7–5.2 nodes in the obturator area [9]. The quality of the pelvic dissection was checked by laparotomy in 68 patients in our earlier surgical work, and no residual positive node was found. In our series of cervical cancer patients, positive nodes were found in 22% of stage IB and 34% of stage II patients. These figures are in the same range as those for lymphadenectomy by open surgery. Fowler *et al.* [10] reported that the accuracy of laparoscopic lymphadenectomy compares favourably with that of laparotomy, but only after several cases have

been performed. In our laboratory it has been shown that experience of 10 cases is enough to reach a plateau in the learning curve for laparoscopic pelvic lymphadenectomy in the pig (see Chapter 6).

Although a high proportion of complications has been observed in the earlier experiences of urological teams [11,12], no visceral injury and no unintended laparotomy were observed in our series. Seven intraoperative complications were observed. One patient did not tolerate the prolonged pneumoperitoneum, and we had to abandon the procedure after the removal of only three nodes. Eight cases of significant intraoperative bleeding (umbilical artery, obturator artery, uterine vein, epigastric vessels) were managed by compression, ligation or bipolar cautery. In one of these cases, control of bleeding at the origin of the obturator artery required a transection of the hypogastric artery with a GIA stapler. Laparoscopically, we have repaired a non-bleeding 2-mm injury of the external iliac vein. Clips may also be used to repair small lateral openings of large veins. Larger laceration of large vessels may have to be managed by laparotomy, but no cases have occurred in our series.

When laparoscopic pelvic lymphadenectomy was performed as the only procedure, the postoperative period was uneventful and the patients were discharged from the surgical ward the following day in all but one case. In this case, a spontaneously resolving pelvic haematoma was observed 5 days after laparoscopic pelvic lymphadenectomy and radium application. Two pelvic lymphocysts were observed.

Later stage results of laparoscopic lymphadenectomy are now available. Dargent [13] reported 51 cases of cervical cancer managed with retroperitoneal lymphadenectomy and radical vaginal hysterectomy. The 3-year survival rate was 95.5% in node-negative stage IB and IIA patients and 80% in node-negative early stage IIB patients.

Results from our series (unpublished results) are available with up to 90 months follow-up for 132 patients with early cervical carcinomas managed with laparoscopic pelvic lymphadenectomy. At the time of writing, the 5-year life-table survival rate is 83% for the whole group, and is similar to the survival of a historical group matched for age, stage and therapy. All recurrences were observed in high-risk patients (young women with bulky tumours or adenocarcinoma). Four recurrences were observed in the lateropelvic area alone in 102 operated node-negative patients. This lateropelvic recurrence rate of 4%, suggesting growth of missed lymph nodes, is similar to the rate observed after laparotomy (5% of 467 patients [14], 2% of 733 patients [15]).

The follow-up of 26 node-positive patients managed by external radiation therapy is available. Only one grade 3–4 complication occurred in this group, compared with six grade 3–4 complications in a matched group of patients in whom node dissection had been performed by laparotomy (*P* < 0.05). The survival was similar in the two groups (48% vs 47%).

Conclusion

Clinical results and evidence from an experimental randomized study from our laboratory [16] show that laparoscopic pelvic lymphadenectomy yields a similar number of nodes compared with laparotomy. The adhesion formation rate [16] and radiation therapy complications are reduced by a minimally invasive procedure which minimizes the surgical trauma.

The procedure is thus safe and accurate, and may be included in the staging and treatment of cervical, ovarian and endometrial cancers.

References

1 Bartel M (1969). Die retroperitoneoskopie. *Zentralbl Chir* **12**:377–383.
2 Giraud B, Dauplat J, Boiteux JP, Franconnet P (1987). Lymphadénoscopie pelvienne. *Chirurgie* **113**:495–498.
3 Wurtz A, Mazeman E, Gosselin B, Woelffle D, Sauvage L, Rousseau O (1987). Bilan anatomique des adénopathies rétropéritonéales par endoscopie chirurgicale. *Ann Chir* **41**:258–263.
4 Dargent D, Salvat J (1989). *L'Envahissement Ganglionnaire Pelvien*. Paris: McGraw-Hill.
5 Querleu D (1989). Laparoscopic lymphadenectomy. In: *Second World Congress of Gynecologic Endoscopy. Clermont-Ferrand, 5–9 June 1989*. Oxford: Blackwell Scientific Publications.
6 Querleu D, Leblanc E, Castelain B (1991). Laparoscopic pelvic lymphadenectomy. *Am J Obstet Gynecol* **164**:579–581.
7 Querleu D (1995). *Techniques Chirurgicales en Gynécologie*. Paris: Masson.
8 Querleu D (1993). Laparoscopically-assisted radical vaginal hysterectomy. *Gynecol Oncol* **51**:248–254.
9 Girardi F, Pickel H, Winter R (1993). Pelvic and parametrial lymph nodes in the quality control of the surgical treatment of cervical cancer. *Gynecol Oncol* **50**:330–333.
10 Fowler JM, Carter JR, Carlson JW *et al* (1993). Lymph node yield from laparoscopic lymphadenectomy in cervical cancer: a comparative study. *Gynecol Oncol* **51**:187–192.
11 Burney TL, Campbell EC, Naslund MJ, Jacobs SC (1993). Complications of staging laparoscopic pelvic lymphadenectomy. *Surg Laparosc Endosc* **3**:184–190.
12 Kavoussi LR, Sosa E, Chandhoke P *et al* (1993). Complications of laparoscopic pelvic lymph node dissection. *J Urol* **149**:322–325.
13 Dargent D (1993). Laparoscopic surgery and gynecologic cancer. *Curr Opin Obstet Gynecol* **5**:294–300.
14 Ng HT, Kan YY, Chao KC, Yuan CC, Shyu SK (1987). The outcome of the patients with recurrent cervical carcinoma in terms of lymph node metastasis and treatment. *Gynecol Oncol* **26**:355–363.
15 Webb MJ, Symmonds RE (1980). Site of recurrence of cervical cancer after radical hysterectomy. *Am J Obstet Gynecol* **138**:813–817.
16 Lanvin D, Elhage A, Henry B, Leblanc E, Querleu D, Delobelle – Deroide A (1997). Accuracy and safety of laparoscopic lymphadenectomy. An experimental randomized study. *Gynecol Oncol* **67**:83–87.

4 Laparoscopic para-aortic lymphadenectomy

Joel M. Childers and Keith M. Harrigill

Introduction

Before the modernization of laparoscopic equipment, operative laparoscopy for patients with gynaecological malignancies was essentially non-existent. However, recent refinement of equipment and skills has led to an increase in the potential uses for laparoscopic intervention in the patients. Laparoscopic pelvic and para-aortic lymphadenectomy are the keystones in the endoscopic management of cervical, endometrial and ovarian cancer.

To date, there are few reports in the literature on the use of transperitoneal laparoscopic para-aortic lymphadenectomy in gynaecological oncology. The first study was reported from the USA in patients with cervical cancer—a series of patients who underwent both laparoscopic pelvic and para-aortic lymphadenectomy in the staging of early or advanced cervical carcinoma [1]. Nezhat *et al.* reported a case in which a low right para-aortic lymphadenectomy was performed in conjunction with a laparoscopic radical hysterectomy [2]. Subsequent reports included patients with endometrial and ovarian cancer. Querleu and Leblanc demonstrated the ability to remove infrarenal lymph nodes in patients with adnexal malignancies [3]. Childers *et al.* reported their combined experience with laparoscopic para-aortic lymphadenectomy in 61 patients, documenting its feasibility, safety and limitations in patients with gynaecological malignancies [4]. Vasilev and McGonigle have reported on four patients who have undergone successful extraperitoneal laparoscopic para-aortic lymph-node dissection [5].

While reports are few, it appears that laparoscopic para-aortic lymphadenectomy meets the oncological standards of most physicians practising gynaecological oncology. However, some oncologists believe that para-aortic lymphadenectomies for patients with adnexal carcinomas should remove all lymphatic tissue, including that tissue underneath the vena cava and aorta. This type of procedure has not been accomplished laparoscopically. However, the standard para-aortic lymph-node sampling performed by most gynaecological oncologists can be accomplished laparoscopically. This includes tissue lateral and superior to the vena cava and aorta. Node counts reported by most authors using this technique are comparable to those via laparotomy. Boike *et al.* performed para-aortic lymphadenectomy, both open and laparoscopically, on patients with endometrial cancer and found no statistical difference in node counts [6]. Spirtos *et al.* performed bilateral pelvic and para-aortic lymph-node sampling on 35 patients with gynaecological malignancies and obtained an average of 28 nodes per patient, which is also comparable to reports using laparotomy [7].

Clearly, the hospital stay and, presumably, the overall recovery time of patients undergoing laparoscopic para-aortic lymphadenectomy is greatly reduced. In a series reported by Childers *et al.*, the average hospital stay for those patients who underwent laparoscopic para-aortic lymphadenectomy without subsequent laparotomy was 2 days [4]. In the series of laparoscopic staging of ovarian cancer reported by Querleu [3], the average hospital stay was 3 days, which is considered short by European standards.

The complication rate appears to be acceptable in experienced hands. Querleu has reported no complications in his experience with low and high para-aortic lymphadenectomy [8]. Boike *et al.* reported one patient with a delayed left lumbar ureteral injury which was managed with a temporary ureteral stent [6]. They also resorted to laparotomy in one patient because of bleeding from a small aortic vessel. Our experience with over 100 para-aortic lymphadenectomies is similar, with three lacerations of the vena cava. The first laceration required laparotomy and transfusion while the others were managed laparoscopically with clips. We also have partially transected the inferior mesenteric arteries in two patients, both of these problems were managed laparoscopically. In addition, we have partially transected one left lumbar ureter and this complication could be repaired laparoscopically. Therefore, despite six potentially serious complications, only one patient (1% of our series) required conversion to laparotomy. Spirtos *et al.* reported a 15% (6/40) major complication rate. Two patients had immediate laparotomy to control bleeding, two patients required delayed laparotomy for bowel herniation at a trocar site and two patients required readmission to the hospital for deep venous thromboses [7].

Para-aortic lymphadenectomy is limited by obesity. Obesity prevented the successful completion of lymphadenectomy in several of Boike's 37 patients [6]. On four of our first 61 patients, the lymphadenectomy could not be completed because of poor exposure secondary to obesity; Spirtos *et al.* limited their procedure to patients with a Quetelet index of less than 30. A good bowel preparation, Trendelenburg positioning and additional laparoscopic ports for bowel retraction may circumvent the problems associated with obesity in some patients. Body weight, height, trunk size and fat distribution are all factors which affect the ability to accomplish the laparoscopic procedure. The size and mobility of the small bowel mesentery also plays an important role. Often the surgeon will not know if the procedure can be accomplished until it is attempted. This should be discussed with the patient preoperatively and contingency plans should be made.

Preoperative considerations

Laboratory evaluation

We routinely obtain a complete blood count with differential, a Chem-20 panel, type and hold, and a urinalysis for our surgical patients. A chest X-ray is also obtained if the patient is over 50 and has not had a chest X-ray taken in the preceding 6 months, has a significant pulmonary history or is at risk from pulmonary metastasis. In addition, obtaining ECGs in patients over 60 or patients with known cardiac disease is worthwhile. A baseline OC-125 is useful in patients with known or suspected ovarian malignancy should postoperative chemotherapy be initiated, and additional studies such as CEA or CA-19-9 may be indicated based on patient history.

Bowel preparation

The laparoscopic approach to the para-aortic lymph nodes is frequently limited by poor exposure caused, in part, by poor bowel preparation. All patients should receive a preoperative bowel preparation. Currently, a liquid diet for 2 days prior to the procedure and the administration of one 240-ml bottle of magnesium citrate for each of those 2 days is used in our centre. A 1-day preparation with macromolecules is an acceptable alternative. Oral or intravenous antibiotics are not used routinely.

Anaesthesia

Following the evaluation of risk factors by an anaesthetist, general anaesthesia is implemented. An endotracheal tube is placed and end-tidal carbon dioxide and cardiac monitoring are carried out. A nasogastric or orogastric tube is inserted to empty the stomach contents prior to the placement of the primary trocar or Veress needle, thereby decreasing the risk of inadvertent viscus perforation. A pulse oximeter is used, and a Foley catheter is placed. The patient's arms are tucked into her sides with her hands in the neutral position, taking care to pad the ulnar nerve. The supine position is preferable, except for those patients in whom vaginal surgery is anticipated. These patients are placed in the dorsal lithotomy position (see 'Special considerations' below).

Because the patient's arms are tucked by her sides to give the surgeon room to manoeuvre, the anaesthetist may prefer to place an arterial or central venous line. The use of hypothermic prevention devices and antithrombotic stockings should be considered.

Operating room and instruments

Surgeons should be familiar with the instruments available at each of the institutions at which they operate. One of the more frustrating problems with laparoscopic procedures is the dependence on the ancillary equipment. Simple problems can result in long delays or abortion of the endoscopic procedure if the surgeon and hospital staff are not familiar with their equipment and with troubleshooting of any problems. A concerted effort should be made to become an expert in this arena, not relying on the nurses or staff. The operative instruments required for laparoscopic para-aortic lymphadenectomy are few and simple, particularly the insufflators, light sources, cameras and telescopes.

Para-aortic lymphadenectomy can generally be accomplished with a few simple instruments. The following are necessary: (i) sharp scissors for monopolar electrocautery—blunt-tipped, curved scissors are ideal; (ii) a large spoon forceps that fits through a 10-mm or 12-mm laparoscopic port; and (iii) a suction irrigator. The spoon forceps is helpful for the extirpation of the lymphatic tissue. A 10-mm 0° laparoscopic telescope is preferable for most cases.

More specialized instruments such as needle drivers, knot pushers, pretied slipknots and stapling devices are not absolutely necessary, but they are useful if complications are encountered or additional procedures are to be performed. On occasion, a laparoscopic clip applier may be indicated, most commonly to occlude perforating veins in the region of the vena cava.

Training

It is best to have advanced laparoscopic training before attempting para-aortic lymphadenectomy. There are several ways to learn the procedure, but the training of the gynaecological oncological laparoscopist is best carried out within a formal course. A course specifically on lymphadenectomy allows the laparoscopist to become familiar with instruments, troubleshooting methods, essential surgical techniques, safety considerations and the avoidance and management of complications. Video-teaching tapes and hands-on operative sessions in the animal model help the beginner to avoid many of the more common pitfalls made while mastering a new procedure. Working one-to-one with an expert is an excellent way to learn this technique.

Operative technique

Instrument insertion

Briefly, we prefer the direct trocar insertion technique. This is accomplished by placing a disposable 10-mm laparoscopic trocar and sleeve through an incision made through the base of the umbilicus. Upward traction to the anterior abdominal wall is applied using towel clips placed on either side of the umbilicus. In many instances, the incision made in the base of the umbilicus will already be into the peritoneal cavity and the laparoscopic sleeve can be placed without a trocar. If a trocar is necessary, it is inserted directly downwards, towards the aorta, taking care to remain superficial. This technique is safe. Considerable time is saved, and there is a lower incidence of annoying preperitoneal insufflation. If the choice is made to insufflate using a Veress needle first, we recommend insufflating to a pressure of 25 mmHg. This allows insertion of the primary umbilical trocar with minimal downward movement of the anterior abdominal wall. After insertion of the trocars, intraperitoneal pressure may be reduced to the normal pressure of 15 mmHg.

In patients with umbilical hernias or abdominal incisions involving the umbilicus, we begin by placing a Veress needle in the ninth or tenth intercostal space in the left upper quadrant and insufflating to a pressure of 25 mmHg. Once an adequate pneumoperitoneum has been established, an incision is made in the midclavicular line just below the costal margin; a 5-mm trocar is then introduced through the incision perpendicular to the plane of the skin. Intraperitoneal pressure is subsequently reduced to 15 mm. A 5-mm telescope is then placed through the sleeve and the subumbilical area is assessed for adhesions. If adhesions are present, ancillary ports are placed, adhesiolysis is carried out, and a 10-mm port is established. It is believed that placement of the primary port lateral to the midline adhesion offers better visualization during adhesiolysis [9].

Three ancillary ports are needed to perform para-aortic lymphadenectomy. The ancillary ports are placed under direct laparoscopic visualization to lessen the risk of bowel or vascular perforation. Five-millimetre ports are placed lateral to the inferior epigastric vessels and the rectus muscles bilaterally in the lower midline. The third port is 12 mm, and is placed in the midline two finger-breadths above the symphysis. This 12-mm port allows easy removal of nodal bundles as well as easy insertion of minilaparotomy pads. Intraperitoneal laparotomy pads are useful—they are excellent for applying pressure to bleeders, cleaning up blood-stained tissues quickly and easily, and they can be used to pack one side while performing lymphadenectomy on the other. All ports are then sutured to the skin. This allows easy insertion of the instruments and prevents the inadvertent removal of the sleeves.

Inspection of the intraperitoneal cavity

Following placement of the laparoscopic ports and before placement of the patient in the Trendelenburg position, it is important to explore the entire intraperitoneal cavity in a systematic fashion. Start at the ileocaecal junction and proceed in a clockwise direction, examining the caecum, appendix, right paracolic gutter, gallbladder, surface of the right lobe of the liver, right hemidiaphragm, falciform ligament, greater curvature of the stomach, anterior surface of the stomach, left hemidiaphragm and its ventricular pulsations, supracolic omentum, transverse colon and infracolic omentum carefully. Then continue with the evaluation of the descending colon and left paracolic gutter before placing the patient in the Trendelenburg position, which facilitates the examination of the pelvis by reducing the bowel into the upper abdomen. Pelvic examination should involve inspection of the bladder, pelvic side walls, rectosigmoid colon and cul-de-sac, as well as the uterus, fallopian tubes and ovaries. It is helpful when examining the pelvic side walls to grasp the utero-ovarian ligament and rotate or lift the ovary so that the ovarian fossa can be seen. Pelvic washings may then be taken.

Packing the bowel

It is mandatory to have the small bowel placed in the upper abdomen during the dissection of the para-aortic lymph nodes. This allows visualization of the operative field and helps to avoid injury to the bowel. To accomplish this procedure first place the patient in the Trendelenburg position (approximately 20°) and place the telescope in the suprapubic port. In obese patients, first flip the omentum over the transverse colon on top of the liver. Then systematically flip the loops of small bowel into the upper abdomen, making sure the mesentery of the small bowel is flipped as well. The time spent in performing the bowel packing is made up during the procedure, when the operative field is unobscured and the bowel is uninjured.

For the patient in whom the above measures are insufficient to gain adequate visualization, additional ports may be placed to retract bowel out of the operative field. Once the bowel is well positioned, several landmarks should be identified. These include the transverse duodenum, which may be seen as it crosses the inferior vena cava and aorta. The aorta, the right common iliac artery, and the right ureter as it crosses the right iliac vessels, should all be inspected before beginning the dissection.

Right-side para-aortic lymphadenectomy

The surgeon begins the procedure by standing on the left side of the patient, using a pair of graspers through the suprapubic port and scissors through the left lateral port. The assistant stands on the right side of the patient and uses graspers in the right lateral port and assumes control of the camera and telescope which is placed through the umbilical port. The camera should be oriented so that the aorta and inferior vena cava are horizontal on the video screen, with the patient's head to the right of the screen. This allows the operating surgeon to be completely oriented.

The procedure begins by incising the peritoneum over the aorta and right common iliac artery. This incision is extended inferiorly along the right common iliac to the right ureter, and superiorly along the aorta to the mesentery of the small bowel or transverse duodenum. The lateral peritoneal edges are then lifted, and blunt dissection is carried out laterally towards the psoas muscle. The right ureter must be identified. Lateral dissection is continued below the ureter and above the vena cava and psoas. The ureter is then elevated and moved out of the way by the assistant, who accomplishes this retraction using a grasper placed through the right lateral port. This improves exposure, prevents ureteral damage and also creates a small tent, which helps prevent small bowel from slipping into the field. The assistant holds the camera and provides exposure while the surgeon performs the lymphadenectomy.

The surgeon then sharply dissects the nodal bundle off the surface of the aorta by working in the adventitial plane of the aorta. This adventitial dissection is extended down the right common iliac artery and up the aorta as far as possible.

The process of unroofing the nodal bundle from the vena cava does not begin until the tissue has been freed from its arterial attachments. The separation of the nodal bundle from the aorta can begin anywhere along the vena cava and is accomplished by grasping and elevating the

nodal bundle. The cava will be tented upwards, so care must be used to stay in the proper plane. Small vessels should be cauterized with the tips of the scissors using monopolar electricity (coagulation current). Even a small amount of bleeding can stain the tissue, obscuring visualization. It is very uncommon to encounter a perforating vessel from the vena cava that cannot be controlled with monopolar electricity. Short bursts of current using a fulguration technique in which sparks are allowed to jump from the electrode to the tissue are completely safe, even using coagulation current.

The nodal bundle is easily separated from its lateral attachments to the cava and psoas using blunt dissection. The bundle is also easily transected at its cephalad and caudad extents with fulgurating monopolar electricity. Electrical effects are greatly enhanced if tension is kept on the tissue. Caution must be used during these transections as the transverse duodenum and the right ureter could be easily damaged if they are not completely seen. The bundle may then be extracted through the lower midline port using the spoon forceps. Haemostasis should be confirmed.

Right common iliac node sampling, if it is to be carried out, may be performed through the same peritoneal incision. The assistant retracts the ureter, atraumatically, towards the pelvis, exposing the nodal bundle over the right common iliac beyond its bifurcation. The dissection proceeds as before down the common iliac artery in the adventitial plane first.

Left-side para-aortic lymphadenectomy

The surgeon, now standing on the right side of the patient, again places graspers through the lower midline port and scissors through the left lateral port. The assistant holds the telescope and attached camera in the umbilical port, taking care to orient the camera properly with the major vessels horizontal on the monitor and the patient's head to the left of the screen. This positioning facilitates the actions of the surgeon, but the monitor will be upside-down for the assistant.

If the peritoneal incision has not already been made, incising the pre-aortic peritoneum is done in exactly the same manner as for the right-side para-aortic lymphadenectomy. This incision is carried as far cephalad as possible, and will eventually be limited by the small bowel mesentery or the distal duodenum. The caudal terminus of the incision should be carried to the proximal left common iliac artery.

The surgeon then dissects in the adventitial plane along the aorta both cephalad and caudad. This dissection should be as extensive as possible to provide maximum room and visualization for the lymphadenectomy. On the left side, the cephalad extent of the nodal dissection will be limitd by the inferior mesenteric artery. Because its origin from the aorta is frequently difficult to visualize, care should be taken to avoid injury to either the aorta or the inferior mesenteric artery. Again, the more extensive the dissection, the better the visibility will be during this portion of the procedure (Fig. 4.1).

Only after the pre-aortic adventitia has been adequately dissected free should lateral dissection along the psoas be carried out. By staying in the previously dissected adventitial plane, the surgeon will be able to safely dissect beneath the left ureter and rectosigmoid mesentery. Note that the sequence of the left-side dissection differs from that of the right, where the lateral dissection is done after the peritoneal incision is made but before the dissection of the pre-aortic adventitia.

Lateral dissection is performed until the psoas muscle and its tendon are clearly identified. The assistant may then place either the irrigator or the grasper into the dissected space beneath the rectosigmoid mesentery and left ureter, retracting to provide maximum exposure to the left-side para-aortic lymph nodes. This exposure is crucial because of the lateral position of the nodes with respect to the aorta.

Once adequate exposure is achieved, the nodal bundle is grasped near the aortic bifurcation and lifted anteriorly, while downward pressure on the aorta is applied with a second instrument. This traction frees the loose attachments between the two structures and aids in the dissection of the bundle. A window should be created bluntly beneath the nodal chain at its caudal end; transection of the bundle may then be carried out using cautery and scissors. Dissection of the bundle then proceeds cephalad using sharp and blunt dissection, with cautery and clips

used as needed for haemostasis. The cephalad end of the nodal chain is transected near the inferior mesenteric artery. The specimen is removed through the lower midline port, haemostasis is confirmed and copious irrigation is carried out (Fig. 4.2).

Infrarenal para-aortic lymphadenectomy

The vena cava and the aorta are separated from the transverse duodenum by blunt and sharp dissection. This dissection is carried cephalad, but lateral dissection is also carried out by sweeping the laparoscopic instruments bluntly toward the psoas muscles. The assistant maintains traction on the transverse duodenum. A fifth port may be needed to aid in the elevation of the duodenum (Fig. 4.3). Anterior retraction is then accomplished through the right lower quadrant and left upper quadrant, with the surgeons facing cephalad. The monitors should be repositioned towards the patient's head. We find it much easier for the surgeon to remove the nodes contralateral to the side on which he is standing; however, this is not absolutely necessary.

After adequate cephalad exposure is obtained, the nodal dissection is continued. On the right side, continue the previously performed lymphadenectomy to the origin of the ovarian vein, which typically enters the vena cava distal to or near the left renal vein (Fig. 4.4). On the left, the surgeon will be limited by the inferior mesenteric artery. By first extending the dissection caudad to the inferior mesenteric artery, enough of the nodal bundle may be freed to allow completion of the dissection of the chain by working cephalad to the artery. To gain adequate exposure, transection of the left ovarian artery may be required. This can be accomplished by using clips placed through the suprapubic port. After placing a clip on the

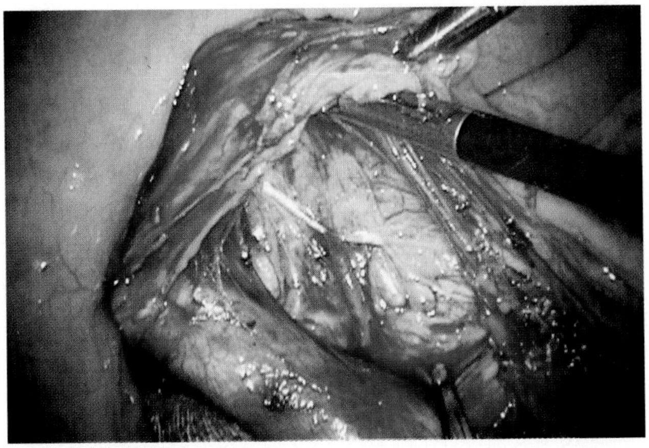

Fig. 4.1 Left aspect of the inframesenteric aorta. The head of the patient is on the left. The posterior parietal peritoneum has been opened. The left lumbar vessels are visible.

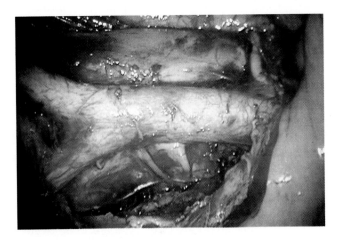

Fig. 4.2 Dissection of the aorta (bottom) and vena cava (top). The aortic bifurcation is seen on the left.

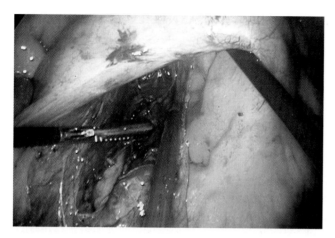

Fig. 4.3 Moving the transverse duodenum in order to reach the upper part of the dissection.

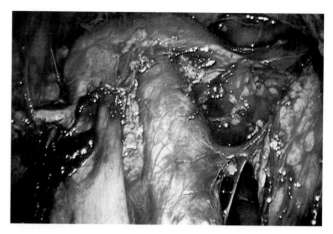

Fig. 4.5 After infrarenal dissection. The left renal vein (top) underlies the aorta. The right ovarian vein (left) floods into the vena cava. The inferior mesenteric artery is skeletonized (right).

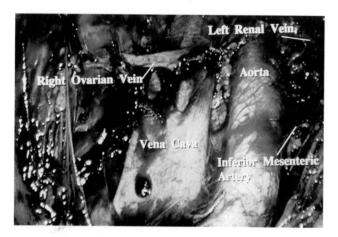

Fig. 4.4 After aortic dissection.

artery, cut the artery and continue the dissection to the renal vessels. Alternatively, monopolar electrocautery may be used to transect the left ovarian artery. The nodal bundle is transected near the left vein as it enters the vena cava (Fig. 4.5).

The peritoneum is not closed, nor are retroperitoneal drains placed. The small bowel mesentery is repositioned over the para-aortic incision site at the end of the dissection and the fascia and skin are closed in the standard way.

Special considerations

Cervical cancer

Patients with cervical cancer tend to fall into two categories. The first group are those who are to be treated with radiotherapy—their radiation fields are based on the findings at surgical staging. The second group involves patients who have already received external therapy and are being admitted for transperineal needle implantation. In this group, laparoscopic para-aortic lymph node dissection is performed and then laparoscopy is used in the placement of the needles. Following this, an omental carpet is created for protection of the pelvic organs.

Remove the proximal and low para-aortic nodes in both groups of patients. Many of these patients require additional procedures such as cystoscopy, proctoscopy and examination under anaesthesia, which should be performed prior to the lymphadenectomy. It is important to remove as much of the air from the rectosigmoid as possible following these procedures, because an air-filled rectosigmoid will make the lymphadenectomy more difficult.

Second-look laparoscopy for ovarian cancer

The intraperitoneal cavity should be carefully evaluated prior to undertaking lymphadenectomy in patients with ovarian carcinoma. Extensive adhesiolysis may be needed for adequate evaluation of residual or recurrent disease if the patient has undergone debulking. If there is no obvious evidence of disease, then washings and multiple intraperitoneal biopsies are taken. The remaining omentum is removed or biopsied, as indicated. Special attention is devoted to evaluation of the right hemidiaphragm; the magnification of modern cameras is especially useful in the evaluation of this high-risk area. If the liver is gently pushed downward with the telescope after placing the patient in a left lateral tilt position, a very different view of the diaphragm may be obtained from that obtained during laparotomy. Laryngeal biopsy forceps work quite nicely for biopsy of the diaphragm.

If all intraperitoneal specimens are negative, then a lymphadenectomy is performed. The lysis of adhesions upon entry into the peritoneal cavity now allows the placement of the bowel into the upper abdomen. Occasionally, there may be enough adhesions to prevent an adequate second look. However, a significant proportion of patients will have positive nodes.

Primary staging of ovarian carcinoma

Primary staging of ovarian carcinoma is possible in patients with presumed stage I disease [10]. Multiple washings should be taken, as well as biopsies from the pelvis and upper abdomen. Careful attention should be paid to the diaphragm in primary staging, as with second-look laparoscopy. In addition, omentectomy is performed along with pelvic and para-aortic lymphadenectomy. Thus far, all of our patients have had unilateral tumours and have therefore undergone unilateral pelvic and para-aortic lymphadenectomy. In these cases, an infrarenal para-aortic node dissection is performed.

Endometrial cancer

A combined laparoscopic and vaginal approach may be used in patients with stage I endometrial cancer. The laparoscopically assisted staging procedure includes intraperitoneal washings, lymphadenectomy and a laparoscopically assisted vaginal hysterectomy. The patients are given prophylactic antibiotics and placed in a dorsal lithotomy position. A uterine manipulator is placed to facilitate the laparoscopically assisted vaginal hysterectomy. Clips are placed across the fallopian tubes to prevent tumour spill during the procedure. Washings are taken and the entire abdominal cavity is carefully and systematically examined. No evidence of extrauterine disease was found in eight out of our first 61 patients, or in 35% (8/23) of patients with grade 2 or 3 lesions [11]. Identification, ligation and transection of the infundibulopelvic ligaments is carried out prior to performing pelvic lymphadenectomy in these patients. This is useful in gaining access to the common iliac nodes, especially on the left side. The surgeon must be familiar with the suturing and stapling techniques described elsewhere in the book.

Our decision to perform lymphadenectomy in these patients depends on the grade of tumour involved as well as the depth of invasion. Patients with grade 1 tumours and invasion to less than one-half of the myometrium do not receive lymphadenectomies.

Conclusion

Operative laparoscopy in gynaecological oncology remains a developing technology, but the ability to incorporate para-aortic lymphadenectomy into the management of their patients should entice some gynaecological laparoscopists to expand their use of the technique. The role of such a procedure has yet to be ultimately determined, although studies are currently underway to determine the utility of laparoscopic para-aortic lymphadenectomy in many gynaecological oncology patients. Our initial work suggests that laparoscopic para-aortic lymphadenectomy is both feasible and safe, even for nodes above the inferior mesenteric artery. However, it is a concern that low complication rates can only be expected when two experienced gynaecological laparoscopists perform the procedure, and that only after they have operated on their first 10–20 cases. This issue, and many others, remains to be resolved.

References

1 Childers J, Hatch K, Surwit E (1992). The role of laparoscopic lymphadenectomy in the management of cervical cancer. *Gynecol Oncol* **47**:38–43.

2 Nezhat C, Burrell M, Nezhat F (1992). Laparoscopic radical hysterectomy with para-aortic and pelvic lymph node dissection. *Am J Obstet Gynecol* **166**:864–865.

3 Querleu D, Leblanc E (1994). Laparoscopic infrarenal para-aortic node dissection in the restaging of carcinomas of the ovaries and fallopian tube. *Cancer* **49**:1467–1471.

4 Childers J, Surwit E, Tran A, Hatch K (1993). Laparoscopic para-aortic lymphadenectomy in gynecologic malignancies. *Obstet Gynecol* **82**:741–747.

5 Vasilev S, McGonigle K (1996). Extraperitoneal laparoscopic para-aortic lymph node dissection. *Gynecol Oncol* **61**:315–320.

6 Boike G, Lurain J, Burke J (1994). A comparison of laparoscopic management of endometrial cancer with traditional laparotomy. *Gynecol Oncol* **52**:105 (abstr).

7 Spirtos N, Schlaerth J, Spirtos T, Schlaerth A, Indman P, Kimball R (1995). Laparoscopic bilateral pelvic and para-aortic lymph node sampling: an evolving technique. *Am J Obstet Gynecol* 1995; **173**:105–111.

8 Querleu D (1993). Laparoscopic para-aortic lymph node sampling in gynecologic oncology: a preliminary experience. *Gynecol Oncol* 1993; **49**:24–29.

9 Childers JM, Brzechffa PR, Surwit EA (1993). Laparoscopy using the left upper quadrant as the primary trocar site. *Gynecol Oncol* **50**:221–225.

10 Childers J, Lang J, Surwit E, Hatch K (1996). Laparoscopic surgical staging of ovarian cancer. *Gynecol Oncol* **61**:315–320.

11 Childers JM, Brzechffa PR, Hatch K, Surwit EA (1993). Laparoscopically assisted surgical staging (LASS) of endometrial cancer. *Gynecol Oncol* **52**:33–38.

5 Retroperitoneal approach for lymph-node sampling and dissection

Daniel Dargent

Introduction

The retroperitoneal approach was first used for laparoscopic assessment of the pelvic lymph nodes in 1986 (author's case). The patient treated had stage IB cervical cancer. She was not suitable for abdominal radical surgery because the cancer had developed on the stump of a supravaginal hysterectomy and she had Wolff–Parkinson–White syndrome. The decision was taken to perform surgery through the vaginal route, after making an assessment of the lymph nodes endoscopically.

At this time urologists had assessed pelvic nodes using a technique derived from that devised by Carlens for the assessment of the mediastinal space. The instrument (the mediastinoscope) and the technique (digital preparation, introduction of the instrument at the contact of the targeted area) were the same. The results were also the same: samples could be taken under direct visualization but the field seen was rather narrow (no more than 2 cm wide — the width of the instrument used).

For the case described above, as a mediastinoscope was not available, a laparoscope was used. A microincision was made in the inguinal area. The retroperitoneal space was entered and prepared with the forefinger along the iliac vessels. The laparoscope was introduced into the prepared space and sutured to the abdominal wall opening by a purse-string suture, in the same way as it is for open laparoscopy. The carbon dioxide was insufflated through the sheath of the laparoscope. A broad overview of the pelvic wall could be made, including the lymph nodes to be sampled. Hence the techniques of 'panoramic retroperitoneal pelviscopy' and the 'endosurgical pelvic lymphadenectomy' came into existence [1].

Some time later Querleu and Leblanc [2] described another technique of endoscopic pelvic lymphadenectomy performed under the guidance of transumbilical transperitoneal laparoscopy. This technique quickly became very popular among gynaecologists, who were more familiar with transumbilical laparoscopy than the variations of the retroperitoneal approach. The urologists soon followed, and used Querleu and Leblanc's technique

[3]. However, the complication rate for the technique in the hands of surgeons who were not familiar with laparoscopy turned out to be very high [4], and many urologists currently use the retroperitoneal approach in preference to the transperitoneal approach [5–7].

Over the years, the choice between the preperitoneal and the transperitoneal approach was made according to the expertise of the surgeon: urologists, who are more familiar with preperitoneal laparotomy, were more inclined to choose this approach for laparoscopy, the gynaecologists did the opposite. Currently, many surgeons are familiar with both approaches (due to the increasing popularity of laparoscopic surgery for stress incontinence). The choice can be made according to the patient's conditions: this fits better with the Mayo's precept — we have to 'adapt the surgery to the patient and not the patient to the surgery'.

General principles

Before describing the technique, some general principles concerning the question of lymph-node involvement in cervical cancer and its management need to be discussed.

Basically lymphadenectomy has two goals: diagnosis and therapy. The assessment of the lymph nodes is of major value in establishing the prognosis of all sorts of epithelial cancer. As therapy, lymphadenectomy enables some patients affected by lymph-node metastasis to remain alive and disease free for a longer time — they certainly would have died if not operated on.

Two points have to be highlighted when considering the therapeutic value of the lymphadenectomy. First, the only cases where a good chance of cure can be expected are those in which the lymph-node involvement is limited (less than three lymph nodes). Second, laparoscopy is not yet acceptable as a surgical approach for debulking procedures. Even if the procedure is technically possible, the feasibility, safety and benefit have not yet been established as there are risks of peritoneal or abdominal tumour seeding. Therefore laparoscopy should be preceded by a complete imaging work-up. In the cases of obvious lymph-node enlargement, percutaneous fine-needle puncture is required. If the puncture is positive, the laparoscopy should be given up.

When using lymphadenectomy in establishing the prognosis, it must be borne in mind that most epithelial cancers involve the lymph nodes step by step. Sentinel lymph nodes may be defined. If they are free of disease, the risk of involvement is very low for the lymph nodes located both upstream and downstream. For example, in cervical cancers, the risk of involvement of the parametrial and aortic lymph nodes is low if the interiliac (obturator and hypogastric) nodes are free of disease. For these reasons, targeted interiliac lymphadenectomy is sufficient in early cervical cancers. Extended and systematic lymphadenectomy have only specific indications.

Standard surgical technique

The extraperitoneal approach can be used both for pelvic and aortic laparoscopic lymphadenectomy. The basic techniques are described here and the variants which can be used will be described later.

For pelvic lymphadenectomy and aortic lymphadenectomy the patient is placed in the classic 'frog leg' position. The instrumentation is basically the same as that used for open laparoscopy. All the instruments used for a minilaparotomy are needed. The disposable 10-mm trocar designed for open laparoscopy (Origin Blunt Tip®) is very useful. The other trocar and instruments are standard, with the exception of the coelio-extractor. This 10-mm instrument is operated by pressing the handle that pushes out a three-finger forceps. The lymph nodes are grasped and taken out without contaminating the abdominal wall (Fig. 5.1).

Interiliac lymphadenectomy

The main port for laparoscopic extraperitoneal pelvic lymphadenectomy is opened in the suprapubic area (Fig.

5.2, port 1). The surgeon stays between the legs of the patient. The skin is incised horizontally on the median line, 3–4 cm above the pubic bone. This incision is just long enough to admit the surgeon's forefinger. The fascia is opened vertically with the knife.

The surgeon introduces a forefinger into the retroparietal space on the median line and pushes a Mayo scissors along this finger. The tip of the scissors is oriented ventrally in order to open the cavum suprapubicum, a space located between the abdominal wall and the fascia parietalis. After entering this space the iliopubic bones can be prepared gently with the finger and the Cooper's ligaments are identified.

Digital preparation of the extraperitoneal space is faster (and cheaper) than the mechanical preparation that can be obtained using inflatable balloons. Also it is no more dangerous if care is taken to stop when any resistance is met. The space that has to be created is not very wide—to be large enough to introduce the laparoscope and two working forceps. The suprapubic forceps is introduced under direct guidance (see later). The other forceps will be introduced through the abdominal wall, about 8 cm cranially to the pubic bone and 3–4 cm laterally to the midline. In order to prepare the introduction of the second forceps, finish the digital preparation of the retroperitoneal space by detaching the peritoneum from the posterior face of the rectus abdominis muscle.

Once the first working space has been created, the laparoscope can be introduced to proceed under visual guidance. Formerly, we used a standard laparoscopic trocar covered by a rubber drain, attached to the abdominal wall by a continuous suture made on the margin of the cutaneous incision. Now we use an Origin Blunt Tip® trocar. The tip of the trocar is introduced into the retroparietal space. The balloon is inflated with 18 ml of saline. The external ring is moved down and locked. The extraperitoneal laparoscopy can now start.

To assess the pelvic wall, move to stand on the side of the patient opposite to the side on which it is intended to

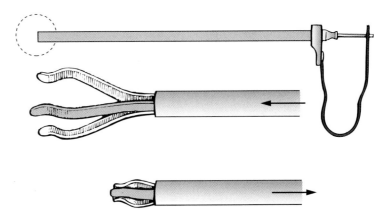

Fig. 5.1 The coelio-extractor.

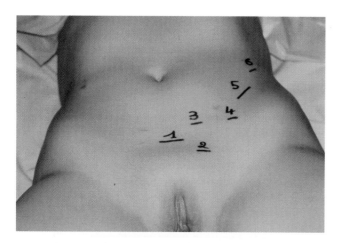

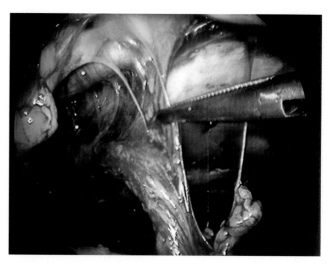

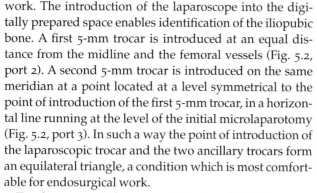

Fig. 5.2 Panoramic retroperitoneal pelviscopy on the left side. The order of placement of the ports: the pelvic dissection (ports 1–3), the common iliac dissection (port 4) and the aortic dissection (ports 5 and 6).

Fig. 5.3 Stretching the connective fibres joining the lymph nodes to the external iliac vein.

work. The introduction of the laparoscope into the digitally prepared space enables identification of the iliopubic bone. A first 5-mm trocar is introduced at an equal distance from the midline and the femoral vessels (Fig. 5.2, port 2). A second 5-mm trocar is introduced on the same meridian at a point located at a level symmetrical to the point of introduction of the first 5-mm trocar, in a horizontal line running at the level of the initial microlaparotomy (Fig. 5.2, port 3). In such a way the point of introduction of the laparoscopic trocar and the two ancillary trocars form an equilateral triangle, a condition which is most comfortable for endosurgical work.

Two laparoscopic forceps are introduced into the operative field by two 5-mm trocars (one grasping forceps and one dissecting forceps: a fine untoothed forceps). First identify the Cooper's ligament. This can be identified easily, even in cases where the alveolar retroperitoneal cellular tissue looks like a 'cobweb', making the anatomical structures impossible to recognize visually. Use the upper forceps as a blind man uses his white stick, slipping downwards along the posterior face of the abdominal wall until the corner of the pubic bone is reached, in the same way as a blind man reaches the corner of the pavement.

Having identified Cooper's ligament, follow it from inside to outside and the external iliac vein will be quickly reached at the point where it crosses the pubic bone. Then following the axis of the iliac vein detach the peritoneal sac from the pelvic wall with the tip of the lower forceps. The upper forceps maintains the obtained result. The lower forceps goes further, and so on until the level of the bifurcation of the common iliac artery is reached. At this point the preparation of the lymph nodes can be started.

The lymph nodes located on the medial face of the external iliac vein in the angle of the arterial bifurcation are prepared first. This is done by bluntly separating them from the vessels with the locked forceps used as a blind dissector. Then the forceps is used as a grasping instrument and the connections tying the lymph nodes to the surrounding structures are dilacerated gently (Fig. 5.3), but not entirely interrupted. The same is done on the obturator lymph nodes. Working on them is easier because the two forceps can be used as they are in conventional surgery. The grasping forceps pulls the lymph nodes and the untoothed forceps dilacerates the connections of the lymph nodes from their surrounding structures. The only danger in this area is the accessory or inferior obturator vein, which is a very frequent anatomical variant and crosses the obturator lymph-node chain and follows an uncertain course. Care must thus be taken while separating the lymph nodes from the caudal face of the iliac vein.

The interiliac lymph nodes—the nodes located around the origin of the hypogastric artery (hypogastric lymph nodes) and the nodes located between the iliac vein and the obturator nerve (obturator lymph nodes)—have then to be taken out. A 10-mm trocar replaces the 5-mm suprapubic trocar, and enables introduction of the coelio-extractor into the operative field. The inferior pole of the obturator group is grasped and pulled into the sheath of the instrument. The connective tissue and lymphatic channels still attaching the lymph nodes to the surrounding structures are interrupted using the dissecting forceps and the lymph nodes are extracted. The same is done for the hypogastric lymph nodes. Finally, the lymph nodes located between the most dorsal part of the external iliac vein and the pelvic wall, the retrovascular obturator lymph nodes, are entirely removed (Fig. 5.4). This step

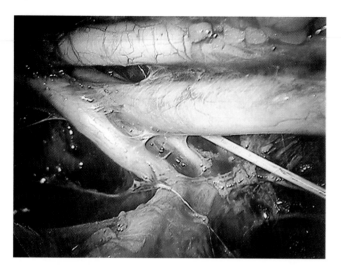

Fig. 5.4 The left pelvic wall after a dissection performed under panoramic retroperitoneal pelviscopy. From top to bottom: external iliac artery, external iliac vein, obturator nerve, internal iliac vein, internal iliac artery and its collaterals (obturator artery, inferior vesical artery and uterine artery).

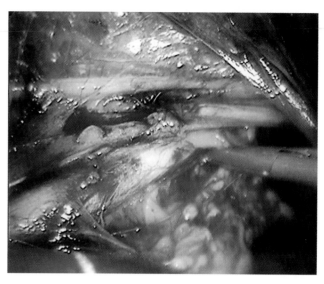

Fig. 5.5 Detaching the lymph nodes between the psoas muscle and the lateral aspect of the aorta. The left ureter and the left ovarian vein are visible above the aorta.

may be easier to perform using the suprapubic approach rather than the umbilical one. It must be emphasized that neither electrocoagulation nor clips are used, as the bleeding is negligible and the leakage of lymph fluid is of no consequence if a prophylactic fenestration of the peritoneum is performed at the end of the procedure (see below).

Common iliac lymphadenectomy

Preparation and extraction of the common iliac lymph nodes are not possible using the plan of action that suits interiliac lymphadenectomy. If the common iliac lymph nodes need to be assessed, the main port (the port used for the laparoscope) has to be the 10-mm inguinal port used for the extraction of the interiliac lymph nodes (Fig. 5.2, port 2). Under laparoscopic guidance, the peritoneal sac is detached from the floor of the iliac fossa while using a forceps introduced through the upper 5-mm trocar (Fig. 5.2, port 3) as a blunt dissection instrument pushing from inside to outside between the external iliac artery and the round ligament. Going further laterally, make free the posterior face of the abdominal wall in the area lying lateral to the inferior epigastric vessels, which makes it possible to introduce another 5-mm trocar just in the middle of the lower quadrant of the abdomen (Fig. 5.2, port 4).

Using the plan described above, the lymph nodes lying either medially or laterally to the common iliac artery can be prepared, including those located between the artery and the psoas muscle. The suprapubic median door is

used for the introduction of the coelio-extractor (Fig. 5.2, port 1) and for the extraction of the lymph-node material.

Aortic lymphadenectomy

If the lymphadenectomy needs to be extended to the aortic lymph nodes while maintaining the extraperitoneal route, opening a new port is mandatory. This opening is made in the McBurney area: a 3–4-cm oblique incision made 3–4 cm medially to the iliac spine (Fig. 5.2, port 5). The fascia and the muscle are divided, as in a classic McBurney incision. The extraperitoneal space is prepared with the finger. A cutaneous microincision (Fig. 5.2, port 6) is made symmetrical to the iliac microincision (Fig. 5.2, port 4), which will be used later for the introduction of a 5-mm trocar. Then the Origin Blunt Tip® laparoscopic trocar can be introduced. The retroperitoneal insufflation can start and the two working forceps are introduced (Fig. 5.2, ports 4 and 6).

The development of the peritoneal sac should not create any problems. The two working forceps are used in a divergent manner, in order to carry on the job initiated by the finger and to detach the peritoneum from the underlying muscle. The ovarian vein and the ureter remain attached to the peritoneal sac. They have to be clearly identified before starting with the preparation of the lymph nodes. The preparation is made in the same way as described earlier for the pelvic lymph nodes, but without detaching the lymph nodes entirely from the surrounding structures (Fig. 5.5).

On the left side the preparation is, at first, done in the

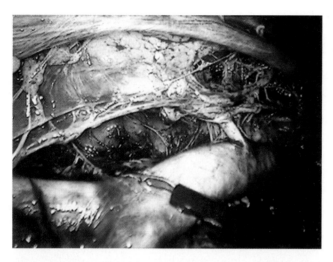

Fig. 5.6 The bifurcation of the aorta after a dissection performed through an extraperitoneal left-side laparoscopic approach. The left ureter is visible at the top and the inferior mesenteric artery in the middle of the figure.

space located lateral to the aorta and lying between it and the psoas muscle (Figs 5.5 & 5.6). The dissection starts at the level of the bifurcation of the aorta and proceeds cranially up to the level where the left renal vein crosses the ventral face of the aorta. After preparation of the latero-aortic lymph-node group, the inferior pole of the nodes is grasped with the coelio-extractor introduced through the suprapubic port (Fig. 5.2, port 2) and the lymph nodes are extracted while dividing the last connections with the dissecting forceps (be careful with the lumbar veins which cross the dorsal face of the aorta).

On the right side do the same with the lymph nodes located laterally to the vena cava and going cranially up to the level of the mouth of the ovarian vein. Then prepare the lymph nodes located on the ventral face of the vena cava and those located in the space between the vena cava and the aorta. The extraction is done in the same way as on the other side. Be careful with a little vein which joins the vena cava to the lymph node situated in front of it at the level of its origin. This vein is almost constant. It is not very significant but it is also very short, and tearing can lead to a lateral injury to the vena cava which can be very difficult to control. This is the only vein that has to be controlled before division. In all other places preventive haemostasis is not necessary if the right dissection plane is worked in!

Complications and problems

The potential complications of the endoscopic approach to the pelvic and aortic lymph nodes are basically the same if either the direct retroperitoneal or the transperitoneal approach are used. Bleeding occurring during the dissection is most common. The obturator vessels are the most endangered. However, the bleeding can usually be controlled laparoscopically.

A specific difficulty of the extraperitoneal approach lies in the problems encountered in opening the extraperitoneal space or in keeping it as a working space. Such difficulties do generally occur in patients previously operated on by laparotomy. In facing such a problem a number of different attitudes can be adopted. In our early experience we turned back to laparotomy. Then we gave up conversion to laparotomy and adopted conversion to transumbilical transperitoneal laparoscopy. Now we deliberately use as first choice transumbilical transperitoneal access for the previously operated patients, reserving the extraperitoneal approach for patients with an untouched abdomen.

The retroperitoneal approach, in addition to being sometimes impossible to perform, gives rise to three main criticisms. First, this approach will not visualize any intraperitoneal disease; consequently its only indication is in cases where the only risk lies in the retroperitoneal area, for example early cervical cancer. However, this drawback can be overcome as a classic diagnostic laparoscopy may be performed before starting with the extraperitoneal approach; moreover, classic laparoscopy can be an excellent guide to the surgeon during the initial steps of the extraperitoneal approach (see below). Second, there is a risk of lymphocyst. Prophylaxis of such a complication can be easily carried out. The pelvic peritoneum along the round ligament is incised at the end of the extraperitoneal procedure, this peritoneotomy is a prophylactic marsupialization of the lymphocyst. Third, using the transperitoneal approach, the cardinal ligaments can be prepared in order to facilitate vaginal radical hysterectomy. Theoretically, this preparation cannot be done if the extraperitoneal approach is used. In fact, the extraperitoneal approach can be used and this is described below.

Variants and prospective

The techniques described above have been carried out on several hundred patients. The techniques described below are more recent, and they are aimed at overcoming the drawbacks of the standard technique.

Comprehensive extraperitoneal approach to laparoscopic and laparoscopic-vaginal surgery for uterine and vaginal cancer

The most significant drawback of the techniques we described above lies in their specificity. Panoramic retroperitoneal pelviscopy is only suitable for assessment of the interiliac nodes. Common iliac lymph-node assessment and aortic lymph-node assessment need more ports. Panoramic retroperitoneal pelviscopy also does not allow for the preparation needed for a vaginal radical hysterectomy. However, other techniques exist which enable one to perform all the manoeuvres needed in the field of laparoscopic-vaginal surgery for uterine and vaginal cancer, while keeping the advantages of the preperitoneal approach. These techniques are described below.

A minilaparotomy is performed 3–4 cm below the umbilicus (transverse cutaneous incision, vertical aponeurotic incision). A transperitoneal open laparoscopy is performed first. After assessment of the peritoneal cavity the peritoneal incision is closed. Then the retroparietal space is prepared with a finger in the median area and in the paramedian area on the left side of the patient (it is assumed that the surgeon is right handed and stands on the left side of the patient). The Origin Blunt Tip® trocar is placed in position. The laparoscope is introduced into the retroperitoneal space. The inferior epigastric vessels on the left side are identified and the 10–12-mm trocar is introduced laterally to them at an equal distance from the umbilicus and left iliac spine. Using a forceps introduced in the operative field through this first lateral port, the posterior face of the abdominal wall right to the median line is bluntly developed and the second 10–12-mm iliac trocardization is performed on the right side. Watching from the infraumbilical minilaparotomy, the suprapubic area is prepared, the Cooper's ligaments are identified and the peritoneal sac is freed from the lateral pelvic walls.

The view obtained on the lateral pelvic wall is exactly the same as that obtained using classic laparoscopy. However, the most dorsal part remains difficult to assess because of the resistance of the round ligaments, which makes pushing up the peritoneal sac difficult. In order to overcome this difficulty the round ligaments are dissected in their retroperitoneal portion and divided near the inguinal canal. After section of the round ligaments, the peritoneal sac can be mobilized dorsally very easily, and the same good panoramic view that is seen while working through the classic umbilical approach is obtained.

The juxtaumbilical retroperitoneal approach enables straightforward dissection of the interiliac lymph nodes, including the lymph nodes located in the bifurcation of the common iliac artery (which are difficult to remove using panoramic retroperitoneal pelviscopy) and the lymph nodes located between the iliac vein and the pelvic wall in the most dorsal part of the obturator area. With a broad access to the dorsal part of the pelvic wall the approach enables us to manage the paracervix as well, in the same way as the classic approach (Fig. 5.7). Finally, it is the best approach to a common iliac and aortic lymph-node assessment.

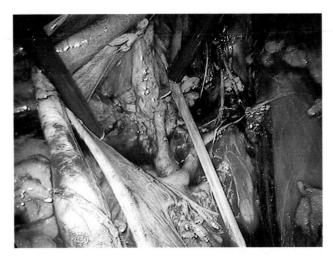

Fig. 5.7 The right pelvic wall after dissection performed under extraperitoneal transumbilical laparoscopy. From left to right: external iliac vessels (pushed medially using a laparoscopic forceps), obturator vessels, obturator nerve, sacrolumbar nerve and psoas muscle.

In order to assess the common iliac and aortic lymph nodes, the endoscope is placed in either of the lateral entry ports. The contralateral port is used to place a laparoscopic retractor (e.g. Auto Suture Endo-retract®). The juxtaumbilical port is used for a dissecting forceps to develop the peritoneal sac laterally. Then a 5-mm trocar can be introduced in the lumbar area. A second dissecting forceps is introduced and the upper lymph-node assessment can start.

Direct extraperitoneal approach to the aortic lymph nodes under transumbilical laparoscopic guidance

When the status of the pelvic nodes is already known or is of no significant value, only the aortic lymph nodes need to be assessed. The targeted area may be reached using minilaparotomy in the McBurney area, digital preparation of the retroparietal space and trocardization. This direct approach is not easy—it failed twice during our first six attempts. Therefore, it is best to start with a transumbilical laparoscopy to assess the peritoneal cavity (this is of great importance in the current indications of the aortic assessment) and to guide the procedure in the retroperitoneal space which is performed by the finger rather than by instruments. A second laparoscope is introduced laterally. The landmarks of the retroperitoneal operative field are identified. The transumbilical laparoscope is removed, the peritoneal cavity is exsufflated and the retroperitoneal aortic lymphadenectomy is carried out.

Extraperitoneal approach without minilaparotomy using trocardization under direct vision

The last variant has only a cosmetic advantage but it deserves to be mentionned: the absence or quasi-absence of scar is one of the great advantages of laparoscopic surgery. In order to avoid the scar left by the infraumbilical minilaparotomy, one can start with direct insufflation of the cranial part of the space of Retzius. The Auto Suture Visiport® device, the Ethicon Optiview® device or the Karl Storz Endotip® can be used. These devices were designed for safe transumbilical transperitoneal trocardization: piercing of the successive sheets of the abdominal wall is performed under direct optical guidance. In fact the retroperitoneal approach represents a logical use of these devices.

A 10-mm transverse cutaneous incision is made immediately under the level of the umbilicus. Subcutaneous adipose tissue and aponeurosis are entered under direct optical guidance. Then the retroperitoneal space is usually entered from behind the fibres of one of the two rectus abdominalis muscles, as it is very rare to work just in front of the linea alba abdominis. Once in the retroperitoneal space the cutting part of the device is withdrawn, the carbon dioxide insufflator is connected on the sheath of the trocar and the laparoscope is placed in position. The goal is to create a small space under the dorsal aspect of the abdominal wall around the midline and to identify the symphysis pubis. A 5-mm trocar is then introduced on the midline midway between the pubis and umbilicus. This trocar accommodates a scissors and mobilization of the peritoneum is undertaken as described above. Two 10–12-mm ports can then be opened in the iliac areas and the pelvic lymphadenectomy can be performed as well as preparation of the paracervix.

Conclusion

The first advantage of the retroperitoneal approach is anatomical—if the structures to be dealt with are retroperitoneal, the logical approach is retroperitoneal. It is the route most urologists use when managing diseases of the urinary tract. Also, the early gynaecological oncologists, such as Taussig and Mitra, advocated pelvic lymphadenectomy by this approach.

The second argument in favour of the retroperitoneal approach is haemodynamic. Retroperitoneal carbon dioxide insufflation has the drawback that there is a higher rate of transfer of carbon dioxide into the blood stream [8]. This rise in gas transfer is linked to the tightness of the space that is worked within. However, the acidosis which is a consequence of the exaggerated carbon dioxide transfer can be easily compensated for by artificial ventilation. Nevertheless, working in a limited space has the advantage of limiting the compression of the large veins and the haemodynamic consequences of this compression. The vena cava is compressed only during the aortic dissection on the right side, but it is interrupted during the whole procedure if transumbilical transperitoneal access is used.

The last and main advantage of the extraperitoneal approach is surgical. Respecting the natural bag that protects the bowel avoids trouble with the gastrointestinal tract during or after surgery. Respecting the peritoneum means that the organs which are attached to its inner surface, ovarian vessels and ureters, are protected. Work can progress without worrying about bowel and ureters. Therefore, postoperative problems with these organs, including intestinal obstruction and ureteric fistulas and/or stenosis, are very unlikely.

References

1 Dargent D (1987). A new future for Schauta's operation through presurgical retroperitoneal pelviscopy. *Eur J Gynaecol Oncol* **8**:292–296.
2 Querleu D, Leblanc E (1991). Laparoscopic pelvic lymphadenectomy in the staging of early carcinoma of the cervix. *Am J Obstet Gynecol* **164**:579–581.
3 Schuessler WW, Vancaillie TG, Reich H, Griffith DP (1991). Transperitoneal endosurgical lymphadenectomy in patients with localized prostate cancer. *J Urol* **145**:988–991.
4 Kavoussi LR, Sosa E, Chandhoke P, Chodak G, Clayman RV (1993). Complications of laparoscopic pelvic lymph node dissection. *J Urol* **149**:322–325.
5 Ferzli G, Raboy A, Kleinerman D, Albert P (1992). Extraperitoneal endoscopic pelvic lymph node dissection vs. laparoscopic lymph node dissection in the staging of prostatic and bladder carcinoma. *J Laparoendoscop Surg* **2**:219–222.
6 Das S, Tashima M (1994). Extraperitoneal laparoscopic staging pelvic lymph node dissection. *J Urol* **151**:1321–1323.
7 Etwaru D, Raboy A, Ferzli G, Albert P (1994). Extra-peritoneal endoscopic gasless pelvic lymph node dissection. *J Laparoendoscop Surg* **4**:113–116.
8 Mullet CH, Vialle JP, Sagnard PE *et al* (1993). Pulmonary CO_2 elimination during surgical procedures using intra or extraperitoneal CO_2 insufflation. *Anesth Analg* **76**:622–626.

6 Experimental laparoscopic lymphadenectomy

Dominique Lanvin, Abdou Elhage, Fabrice Lecuru,
Eric Le Goupils, Eric Leblanc and Denis Querleu

Introduction

The role of animal or cadaver experiment is critical in training for laparoscopic surgery. Reliable models for lymphadenectomy are readily available. Experiments on human cadavers are difficult to carry out, do not involve the standard conditions of surgery on the living subject, but they do reproduce the exact anatomical setting. Experiments on animals with an anatomy that is similar have the advantage of reproducing the stress and conditions of surgery on the living subject.

From a scientific point of view, experimentation is the only ethically acceptable tool to: (i) assess the learning curve of the individual surgeon; and (ii) compare laparoscopic techniques to laparotomy in randomized studies.

The authors of this chapter completed a series of experiments during the past 2 years. The experiment on human cadavers was performed by one of us (F.L.) at the University of Paris. The experiments on the pig model were performed in the animal laboratory of the Faculté de Médecine de Lille, France, and supported by a grant from the Délégation à la Recherche, CHRU, Lille, France.

These experiments will be reviewed in detail. All the experiments have been published or submitted for publication.

Some papers published in the literature deal with the development of a technique in experimental settings. Only the comparative trials completed in other laboratories, one in Belgium [1] and the other in the USA [2], will be detailed in this chapter. Both complement our research work, and give results consistent with our findings.

Laparoscopy and laparotomy for pelvic lymph-node dissection in human cadavers [3]

Materials and methods

Non-embalmed human cadavers were used. This anatomical model was preferred to the animal because the anatomy of the pelvic anatomy is rather different: pelvic vessels and lymph-nodel tissue do not have the same size, structure and relationship. Finally, extrapolation of animal studies to humans could be hazardous.

This study aimed to compare the effectiveness of pelvic lymphadenectomy using laparoscopy and laparotomy in the same subject. Secondary goals were assessment of the radicality and the operative morbidity of the laparoscopic dissection compared with laparotomy.

The anatomical models were placed in the Trendelenburg position. The side of the laparoscopic lymphadenectomy was randomly decided. Three-port laparoscopic access with disposable tools was used (Ethicon Ethnor Endosurgery). One was placed transumbilically (12-mm diameter), one was in a medial suprapubic position and one was lateral to the epigastric vessels. This installation was sufficient to perform a unilateral dissection. A 15-mmHg pneumoperitoneum was created using a high-flow insufflator (Olympus). A 10-mm laparoscope attached to a video camera gave a panoramic vision.

Lymphadenectomy was then performed using grasping forceps and scissors. Dissection was carried out between the external iliac artery laterally, the obliterated umbilical artery medially and the obturator nerve at the bottom of the obturator fossa. The lymphatic tissue removed between these boundaries was placed in the pouch of Douglas. Then a large transverse laparotomy was performed. Residual tissue in the area of the laparoscopic dissection was assessed. The surgical site and the whole abdomen were closely examined to look for any complication resulting from the laparoscopy. An open lymphadenectomy was performed on the opposite side, using the same margins. Each sample of tissue was placed in an anonymous pot containing a 10% formalin solution. Finally, a careful inspection controlled the quality of the dissection limits and noted any complications that might have occurred during the open procedure.

Lymphatic tissue was sent to a pathologist who examined it under light microscopy after fixation and staining with haematoxylin and eosin. The pathologist counted the number of lymph nodes in each lymphadenectomy specimen without any knowledge of the procedure used for each sample. The statistical analyses used were the paired chi-square test, Student *t* test or non-parametric tests.

Results

Thirty-three non-embalmed cadavers were used. Three cases had to be excluded from further analysis. Laparoscopy had to be aborted in one case because of an abundant ascites in an obese woman. Lymphatic tissue in another two subjects was poorly preserved, which prevented a correct evaluation by the pathologist. Once the dissection had begun, no laparoscopic lymphadenectomy had to be aborted.

The subjects were principally postmenopausal women. Their mean age was 77.6 years (SD = 9.8, range = 49–96). Twenty-three per cent of the women were obese (weight over 90 kg) and 23.3% had a history of laparotomy.

Fifteen laparoscopic lymphadenectomies were performed on the right side and 15 on the left side. Laparoscopy retrieved 112 lymph nodes (mean = 3.73, SE = 2.9). The average number was 3.3 ± 2.9 (range 0–11) on the right side and 4.1 ± 2.9 (range 0–11) on the left side (NS). Eighty-four lymph nodes were obtained with the open technique (mean 2.77, SE = 2.06). The average number was 1.73 (range 0–6) on the right side and 3.8 (range 0–6) on the left side. Laparoscopy harvested more nodes than laparotomy, but the difference was not significant (*P* = 0.1). The completeness of dissection was not significantly different in the initial 10 procedures than in the second 10 or the last 10 procedures (Wilcoxon *T* test and linear regression). The number of lymph nodes retrieved by laparotomy increased significantly from the begining to the end of the study (*P* < 0.006), although the open dissections were complete in all cases.

The effectiveness was lower for laparoscopy and open surgery in subjects with previous history of laparotomy or pelvic surgery, but this variation was not significant (respectively 4.04 ± 3.05 and 2.8 ± 1.96 vs 2.7 ± 2.2 and 2.5). The number of harvested lymph nodes increased with the corpulence of the cadavers for the two techniques (not significant).

Residual tissue was found after laparoscopy in 13.3% of the procedures. In three cases (10%) fatty tissue remained in the area of the common iliac artery bifurcation, and in one case (3.3%) near the femoral canal. Half of these failures were observed among the first 10 cases and 75% among the first 15 cases. This residual tissue did not contain any lymph node, but it could have contained some. Incomplete laparoscopic lymphadenectomies were more frequent in obese compared to 'normal' subjects (40% vs 7%) and also in subjects with a previous history of pelvic surgery, but differences were not significant

(Fisher test). Open lymphadenectomies were judged to be anatomically complete in 100% of cases.

Two complications occurred during the laparoscopic procedures (6.7%) and none during the open lymphadenectomies (NS). The two complications, an external iliac vein injury and section of a venous anastomosis between the obturator and the external iliac veins, occurred during the first 10 cases. A history of pelvic surgery significantly increased the complication rate (40% vs 0%, *P* < 0.05 Fisher test). Conversely, corpulence had no significant influence on morbidity.

Conclusion

This trial confirmed that pelvic lymph-node dissection could be performed by laparoscopy or laparotomy with the same effectiveness. A similar number of nodes was retrieved by both techniques. A learning curve was not recorded, probably because we have had previous experience in the technique. The effectiveness of laparoscopy did not vary significantly between obese and normal subjects, or between those with or without a prior history of laparotomy. Thus laparoscopic lymphadenectomy probably is effective in a routine situation, despite the characteristics of the patients.

The sensitivity of laparoscopy reaches 96.5% if it is postulated that open dissections are always complete; however, this is not true in clinical practice. The complication rate is very low and does not differ significantly for the two approaches. No complications were recorded due to the laparoscopic access, only operative incidents.

Non-embalmed cadavers are an interesting model for anatomical investigation and training. However, the operative conditions will differ from that in surgery on living patients. Dissection is made easier, but the recognition of some complications is impossible, and assessment of the postoperative period is obviously not feasible. For these reasons, animal models should be used in these situations.

Learning curve for pelvic and para-aortic lymphadenectomy [4]

Materials and methods

Three surgeons were involved in this study. One of them (A.E.) was an assistant experienced in transperitoneal laparoscopic pelvic lymphadenectomy but not in para-aortic lymphadenectomy. This surgeon completed a para-aortic lymph-node dissection for each animal. The two others were residents (B.H. and D.L.) who were trained in basic surgical techniques in laparoscopy. They were not experienced in transperitoneal laparoscopic pelvic lymphadenectomy. These surgeons performed a pelvic lymph-node dissection for each animal. One of them worked on one side, the second surgeon on the other side. The side (left or right) and the surgeon who began were randomly distributed. Twenty adult female hogs were used for the study (Figs 6.1–6.3). The dissection started at the bifurcation of the vena cava and extended to the left renal vein. The lymph nodes between the aortic bifurca-

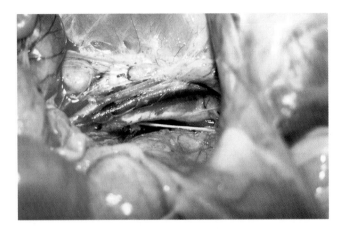

Fig. 6.1 Anatomy of the external iliac vessels and obturator nerve in the pig (right side).

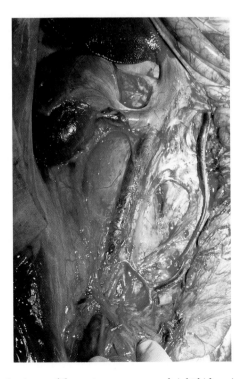

Fig. 6.2 Anatomy of the aorta, vena cava and right kidney in the pig.

tion and the left renal vein were retrieved. A bilateral pelvic lymph-node dissection was then performed. The lymphatic tissue along the external and internal vein, as well as the obturator space, was removed. All tissue material was examined histopathologically and the lymph nodes were counted independently for each case by a pathologist. The operating times were reviewed and included all the procedures performed. The intraoperative complications were noted. An exploratory laparotomy through a vertical midline incision was performed on all animals for noting the residual lymph-node counts. Twenty hogs were operated upon laparoscopically, and between none and six lymph nodes and between five and 26 lymph nodes were retrieved from each pelvic and para-aortic area, respectively.

Results

The learning curve of surgeons B.H. and D.L. were assessed separately. Between none and six lymph nodes were removed from each interiliac space. The number of residual lymph nodes removed at laparotomy by surgeon B.H. was between none and one from one pelvic side (left or right). After the first six cases, no residual lymph-node tissue remaining after laparoscopic pelvic lymphadenectomy was found at laparotomy. The time required for operation was between 12 and 60 minutes. Two complications were observed in 20 animals; haemorrhage occurred in the second and sixth procedure. A bladder artery was transected, but the bleeding could be controlled by cautery. A right internal iliac vein was injured by a grasping forceps and the injury was repaired laparoscopically.

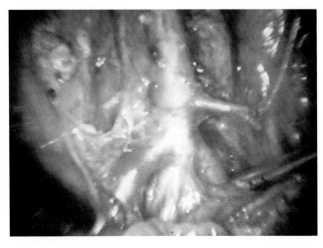

Fig. 6.3 Transperitoneal dissection of the aorta in the pig. The inferior mesenteric artery is visible on the right, the division of the aorta into three branches is at the bottom.

Surgeon D.L. removed between none and three lymph nodes from each interiliac space. The number of residual lymph nodes removed at laparoscopy was between none and two from one pelvic side (left or right). After the first nine cases, no residual lymph-node tissue was found after laparoscopic pelvic lymphadenectomy. The time required for operation was between 10 and 45 minutes. Two minor complications were observed in the fourth and fifth procedure. Inferior epigastric vessels were injured during a 5-mm trocar insertion but without significant blood loss. A parietal haematoma of the external iliac artery occurred during dissection, but without haemorrhage.

Between five and 26 lymph nodes were removed from the para-aortic area by surgeon A.E. The number of residual lymph nodes removed at laparotomy was between none and eight. The residual lymph-node number fell to under 5% after the first 14 cases. The time required for completion of the procedure was between 50 and 100 minutes. Four complications occurred in 20 animals in the second, fourth, eighth and 13th procedure. Three of the four complications were managed laparoscopically. Respectively, the caudal mesenteric artery was transected and a laparotomy was required to control the bleeding. The dissection was not complete. Bleeding from a gonadic vein was controlled by electrocautery. A lumbar artery was cut open, and haemostasis was achieved with a bipolar electrocoagulating forceps. A caudal mesenteric artery was transected, and the bleeding could be controlled by cautery.

Conclusion

It can be concluded that a learning curve for laparoscopic pelvic and para-aortic lymphadenectomy does exist. Ten procedures for pelvic lymphadenectomy and 15 procedures for para-aortic lymphadenectomy are necessary to performing these laparoscopic procedures effectively.

Laparoscopy and laparotomy for pelvic and para-aortic lymph-node dissection [5]

Materials and methods

Fifteen adult, female hogs underwent lymph-node dissection by laparoscopy and 15 underwent laparotomy. A complete pelvic and para-aortic lymphadenectomy was performed in each animal by an experienced surgeon. Lymph-node counts were performed for each case. The operating times were reviewed and included all the procedures performed. The intraoperative complications were noted. Four weeks after the lymphadenectomy, the animals underwent exploratory laparotomy and the adhesions were quantified.

Results

Thirty animals were evaluated. One animal died from the effects of anaesthesia. Another animal from the laparoscopy group died on postoperative day 12 from a small bowel obstruction resulting from herniation of the small bowel through a 5-mm trocar site. Haemorrhage occurred in three animals from the laparoscopy group. In one of the first procedures, a branch of the renal artery was transected, but the bleeding was controlled by electrocautery. Bleeding from an ovarian artery could be controlled in two other cases. There were no intraoperative complications in the laparotomy group. The average total number of lymph nodes retrieved by laparoscopy was 16.9 ± 3.8, which was not statistically different ($P = 0.77$) from 16.5 ± 4.9 nodes retrieved by laparotomy. The average operating time for laparotomy was 60 ± 16 minutes, compared with 128 ± 24 minutes for laparoscopy. Twenty-eight animals were evaluated for adhesion formation. The average adhesion scores observed in different locations of the pelvis and abdomen after laparoscopy were uniformly lower than after laparotomy. The average adhesion scores in the laparoscopy group (anterior abdominal wall 1.86 ± 1.51; para-aortic 29 ± 1.07; right interiliac space 0; left interiliac space 0) were lower than in the laparotomy group (anterior abdominal wall 5.14 ± 2.77; para-aortic 3.14 ± 2.48; right interiliac space 1.71 ± 2.46; left interiliac space 1.29 ± 2.13).

Postoperative complications were noted. One animal (7%) in the laparoscopy group had a wound infection, whereas three (21%) had a wound infection in the laparotomy group. The incidence of wound dehiscence was lower in the laparoscopy group (7%) than in the laparotomy group (21%). Four lymphoceles (28%) were observed in the laparotomy group only.

Conclusion

This study provides evidence that laparoscopic pelvic and para-aortic lymphadenectomy is safe and effective compared with the open procedure. The node yield is similar for both approaches. The transperitoneal laparoscopic pelvic and para-aortic lymphadenectomy may not induce the same degree of adhesion formation associated with laparotomy.

Transperitoneal and retroperitoneal endoscopic approaches for lymph-node dissection [6]

Materials and methods

Twenty adult female hogs were used for the study. Hogs

were randomly selected to undergo either a transperitoneal ($n = 10$) laparoscopic para-aortic lymphadenectomy or an extraperitoneal endoscopic ($n = 10$) para-aortic lymphadenectomy (Fig. 6.4). Two surgeons had been trained in laparoscopic surgery in clinical practice and also had previously performed 10 transperitoneal laparoscopic or extraperitoneal endoscopic para-aortic lymphadenectomies in pigs. Each surgeon was randomly assigned to perform a transperitoneal laparoscopic ($n = 5$) or an extraperitoneal endoscopic ($n = 5$) para-aortic lymphadenectomy.

Lymph-node counts were performed for each case. The operative times were reviewed and included all the procedures performed. The intraoperative and postoperative complications were noted. Four weeks after the lymphadenectomy, an exploratory laparotomy was performed on all animals for para-aortic, anterior abdominal wall adhesion scoring, late complications and residual lymph-node count. The adhesions were scored for their extent and tenacity. Retroperitoneal fibrosis was evaluated by scoring the difficulty of dissection and the assessment of the number of vascular injuries occurring during the dissection of the para-aortic area at the second-look procedure.

Results

The average operating time in the transperitoneal laparoscopic group was 83 ± 13 minutes, compared with 90 ± 21 minutes in the extraperitoneal endoscopic group. The average total number of lymph nodes retrieved by transperitoneal laparoscopy was 18 ± 9, which was not statistically different ($P = 0.67$) from 16 ± 7 nodes in the extraperitoneal endoscopic group. The average number of residual lymph nodes in the transperitoneal laparoscopic group (3 ± 2) was not statistically different from 6 ± 7 in the extraperitoneal endoscopic group ($P = 0.77$).

There were no intraoperative complications for either procedure. Postoperative complications were observed. One animal in the transperitoneal laparoscopic group (10%) had a peritonitis on the fifth postoperative day; there was no bowel injury. Another animal from this group died on postoperative day 25 with small bowel obstruction resulting from adhesion formation. One animal from the extraperitoneal endoscopic group died on postoperative day 5 with small bowel obstruction resulting from herniation of the small bowel through a large peritoneal gap. This gap was an injury that had occurred during the lymphadenectomy and had not been closed. Two animals (20%) in the extraperitoneal endoscopic group and three animals (30%) in the transperitoneal laparoscopic group had anterior abdominal wall adhesions. Two lymphocysts (20%) in those animals undergoing endoscopy and one lymphocyst (10%) in those undergoing laparoscopy were noted.

Both approaches induce a similar amount of retroperitoneal fibrosis. Adhesion formation was noted to occur less frequently after extraperitoneal dissection. However, the difference was not significant. For that reason, the experiment is being completed to increase the power of statistical tests.

Conclusion

These preliminary results show that the number of lymph nodes removed, the number of residual nodes and the operating time were similar in both groups. These data do not prove the benefit of extraperitoneal endoscopy over transperitoneal laparoscopy in terms of adhesion formation, but this remains to be confirmed in a larger study.

Nodal yield in endoscopic and open pelvic and para-aortic lymphadenectomy [1]

Twenty-one piglets were subjected to endoscopic lymphadenectomy. They were divided into two groups: 'early' (first 10 animals) and 'late' (subsequent animals). The instrumentation consisted of a 10-mm 0° scope connected to a single chip CCD camera, four trocars, two grasping forceps and a monopolar 5-mm scissors. In case of bleeding, visualization was enhanced by the use of regular swabs, introduced through the ports. Four lymph-node stations were discerned bilaterally: obturator fossa, external iliac, para-aortic and internal iliac. All visible nodes and fat tissue were removed between predefined margins, without attempting to dissect under the vessels. This pro-

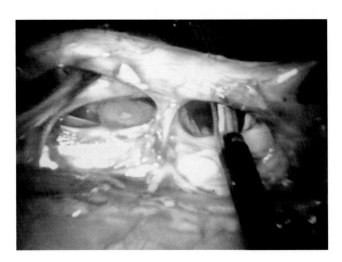

Fig. 6.4 Extraperitoneal dissection of the aorta in the pig. The aorta (top) has been separated from the prevertebral fascia (bottom). Three lumbar pedicles (left, middle and right) are visible.

cedure was repeated afterwards by laparotomy for resection of the remaining lymph nodes. The operating time (first incision to last stitch) and the number of lymph nodes removed by laparoscopy were noted. The nodal yield was defined as the number of nodes retrieved during laparoscopy divided by the total number obtained at both operations. Two major complications occurred: one ureter lesion and one bladder injury. Laparoscopic pelvic and para-aortic lymphadenectomy is feasible in pigs. A learning curve is suggested by a decrease in the operating time (91 ± 31 minutes in the early group vs 84 ± 10 minutes in the late group), but the nodal yield did not increase significantly over time (82 ± 10% in the early group vs 86 ± 7% in the late group.

This work confirms our findings on the node yield of laparoscopic lymphadenectomy compared with the same procedure completed via laparotomy. It includes performance of para-aortic lymphadenectomy. Although follow-up information is lacking, it also provides interesting information about the learning curve. The learning-curve process is found to be different in the Belgian experience, with only a limited improvement in the operating time and no increase in the node yield. This finding may reflect the relatively low node yield in this work.

Transperitoneal laparoscopy and extraperitoneal laparotomy for pelvic lymphadenectomy [2]

Pelvic adhesion formation was investigated in a porcine model after pelvic lymphadenectomy performed either via transperitoneal laparoscopic lymphadenectomy or via extraperitoneal laparotomy. The animals underwent second-look laparotomy, and the postoperative adhesions were quantified. Two groups of 10 animals were used; 10 animals were evaluated in the laparoscopy group, nine in the laparotomy group. No *de novo* adhesion was found in 80% of the laparoscopy animal group, vs 56% in the laparotomy group. The adhesion scores (mean 0.075 in the laparoscopy group vs 0.28 in the extraperitoneal laparotomy group) were not significantly different.

This work provides complementary evidence to our data, and shows that laparoscopic lymphadenectomy is not only superior to the open procedure performed via laparotomy, but also to the open procedure performed via an extraperitoneal approach. As the extraperitoneal

approach has been found to be associated with a lower frequency of postirradiation complications compared with laparotomy, further evidence that laparoscopy induces a minimum of *de novo* adhesions is given. Unfortunately, only pelvic dissections were performed in this research work.

Conclusion

Evidence is given that pelvic and para-aortic lymphadenectomy are safe and accurate, provided they are performed by experienced surgeons skilled in laparoscopic surgery techniques. The learning curve can be defined, and approximately 10 cases of pelvic and 20 cases of para-aortic dissections under supervision are required for the solo performance of the technique. The level of scientific evidence needs to be high because of the randomized design of the experiments, which would be ethically and practically difficult to carry out in living humans. The similarity between surgery on the living human and operative experimental conditions makes acceptable an extrapolation of the experimental results on the pig [1,2,4–6], considering that similar results have been obtained in a human anatomical model [3].

References

1 Deprest J *et al* (1997). Comparison of nodal yield between endoscopic and open pelvic and para-aortic lymphadenectomy in the porcine model. (Personal communication.)

2 Fowler JM, Hartenbach EM, Reynolds HT *et al* (1994). Comparison between transperitoneal laparoscopy and extraperitoneal laparotomy for pelvic lymphadenectomy. *Gynecol Oncol* **55**:25–28.

3 Lecuru F, Robin F, Neji K *et al* (1997). Randomized study comparing laparoscopy and laparotomy for pelvic lymph node dissection. *Eur J Obstet Gynecol Reprod Biol* **72**:51–55.

4 Querleu D, Lanvin D, Elhage A, Leblanc E (1998). Assessment of the learning curve for pelvic and para-aortic lymphadenectomy. *Eur J Obstet Gynecol Reprod Biol* (in press).

5 Lanvin D, Elhage A, Henry B, Leblanc E, Querleu D, Delobelle-Deroide A (1997). Accuracy and safety laparoscopic lymphadenectomy. An experimental prospective randomized study. *Gynecol Oncol* **67**:83–87.

6 Lanvin D, Le Goupils E, Leblanc E, Querleu D (1997). Randomized study comparing transperitoneal and retroperitoneal endoscopic approaches for lymph node dissection. MD thesis, Eric Le Goupils, Lille, France.

Section 2
Technique of Laparoscopic Surgery in Gynaecological Cancers

7 Laparoscopic modified radical hysterectomy

Denis Querleu and Eric Leblanc

Introduction

Stage I endometrial, microinvasive cervical and possibly early ovarian cancers may be treated with a combination of a laparoscopic staging procedure and vaginal or laparoscopic simple hysterectomy. When radical hysterectomy is required, in particular for cervical cancer, radical vaginal surgery may follow laparoscopic staging in the same session [1]. Techniques of laparoscopic or laparoscopically assisted radical hysterectomy have also been described. These techniques for radical surgery of cancer are still under investigation, but their feasibility has been demonstrated by several teams [2–9].

The term 'radical' hysterectomy includes many different operations. An attempt at classification has been published by Piver et al. [10]. However, this classification is not clear, and simultaneously takes into account the extent of removal of the cardinal ligaments (paracervix), of the uterosacral ligaments and of the vagina. We use only two terms, referring to two operations that are different in radicality. The only criterion used is the extent of removal of the cardinal ligaments (Fig. 7.1), taking into account that the lateral extent is the main source of complications, including fistula formation and long-term voiding difficulties. 'Proximal' or 'modified' radical hysterectomy refers to those procedures in which only the proximal part of the parametria is excised medially to the level of the ureters, and corresponds to the Piver type 2. The uterosacral ligaments are also removed in their mid portion proximal to the uterus. The vagina is incised to leave a 2-cm margin. 'Distal' or 'classic' radical hysterectomy is the procedure which removes the entire parametria, up to their insertion to the pelvic side wall, and corresponds to the Piver type 3 or 4. The uterosacral ligaments are removed in toto. Again, the vagina is incised with a 2-cm margin.

This classification is much simpler than the Piver and Rutledge classification, and may help to compare the results of different papers as far as the technique of radical hysterectomy is concerned. It is also more versatile, leaving the extent of removal of vagina dependent only on the extent of tumour. It takes into account asymmetrical operations, proximal on one side, distal on the other.

Only the technique of modified radical hysterectomy will be addressed in this chapter. 'Proximal' or modified radical hysterectomy is indicated for early stage IB, less than 2 cm in diameter or not exceeding $10\,cm^3$, or after primary brachytherapy. Different approaches have already been described for modified radical hysterectomies. Wertheim [11] described in 1900 what is now the standard modified abdominal operation. In 1928 Stoeckel described [12] a modification of the Schauta operation, that referred to as the Schauta–Stoeckel operation. Obviously, the vaginal approach does not allow lymph-node dissection to be performed, and it has been abandoned for that reason. Mitra described in 1959 [13] a combination of abdominal and vaginal surgery in which pelvic lymphadenectomy and section of the uterine vessels are performed abdominally by a retroperitoneal approach, then incision of the vagina and division of the cardinal ligaments are performed vaginally. However, this technique implies two large inguinal incisions, and it is not clear whether it involves less complications than the standard abdominal approach. For all these reasons, the abdominal approach has remained the only widely accepted approach for the completion of modified radical hysterectomy and lymph-node dissection.

The introduction of laparoscopic surgery in gynaecological oncology has had two consequences. First, it elicited a revival of radical vaginal hysterectomy, giving birth to new variants of radical hysterectomy. Second, procedures similar to the standard surgery were described, challenging the supremacy of abdominal surgery. The first historical application of panoramic endoscopic surgery in the field of gynaecological oncology was interiliac lymphadenectomy by a retroperitoneal approach [14]. Daniel Dargent, the 'father' of this approach, started with the idea of the addition of endoscopic lymphadenectomy to a classical (distal) Schauta operation or a modified (proximal) Schauta operation, to overcome the undertreatment secondary to the lack of lymph-node dissection in the vaginal procedure. The transumbilical approach was

49

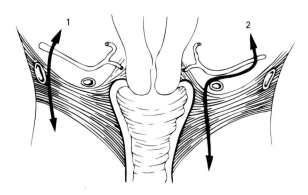

Fig. 7.1 Definition of radical hysterectomies: 1, proximal ('modified') type; 2, distal ('classic') type. (Redrawn from Querleu [28] with permission.)

pioneered by our group (see Chapter 3). A few years later, leading teams in advanced laparoscopic surgery attempted radical operations using laparoscopic techniques [2,4]. Later, we invented the idea that vaginal radical hysterectomy, and specially the more difficult Schauta–Stoeckel variant, could be prepared with the help of laparoscopic surgery [5]. Different variants according to the 'blend' of use of laparoscopic and vaginal surgery have recently been developed.

Routes for modified radical hysterectomy

Two major variants of modified radical hysterectomy using laparoscopic surgery have been described. The 'full' laparoscopic modified radical hysterectomy will be referred to as the Canis (1990)–Nezhat (1992) technique [2,4]. The two names are combined in this chapter, as both groups claim to have developed the technique. The laparoscopic-vaginal modified radical hysterectomy will be referred to as the Querleu technique [6,15] in its first version, and the Querleu–Dargent technique in its second version (D. Querleu & D. Dargent, unpublished data).

In the first cases of laparoscopic modified radical hysterectomy presented in the literature, early (stage IA) cervical cancers were removed by a procedure reproducing abdominal modified radical hysterectomy [2,4]. A pelvic lymphadenectomy was performed, with or without limited para-aortic node sampling. The ovarian, uterine and cervical vessels were desiccated with bipolar current and divided with the carbon dioxide laser or with scissors. The ureters were unroofed, the rectovaginal and vesicovaginal spaces were developed, the parametria were divided laparoscopically. The vagina and some part of the remaining paracolpos was incised vaginally. Later on, a technique including laparoscopic incision of the vagina was described [16]. In these techniques, the laparoscopic approach effectively follows the steps of the technique used at laparotomy. The only basic difference between the two techniques is in the way haemostasis is achieved. Bipolar cautery or stapling devices simply replace the clamps. The first videos presented by the pioneers of this technique were not really convincing, but later the Clermont-Ferrand team showed videos of indisputable radical hysterectomies.

Laparoscopic-vaginal modified radical hysterectomy is another concept. In the historical description of our operation (original version), the uterine arteries were divided and the terminal ureters fully dissected laparoscopically. The operation was completed vaginally with the transection of the cardinal ligament; the placement of clamps on the cardinal ligament was made with the assumption that the ureters were displaced far enough from the operative field. However, our technique has evolved, and a new version of this operation, which differs on some points from the original technique, will be described in this chapter under the name of the Querleu–Dargent technique. At this time, it is felt that preparation for vaginal surgery by the opening of the lateropelvic spaces and by the division of the uterine artery is enough in the majority of cases; as a consequence, we dissect the ureters vaginally, pull the already divided uterine arteries out and place the clamps on the cardinal ligaments under direct vision of the knee of the ureters. Credit has to be given to Daniel Dargent for having taught us the technique of vaginal dissection of the ureter and to have imagined that uterine arteries could be simply pulled out vaginally after their laparoscopic division.

Whatever the blend of vaginal and laparoscopic techniques, the rationale of laparoscopic-vaginal modified radical vaginal hysterectomy is that an oncological surgeon familiar with both laparoscopic surgery and radical vaginal hysterectomy is able to take advantage of the benefits of both routes in the same patient. The advantages of laparoscopic surgery are: (i) it is well suited to lymph-node dissection; and (ii) it gives a direct access to the origin of the uterine arteries. The drawbacks are: (i) a long operating time; and (ii) blind vaginal incision. Vaginal surgery: (i) provides a precise incision of the vaginal cuff; (ii) ensures a modified radical hysterectomy with a minimum of operating time; and (iii) has the unmatched advantage of a very limited dissection of the ureter.

Both routes may be used for the section of parametria at the appropriate level, but the experienced vaginal surgeon will find that the vaginal route is shorter and requires less ureteral dissection. The vaginal approach gives a direct access to the middle part of the cardinal ligament, at the exact place where a clamp has to be placed. The ureter crosses the cardinal ligament exactly where the tip of the clamp has to be placed. As a consequence, only a dissection of the ureter limited to this point ('knee' of the ureter, that means the most caudal point of the pelvic ureter) is required.

Combining the two approaches means combining the advantages and eliminating the drawbacks. In addition, starting surgery with the laparoscopic procedure makes vaginal surgery easier. The development of lateropelvic spaces improves uterine mobility, even if the cardinal ligaments are not divided laparoscopically. The laparoscopic division of the uterine artery ensures a relatively bloodless vaginal operating field. Both factors make easier the vaginal identification of surgical planes and of major landmarks, especially the knees of the ureters. The combination of the two 'minimal incision' approaches may thus be the most logical technique for surgical therapy of cervical carcinomas in the future, avoiding the discomfort of both laparotomy and of perineotomy, while reducing the excessively long operating time of laparoscopic surgery, and adding accuracy to the placement of the vaginal incision.

Using concurrent laparoscopic and vaginal approaches means the best route for each has to be chosen. Lymphadenectomy can only be performed laparoscopically. The preferential use of either route for other steps may depend on the training of the surgeon or of individual features of the patient. The upper pedicles of the uterus (ovarian or utero-ovarian vessels) may be controlled laparoscopically or vaginally. Division of the uterine artery at its origin is more precisely accomplished laparoscopically. Laparoscopic unroofing of the ureter is unnecessary if no superficial uterine vein crosses the ureter along with the uterine artery, as the uterine artery will only have to be pulled vaginally. On the other hand, superficial uterine veins may bleed during the process of pulling the stump of the uterine artery from below, and should be controlled laparoscopically, which means unroofing the ureter. Full dissection of the ureter in the vesicouterine ligament may be accomplished, as described below, laparoscopically or vaginally. Ureteral dissection is best performed vaginally by an experienced vaginal surgeon, but laparoscopic ureteral dissection may at times be easier than vaginal dissection in patients with a very narrow vagina. Finally, the main difference between laparoscopic modified radical hysterectomy and laparoscopic-vaginal modified radical hysterectomy is that the proximal parametria are divided and the vagina incised laparoscopically in the former and vaginally in the latter technique.

The use of a transperitoneal or retroperitoneal approach is a question of surgeon's preference. Lymphadenectomy, preparation of the lateropelvic spaces and division of the uterine arteries may be completed using both approaches. In an intermediate analysis of an experimental study carried out on pigs in our laboratory, the retroperitoneal approach induces less adhesions and more lymphoceles, but these findings have to be confirmed in a larger experiment (see Chapter 6). Obviously, a retroperitoneal approach is excluded if the surgeon wishes to divide the upper pedicles of the uterus laparoscopically.

Technique of laparoscopic modified radical hysterectomy: common steps

Several steps are common to all techniques of modified hysterectomy involving a full or partial laparoscopic approach: installation, lymph-node dissection, and division of the uterine artery.

Installation

The patient is lying flat, with no abduction of the legs. However, Allen stirrups will be used as soon as the vaginal step of the operation begins. In all techniques, the uterus is taken out vaginally. The laparoscopic approach is standard. Two 5-mm portals and one 10-mm portal, or one 5-mm and two 10-mm, are necessary. Two portals are usually placed in the inguinal areas, respectively on the right and left side, lateral to the epigastric arteries, 5 cm above the inguinal rings. The third trocar is placed in the midline, halfway between the umbilicus and the symphysis pubis. The 5-mm ports are used to accommodate standard instruments (bipolar cautery, forceps, scissors). The 10-mm portals are used to accommodate clips or EndoGIA stapling devices and to take out nodes. No uterine cannulation is used, to avoid unnecessary trauma to the cervical tumour. Other instruments such as lasers [4] and argon beam coagulators [9] are, in our opinion, no more than gimmicks.

Lymph-node dissection

The technique of lymph-node dissection depends on the conviction of the surgeon. Briefly, some groups advocate a full pelvic and low (and even high) para-aortic dissection, while some groups prefer a dissection limited to the interiliac area. The reasons leading to the choice of the modified operation are exactly the same as the two reasons that justify the removal of the interiliac sentinel lymph nodes: the low risk of involvement of both the higher nodes [14] and of the lateral parametrial nodes [17,18] if the interiliac nodes are free of disease. However, systematic dissection is required in a case of interiliac node metastasis.

Bilateral pelvic lymphadenectomy and, when required, para-aortic dissection are performed first. The portals for this part of the operation will be used for the preparation of the vaginal radical hysterectomy.

Division of the uterine artery

The ureter is identified at the point where it crosses the iliac vessels. The ovarian ligaments (in the case of salpingo-oophorectomy) or the utero-ovarian vessels (in the case of ovarian conservation) and the round ligaments are controlled and cut. Haemostasis of the upper pedicles is achieved by the use of bipolar cautery, stapling devices or extracorporeal knots, according to the surgeon's preference. Alternatively, they may be left intact for later laparoscopic or vaginal management, helping to contain the bowel loops during laparoscopic surgery. We favour the cheaper and faster vaginal management of utero-ovarian vessels; the management of the ovarian vessels may be performed laparoscopically (at the end of the laparoscopic step) or vaginally, depending on the laxity of the ligament. The ureter is identified from the pelvic brim to the level of the uterine artery. For this purpose, the incised broad ligament is grasped and brought medially, showing the ureter running on its deep surface. The ureter is left attached to the undersurface of the peritoneum to avoid impairing its vascular supply. The pararectal space is entered, but not fully developed (Fig. 7.2). The opening of the pararectal space is found between the ureter medially and the hypogastric artery medially. The opening of the pararectal space delineates the anterior trunk of the internal iliac artery, which is located between the paravesical and pararectal spaces. The origin of the uterine artery is easily identified (Fig. 7.3). It is skeletonized by blunt dissection, then controlled by bipolar cautery using 3-mm broad forceps (Fig. 7.4) or by clips. Superficial uterine veins may overlie the uterine artery, and have to be managed with

preventive haemostasis and section. In the same way, superficial uterine veins crossing the ureter close to the ureteral tunnel may have to be controlled. To identify these veins, it is advisable to grab the visceral stump of the uterine artery in order to lift it and to discover the ureteric tunnel. A good magnified view of the posterior opening of the ureteral tunnel is usually obtained. The ureteric artery coming from the uterine artery may be made visible (Fig. 7.5), as well as superficial uterine veins crossing the ureter. When they are present, the ureteric artery and the superficial uterine veins are desiccated by bipolar cautery then divided, taking care not to jeopardize the ureter by thermal or mechanical injury.

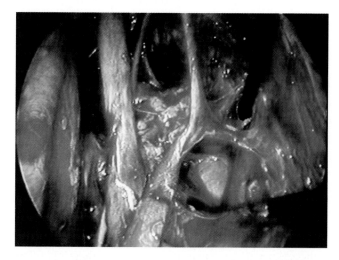

Fig. 7.3 Skeletonizing the left uterine artery. The left pararectal space is opened, the left ureter and lateral face of the rectum are pushed medially (bottom right). The instrument coming from top right separates the uterine artery from the inferior vesical artery.

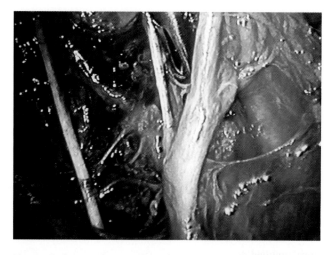

Fig. 7.2 Left ureter (bottom right), identified down to the point where it is crossed by the uterine artery. The division of the anterior branch of the internal iliac artery (from left to right: obturator, superior vesical, uterine arteries) has been dissected. The obturator nerve is seen on the left.

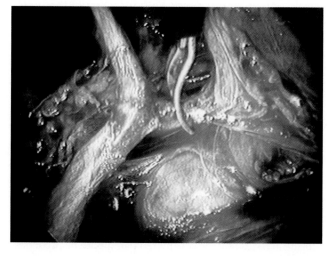

Fig. 7.4 Division of the origin of the left uterine artery after bipolar cautery.

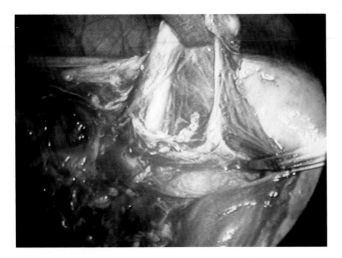

Fig. 7.5 Unroofing the right ureter. The divided uterine artery is grabbed and lifted. The ureter is gently pushed down. A ureteric artery is stretched before division. The bladder end of the ureter is on the right side of the picture.

Only at this point will the full laparoscopic operation (laparoscopic modified radical hysterectomy) differ from the laparoscopically assisted variant (laparoscopic-vaginal modified radical hysterectomy, see the following section).

Technique of laparoscopic modified radical hysterectomy: Canis–Nezhat procedure

To complete the operation laparoscopically, the ureter must be dissected from the bladder pillar, the cardinal and uterosacral ligaments have to be divided, then the vagina has to be incised.

Dissection of the ureter

After unroofing, further separation of the ureter is obtained by section of the cephalic part of the vesicouterine ligament. The vesicouterine fold is incised with scissors or unipolar cautery. The vesicouterine ligament is separated from the ureter with the help of an endoscopic curved dissector or by gradual preventive haemostasis and section. The bladder base and the terminal ureter are then freed from the cervix by blunt dissection. Finally, the ureter is further mobilized from the cervix and vagina by blunt dissection. It must be entirely freed from the vaginal wall.

According to the circumstances, the uterosacral or the cardinal ligaments may be divided first. Transection of either of these ligaments helps to elevate the uterus and facilitates the next step.

Division of the uterosacral ligaments

Laparoscopic division of the uterosacral ligaments is ideally performed after a thorough identification of this ligament to avoid injury to the ureter or rectum. The lateral aspect of the uterosacral ligament is freed by blunt dissection. The pararectal space is partially opened to separate the cardinal ligament from the ureter. Access to the medial aspect of the uterosacral ligament is obtained by opening the rectovaginal septum. To achieve this, the peritoneum of the pouch of Douglas is incised right under the level of the insertion of the uterosacral ligaments. Sharp dissection is necessary to open the rectovaginal space, then blunt dissection is used to develop that space as low as necessary. The uterosacral ligaments are delineated between the pararectal and rectovaginal spaces, separated from the rectum medially by further blunt dissection and can be divided at the required level after haemostasis. We favour bipolar cautery and section, but some surgeons will use the stapler devices.

Division of the cardinal ligaments

To divide the cardinal ligaments, the ureter is reflected laterally or medially. The point where the cardinal ligament has to be divided is therefore shown, and haemostasis can be applied without injury to the ureter. This point is usually midway between the cervix and the pelvic wall, 2 cm away from the cervix, but the distance may be adapted to the size of the primary tumour. The cardinal ligament is gradually electrodesiccated and cut or divided with an EndoGIA stapler. The section of the cardinal ligament is completed as low as necessary to remove the desired vaginal cuff. Further laparoscopic separation of the bladder by electrodesiccation and division of the caudal part of the vesicouterine ligament may be necessary if a large vaginal cuff excision is required.

Incision of the vagina

The vagina may be opened laparoscopically. If a very high flow carbon dioxide insufflator is not available, the vagina must be obturated by a sponge or an inflated balloon. Vaginal and/or rectal probes may be useful to delineate the vagina or rectum. The specimen is removed vaginally and the vaginal obturator is replaced. Haemostasis is checked. Residual bleeders are controlled by bipolar cautery or clips. The vaginal cuff may be left open or closed with the help of endoscopic sutures or sewing devices. A needle-holder and a standard size 1 Vicryl suture may be used. In the same way, the peritoneal edges may be approximated in the midline or not. We usually close the vagina but not the peritoneum. If postoperative irradiation is anticipated in a young woman, lateral transposition of the ovaries is performed. The lateral pelvic spaces are left open to provide drainage of lymph fluid into the peritoneal cavity. The pelvis is washed. No drain is left in the peritoneal cavity.

An alternative technique to complete the procedure is to incise the vagina to remove the specimen and, optionally, to close the vagina from below. Peritoneal closure in the midline is optional, and may also be performed vaginally. It is advisable to check the haemostasis and to wash the operative field laparoscopically after completion of the procedure.

Technique of laparoscopically assisted modified radical hysterectomy: Querleu procedure, original version [5]

The description starts after completion of the common steps (see above). In this first version of the operation, the anterior cul-de-sac was opened, the vesicouterine space was developed then the ureters were freed laparoscopically as described previously. The goal of the laparoscopic assistance was to fully mobilize the bladder base and the terminal ureters from the vagina and from the proximal part of the cardinal ligament to ensure the safety of the vaginal step of the operation. Indeed, only the properly freed terminal ureters can be moved away vaginally by a retractor placed under the bladder base.

The vaginal step was then started, making the vaginal cuff according to the Schauta technique (Figs 7.6–7.11), with a limited opening of the paravesical space. The transection of the cardinal ligament was performed vaginally,

with no direct vision of the ureter, with the assumption that it was moved away by the help of the retractors.

After laparoscopic preparation of the ureter and of the bladder, the standard Schauta technique is modified as follows. The ureter cannot be palpated. As it is detached from the vagina and from the uterus, traction on the vaginal cuff does not attract it as in the standard technique. On the contrary, palpation is used to identify the part of the bladder pillar that can be safely incised. Indeed, the part of the bladder pillar where the ureter cannot be palpated can be divided without any danger, provided that the surgeon is experienced enough in radical vaginal surgery to be able to exclude the presence of the ureter in a specific part of the bladder pillar. This incision is placed

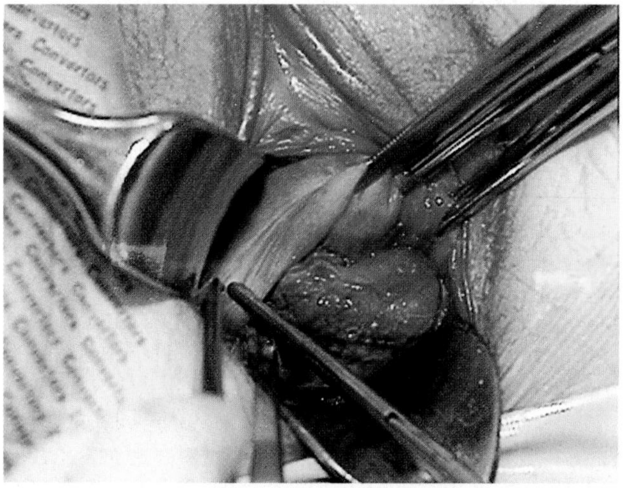

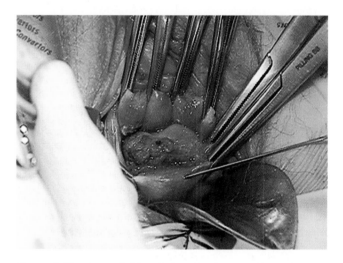

Fig. 7.7 Infiltration with diluted adrenaline between the two layers of the vaginal wall.

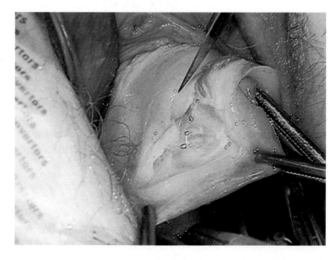

Fig. 7.8 Anteriorly, incision of the full depth of the external layer of the vaginal wall.

Fig. 7.6 Making an adequate vaginal cuff using straight Kocher forceps. The tumour is visible and the vaginal incision will be placed as precisely as possible.

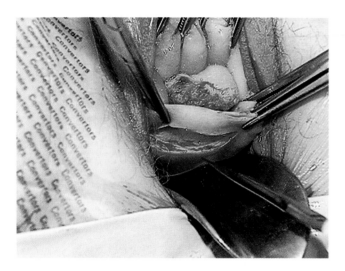

Fig. 7.9 Posteriorly, incision of the full depth of the external layer of the vaginal wall.

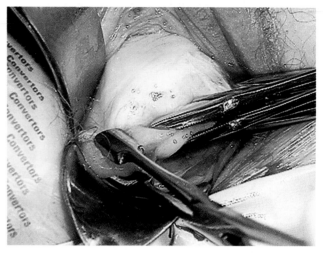

Fig. 7.11 Closure of the vaginal cuff using Chroback forceps.

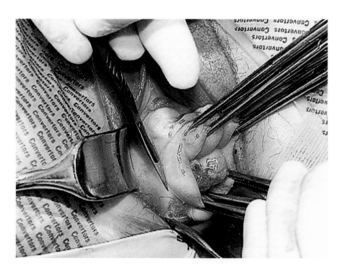

Fig. 7.10 Laterally, superficial incision of the external layer of the vaginal wall.

without preventive haemostasis with clamps. The parietal stump of the ligament will be taken only after incision and tied. After this step, the left ureter is fully separated from the medial part of the cardinal ligament. It is not identified, but reflected with a retractor placed under the left side of the bladder base. The anterior aspect of the cardinal ligament is then freed, and it can be clamped at the level of its medial mid-portion. Two clamps are placed. The cardinal ligament is divided. The parietal stump is tied. The clamp on the uterine side is kept to ensure further traction on the uterus. The left uterine artery is identified then only gently pulled up to the point where it is completely detached, and its coagulated origin visible. This step is made possible due to the division of the

uterine artery during the laparoscopic step of the operation. The same steps are performed on the right side.

The operation was logically finished vaginally, with incision of the peritoneal cul-de-sacs, division of the upper pedicles and closure of the vagina. The rationale for this technique was the fact that in the Schauta technique, vaginal identification and mobilization of the ureters is the most difficult part of the operation, especially in patients with a narrow vaginal access. As a consequence, this version of the operation is still used in patients with a narrow vagina in whom laparoscopic assistance may spare them a perineotomy.

Technique of laparoscopically assisted modified radical hysterectomy: Querleu–Dargent procedure (Figs 7.6–7.24)

The vaginal step of the operation starts immediately after transection of the uterine arteries (Dargent's variation) or after limited unroofing of the uterus involving section of the superficial uterine veins and/or ureteric artery (our variation). It differs from the original version in that, similar to the classic Schauta–Stoeckel technique, it involves a vaginal dissection of the ureters.

Making the vaginal cuff is now described in detail. The vaginal operation begins with incision of the vagina. No perineal incision is required. Infiltration of the vaginal cuff with 2% adrenaline is advised. The vagina is grasped with forceps and incised circumferentially 2–3 cm from the fornices or at the level required by the lesion. The normal vagina can be delineated by iodine application. The vaginal incision is deep, dividing all the layers, anteriorly and posteriorly. Laterally, it is advised not to incise too deeply, in order to leave the cardinal ligament attached

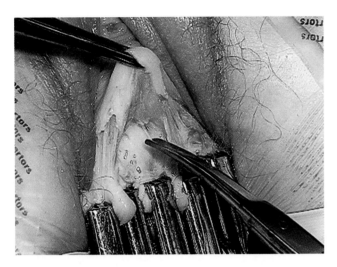

Fig. 7.12 The vesicouterine space is entered by sharp dissection, taking care not to injure the bladder.

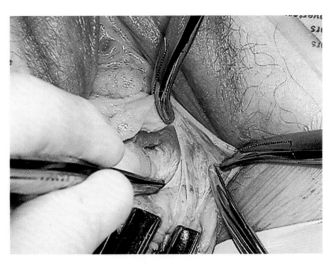

Fig. 7.14 Two forceps are placed at the 1 and 3 o'clock position, respectively, showing the point where the left paravesical space can be opened, at the deep surface of the vagina.

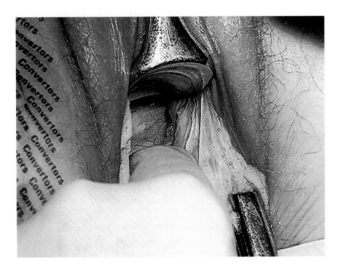

Fig. 7.13 The vesicouterine space is developed, the broad ligament is reached laterally.

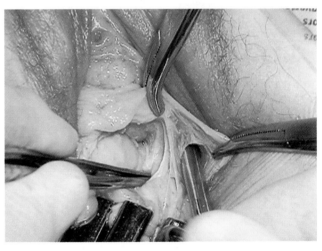

Fig. 7.15 The paravesical space is reached after perforation of the endopelvic fascia with the tip of scissors.

to the vaginal cuff. This part of the cardinal ligament will be later included in the operative specimen and must not be separated from the vagina. A vaginal cuff is formed with a bunch of Chrobak forceps, as described for classic vaginal radical surgery [19]. The vaginal cuff is pulled upwards.

The rectovaginal space is easily reached and developed by blunt dissection with the tip of scissors. The opening of the pararectal space is found at the deep surface of the vagina between the 3 and 4 o'clock direction on the left side and the 8 and 9 o'clock direction on the right side. The pouch of Douglas is then incised and the peritoneal cavity is entered. The uterosacral ligaments are then identified

lateral to the peritoneal opening and medial to the pararectal space. They are divided with scissors. Section of the uterosacral ligaments improves the mobility of the cervix and provides access to the pararectal spaces. The pararectal spaces are partially developed to gain access to the posterior aspect of the cardinal ligaments.

It is then necessary to reach and to develop the vesicovaginal and vesicouterine space. The vaginal cuff is pulled downwards. The fibres connecting the bladder base to the vagina are put in tension by a retractor placed on the anterior vaginal wall. The connective tissue is divided in the midline, taking care not to injure the bladder: when a vaginal cuff has been made, the bladder is

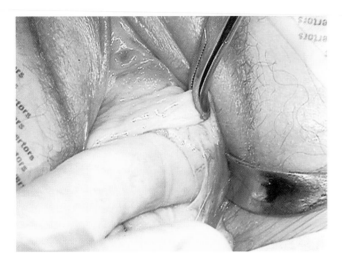

Fig. 7.16 A retractor is placed in the paravesical space. The ureter is palpated in the bladder pillar.

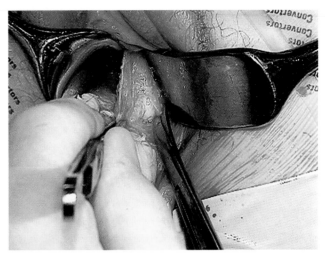

Fig. 7.18 The left ureter is found.

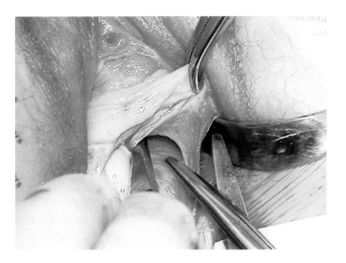

Fig. 7.17 The lateral fibres of the bladder pillar are divided.

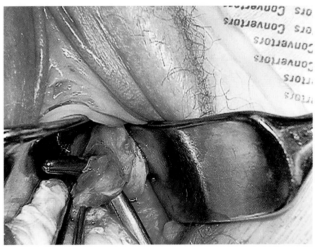

Fig. 7.19 The left uterine pedicle is found, coming from the knee of the ureter, skeletonized using a right-angle dissector. It will be controlled and divided as high as possible.

attached in the midline in a different manner than it is during a simple hysterectomy.

The paravesical spaces are then entered and developed on each side, starting on the left side. The edge of the vaginal incision is grasped with two Allis forceps in a 2 and 3 o'clock position. The deep surface of the vagina is freed with scissors to find the opening of the paravesical space. The space is developed by blunt dissection with the tips of the scissors. Only a limited opening is necessary for modified radical hysterectomy. The dissection is considered to be satisfactory when a 2-cm-wide retractor or a finger can be placed in the paravesical space.

The operation continues with the identification of the ureter. The ureter can be palpated in the bladder pillar between two fingers, one placed in the paravesical space,

the second finger in the vesicovaginal space. Alternatively, the ureter can be palpated in the bladder pillar using a retractor placed in the corresponding paravesical space and a finger placed in the vesicouterine space and used as a hook to explore the medial aspect of the bladder pillar. The lowest point of the ureter is palpated, and will be referred to as the 'knee' of the ureter. The lower (caudal) part of the vesicouterine ligament is then safely divided under the level of the ureteral knee. It is advisable to open this caudal part of the bladder pillars in two parts, one medial, one lateral, with scissors, to check again for the ureters by palpation, then to divide gradually either of the two parts. Finally, the knee of the ureter is made visible

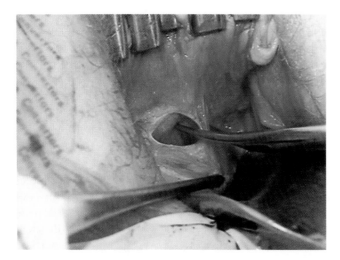

Fig. 7.20 The pouch of Douglas is entered.

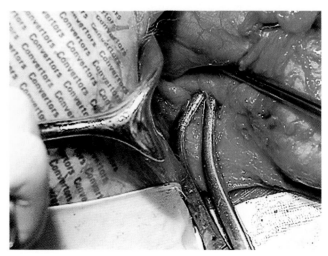

Fig. 7.22 The right cardinal ligament is clamped. The tip of the clamp is placed close to the ureter.

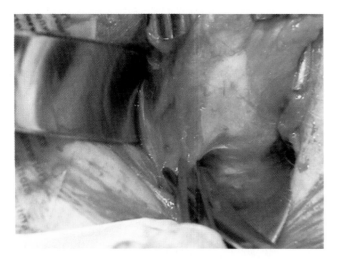

Fig. 7.21 The right rectovaginal ligament is divided.

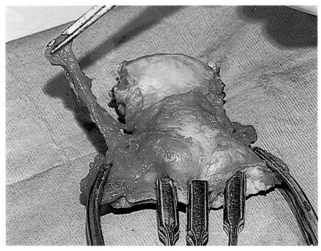

Fig. 7.23 The operative specimen.

and freed over a 2-cm distance. The uterine artery is gently pulled and detached (Fig. 7.24). This is enough to place a clamp on the cardinal ligament at the level of the knee of the ureter, that is approximately 2 cm lateral to the cervix, the tip of the clamp being placed right under the knee of the ureter. A second clamp is placed slightly more laterally, and the cardinal ligament is divided between the two clamps and tied.

The right paravesical space is entered and developed symmetrically, between the 9 and 10 o'clock position. The right bladder pillar and ureter are managed symmetrically.

After the two cardinal ligaments have been divided, the specimen is detached by incision of the peritoneum of the caudal part of the posterior leaf of the broad ligament, then of the vesicouterine fold. If the upper pedicles have

already been detached laparoscopically, the specimen is pulled out. If not, the round ligaments, the utero-ovarian vessels or the ovarian vessels have to be clamped and divided. The haemostasis is checked. The peritoneum may be approximated in the midline, but peritoneal closure is not advised. The vagina is closed transversely by approximation of the anterior and posterior edge of the incision. In some cases, a rubber drain may be placed in either or both the paravesical spaces, but we do not leave a drain routinely. The operation is now completed, but the surgeon may find it reassuring to check the haemostasis and the integrity of the ureter laparoscopically. For this purpose, the trocars have been left in place. The laparoscopic openings will be closed later, taking care to close

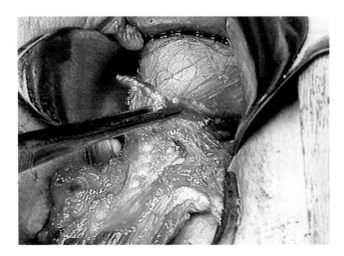

Fig. 7.24 After completion of the first steps of the radical vaginal operation, the stump of the uterine artery, already controlled and divided laparoscopically, is pulled.

Table 7.1 Operative data (33 patients).

Average duration of operation	240 min
Average duration of lymph-node dissection	69 min
Average number of righ pelvic nodes	9.6
Average number of left pelvic nodes	8.0
Average blood loss	372 ml
Average haemoglobin loss	2.6 g/dl

the 10–12-mm openings in order to avoid the occurrence of incisional hernias.

Finally, the only difference between the original version and this version is the way in which the ureter is dissected. Whenever possible, we prefer this version, for two reasons.

1 Direct vision of the ureter makes placing of the clamps safer.

2 The ureter is dissected only over a limited length, thus reducing the unnecessarily wide dissection of the abdominal approach.

Results

Nezhat *et al.* have reported their experience of 19 cases, including 10 stage IA2 cervical cancers, and also eight stage IB and one stage IIA patients [15]. They used a full laparoscopic technique, with some amount of vaginal surgery at the end of the procedure. One procedure was converted to laparotomy. The average operative time was 315 minutes for laparoscopic modified radical hysterectomy and 163 minutes for laparoscopic-vaginal modified radical hysterectomy, suggesting that this method is probably the best choice for modified radical hysterectomies. There were two minor postoperative complications (one urinary tract infection, one incisional bleeding). The postoperative hospital stay averaged 2.1 days.

The Clermont-Ferrand team has operated on patients with a laparoscopic modified radical hysterectomy technique, with incision and closure of the vagina from below (G. Mage *et al.*, personal communication), with no complication requiring laparotomy. The results are similar to those reported in the other two series.

Querleu has performed eight laparoscopic-vaginal radical hysterectomies between November 1990 and December 1992 [6]. In these cases he divided the uterine arteries and dissected the ureters laparoscopically, then transected the cardinal ligaments vaginally. Four of these operations may be classified as modified radical hysterectomies. A perineal incision was avoided in all cases. The operative blood loss was less than 300 ml in the four cases. No unintended laparotomy was required. The average operating time was 182 minutes, including lymphadenectomy, frozen section examination and radical hysterectomy. The average postoperative stay was 3.5 days. No major complication, and particularly no lymphocyst, no ureteral injury and no urinary retention of more than 3 days' duration occurred. Since the publication of these results, further follow-up information on these patients has become available. All four patients are doing well, with a minimum follow-up of 5 years.

Additional personal, yet unpublished, data is available. Thirty-three patients underwent a laparoscopic-vaginal modified radical hysterectomy in our department before the end of June 1996 for stage IB–IIA cervical carcinoma, and have been followed up for a minimum of 2 years. The operative data are shown in Table 7.1. Twenty-five of the patients had tumours of less than 2 cm diameter. The only significant complication (injury to the inferior epigastric artery) did not require laparotomy. One patient only had a blood transfusion. Nine of these patients had an additional paracervical lymphadenectomy, with an average node yield of 2.2. The pathological examination found microscopic involvement of the cardinal ligament in two cases (clear margins in both cases) and disease in the vaginal cuff in five patients (one with diseased margins). Three patients underwent adjuvant radiotherapy for vaginal or parametrial disease. The long-term urinary dysfunction rate is 12%. One patient (4%) in the group of 25 patients with a tumour diameter of less than 2 cm and one patient in the group of eight patients with a tumour diameter larger than 2 cm recurred. These results are encouraging.

Schneider *et al.* [8] have reported recently on an operation that is quite similar to the Querleu–Dargent version of the operation, although they divided the cardinal ligament laparoscopically at the pelvic side wall. Therefore it is an example of a laparoscopic distal and a vaginal proximal radical hysterectomy.

Discussion

The place of laparoscopic surgery in radical hysterectomy is not yet well established. The abdominal approach remains the standard operation for radical hysterectomy. However, we must keep in mind that in experienced hands, vaginal surgery is efficient and at the same time safer and more comfortable for the patient than abdominal surgery. As the accuracy of laparoscopic node dissection has been recently demonstrated, we can infer that a combination of laparoscopic and abdominal surgery is as effective as the abdominal approach. In the same way, laparoscopic modified radical hysterectomy is acceptable only if it strictly mimics open abdominal surgery.

Whenever possible, we favour the vaginal approach, as vaginal surgery is shorter and cheaper than laparoscopic surgery, especially when disposable instruments are used for laparoscopic surgery. In other situations, the laparoscopic approach should be continued only to the point at which vaginal access becomes possible. This point depends on the particular case. In some patients, i.e. multiparas, vaginal access is easy and does not require a Schuchardt incision. In these cases, laparoscopic lymphadenectomy may be associated with a vaginal modified radical hysterectomy, but laparoscopic preparation makes this easier. In such cases, the Querleu–Dargent version of the operation is indicated. In other groups of patients, where vaginal surgery is possible, it would be made easier and safer by using an additional perineal incision. In these cases, a more extensive laparoscopic preparation of the vaginal operation spares the patient the painful perineal incision, and the original Querleu (laparoscopic-vaginal modified radical hysterectomy) procedure is indicated. Finally, when the vaginal access may be quite inadequate for easy vaginal surgery, or when the surgeon does not feel comfortable with radical vaginal surgery, the Canis–Nezhat procedure (laparoscopic modified radical hysterectomy) is the best choice.

Ideally, the operative technique should be adapted to the individual patient and not to the surgeon's preference. The available techniques should be combined to provide the best management at the lowest cost in operating time and use of instruments. This policy has been found to be efficient in the case of hysterectomy for benign conditions [16,20], and it is probably the most logical for radical hysterectomy. However, this policy requires full training in radical vaginal surgery as well as in advanced laparoscopic surgery. More and more gynaecological oncologists are willing to invest time and money to train in laparoscopic surgery, but they are reluctant to learn vaginal surgery. Hopefully they will understand that as far as hysterectomy, radical or simple, is concerned, it is illogical to train only in laparoscopic surgery. Some steps may be difficult to accomplish laparoscopically, and vaginal surgery may be required to avoid an unintended conversion to laparotomy. Furthermore, vaginal surgery may safely fulfil the same goals as a laparoscopic approach in a shorter operative time, with a similar level of comfort for the patient.

There are few long-term follow-up studies on laparoscopic or laparoscopic-vaginal radical hysterectomy in stage IB2 cervical cancers. Indeed, in a majority of the published or unpublished cases (10 out of 18 in the Atlanta series [15], six out of nine in the Clermont-Ferrand series (unpublished data)), including the two principle reports of laparoscopic modified radical hysterectomy [2,4], modified radical hysterectomies have been performed for stage IA2 cervical cancers. In such cases, wide removal of the parametria is unnecessary, and the prognosis is good even after simple hysterectomy. The good results obtained in our unpublished series of frankly invasive cancer demonstrate the efficacy of the laparoscopic approach.

This option may be acceptable for clinical trials as it mimics standard open abdominal surgery and a similar degree of radicality is reached. It is mandatory to obtain operative specimens similar to those obtained at standard abdominal and vaginal surgery. In our series we feel that these criteria have been fulfilled in every case. However, cost and quality-of-life data are still needed to show that minimal access surgery is successful for radical hysterectomy. Nevertheless, this should not discourage the use of minimal access surgery for this indication. A continuing effort to refine the technique, to assess the short- and long-term results and to teach advanced laparoscopic as well as vaginal surgery to gynaecological oncologists is warranted.

The indication for proximal versus distal radical hysterectomy is probably underestimated. Classic (distal) radical hysterectomy is followed by a high complication rate compared to the modified (proximal) type [21,22]. On the other hand, the results of modified versus distal radical hysterectomy in early cervical cancers less than $50\,cm^3$ are similar [22,23]. As the difference between the distal and proximal type is only in the removal of the distal part of the cardinal ligament, it is logical to try to predict the risk of involvement of this anatomical structure.

Three predictive factors can be identified: tumour volume, pericervical extension and pelvic node involvement. Data from pathological study of radical hysterectomies [24,25] show that parametrial disease is uncommon in tumours less than 2 cm in diameter. Data from serial study of giant sections [18] show that the risk of involvement of the cardinal ligament is correlated with the presence of anterior or posterior pericervical involvement. The involvement of the distal part of the cardinal ligament is correlated with involvement of the proximal part. It can be computed from the data of Girardi *et al.* [17] that the risk of involvement of the distal part of the cardinal ligament is 28% (11 out of 39) when the proximal part is involved, compared with 7.5% (24 out of 320) when the proximal part is not involved. The third predictive factor is the involvement of iliac nodes. When the pelvic parietal nodes are involved, the risk of pathological involvement of the cardinal ligament is found to be 46–61%, compared with 5–13% when the parietal nodes are free of metastatic disease [17,18,26,27]. Interestingly, all three predictive factors can be investigated preoperatively with MRI or peroperatively with frozen section of the iliac nodes.

Our new approach to the distal cardinal ligament (see Chapter 3) takes into account this knowledge and may further modify surgical strategies. In fact, the combination of a vaginal proximal radical hysterectomy with laparoscopic removal of the distal part of the cardinal ligament is similar to a classic distal hysterectomy, with a reduced risk of urinary complication. If our early results are confirmed, the proximal type may become the only type of radical hysterectomy used in the future, at least for tumours smaller than 4 cm which can be removed vaginally. Our present policy is to combine a proximal radical hysterectomy with paracervical lymphadenectomy when the risk of involvement of the distal part of the cardinal ligament is significant. Briefly, the risk is minimal in pathological stage IB cases less than 2 cm in diameter with no parietal node involvement [17,18,24]. As a consequence, when MRI measurement of the tumour is less than 2 cm or 10 cm³, and when no pericervical extension is suspected at MRI, and when no diseased pelvic node is identified at frozen section, no extension of surgery is necessary.

In more advanced cases, more radical surgery is required, and the place of paracervical lymphadenectomy is under investigation in our group, especially in the group of patients in whom the risk of involvement of the distal part of the cardinal ligament is significant but low (tumours 2–4 cm in diameter with no pericervical extension at MRI and no positive pelvic nodes at frozen section). The combination of laparoscopic removal of the distal part of the cardinal ligament with a proximal radical hysterectomy may provide, in the future, a compromise between radicality and quality of life.

References

1 Dargent D (1993). Laparoscopic surgery and gynecologic cancer. *Curr Opin Obstet Gynecol* **5**:294–300.
2 Canis M, Mage G, Wattiez A, Pouly J-L, Manhes H, Bruhat M-A (1990). La chirurgie endoscopique a-t-elle une place dans la chirurgie radicale du cancer du col utérin? (letter). *J Gynecol Obstet Biol Reprod* **19**:921.
3 Dargent D, Mathevet P (1992). Hystérectomie élargie laparoscopico-vaginale. *J Gynecol Obstet Biol Reprod* **21**:709–710.
4 Nezhat CR, Burrell MO, Nezhat FR, Benigno BB, Welander CE (1992). Laparoscopic radical hysterectomy with paraaortic and pelvic node dissection. *Am J Obstet Gynecol* **166**:864–865.
5 Querleu D (1991). Hystérectomies de Schauta–Amreich et Schauta–Stoeckel assistées par coelioscopie. *J Gynecol Obstet Biol Reprod* **20**:747–748.
6 Querleu D (1993). Laparoscopically-assisted radical vaginal hysterectomy. *Gynecol Oncol* **51**:248–254.
7 Sedlacek TV, Campion MJ, Reich H, Sedlacek T (1995). Laparoscopic radical hysterectomy: a feasibility study. *Gynecol Oncol* **56**:126 (abstr).
8 Schneider A, Possover M, Kamprath S, Endisch U, Krause N, Nöschel H (1996). Laparoscopic assisted radical vaginal hysterectomy modified according to Schauta–Stoeckel. *Obstet Gynecol* **88**:1057–1060.
9 Spirtos NM, Schlaerth JB, Kimball RE, Leiphart VM, Ballon SC (1996). Laparoscopic radical hysterectomy (type III) with aortic and pelvic lymphadenectomy. *Am J Obstet Gynecol* **174**:1763–1768.
10 Piver MS, Rutledge F, Smith JP (1974). Five classes of extended hysterectomy for women with cervical cancer. *Obstet Gynecol* **44**:265–272.
11 Wertheim E (1900). Zur Frage der Radikaloperation beim Uteruskrebs. *Arch Gynakol* **61**:627–668.
12 Stoeckel W (1928). Die vaginal Radikaloperation des Collumkarzinoms. *Zentralbl Gynakol* **1**:39–63.
13 Mitra S (1959). Extraperitoneal lymphadenectomy and radical vaginal hysterectomy for cancer of the cervix (Mitra technique). *Am J Obstet Gynecol* **78**:191–196.
14 Dargent D (1987). A new future for Schauta operation through presurgical retroperitoneal laparoscopy. *Eur J Gynaecol Obstet* **8**:292–294.
15 Nezhat CR, Nezhat FR, Burrell MO *et al* (1993). Laparoscopic radical hysterectomy and laparoscopically assisted vaginal radical hysterectomy with pelvic and paraaortic dissection. *J Gynecol Surg* **9**:105–120.
16 Querleu D, Cosson M, Parmentier D, Debodinance P (1993). The impact of laparoscopic surgery on vaginal hysterectomy. *Gynaecol Endosc* **2**:89–91.
17 Girardi F, Lichtenegger W, Tamussino K, Haas J (1989). The importance of parametrial lymph nodes in the treatment of cervical cancer. *Gynecol Oncol* **34**:206–211.
18 Landoni F, Bocciolone L, Perego P, Maneo A, Bratina G, Mangioni C (1995). Cancer of the cervix, FIGO stages IB and IIA: patterns of local growth and paracervical extension. *Int J Gynecol Cancer* **5**:329–334.
19 Reiffenstuhl G, Platzer W (1975). *Atlas of Vaginal Surgery*, Vol 1. Philadelphia: WB Saunders.
20 Richardson RE, Bournas N, Magos AL (1995). Is laparoscopic hysterectomy a waste of time? *Lancet* **345**:36–41.
21 Magrina JF, Goodrich MA, Weaver AL, Podratz KC (1995). Modified radical hysterectomy: morbidity and mortality. *Gynecol Oncol* **59**:277–282.
22 Stark G (1987). Zur Operativen Therapie des Collumkarzinoms Stadium Ib. *Geburtshilfe Frauenheilkd* **47**:45–48.
23 Burghardt E, Baltzer J, Tulusan AH, Haas J (1992). Results of

surgical treatment of 1028 cervical cancers studied with volumetry. *Cancer* **70**:648–655.

24 Kinney WK, Hodge DO, Egorshin EV, Ballard DJ, Podratz KC (1995). Identification of a low-risk subset of patients with stage IB invasive squamous cancer of the cervix possibly suited to less radical surgical treatment. *Gynecol Oncol* **57**:3–6.

25 Sartori E, Fallo L, Bianchi UA, Pecorelli S (1995). Extended radical hysterectomy in early-stage carcinoma of the uterine cervix: tailoring the radicality. *Int J Gynecol Cancer* **5**:143–147.

26 Bleker OP, Ketting BW, Van Wayjen-Eecen B, Kloosterman GJ (1983). The significance of microscopic involvement of the parametrium and/or pelvic lymph nodes in cervical cancer stages IB and IIA. *Gynecol Oncol* **16**:56–62.

27 Inoue T, Okumura M (1984). Prognostic significance of parametrial extension in patients with cervical carcinoma stages IB, IIA, and IIB. A study of 628 cases treated by radical hysterectomy and lymphadenectomy with or without postoperative irradiation. *Cancer* **54**:1714–1719.

28 Querleu D (1995). *Techniques Chirurgicales en Gynécologie*. Paris: Masson.

8   Laparoscopically assisted radical hysterectomy (distal 'coelio-Schauta' procedure)

Daniel Dargent

Introduction

When our centre started using laparoscopy in gynaecological oncology, assistance to radical hysterectomy was our first aim [1]. It remains a major justification for this still controversial practice.

Radical hysterectomy is the most cost-effective treatment for early cervical cancer (stage IB and early stage II). However, although results are excellent for node-negative patients (about 90% 5-year disease-free survival), they are less favourable for node-positive patients: 50–60% 5-year survival is expected if one or two lymph nodes are involved compared with 0–15% if three or more lymph nodes are involved [2]. This knowledge was the basis of the concept of 'staging laparotomy' introduced by Nelson *et al.* [3]. Staging laparotomy for patients with advanced disease was popular during the 1970s and early 1980s. Because of the selection made by staging laparotomy (the lymph-node-positive patients were not submitted to radical surgery but were referred to the radiotherapist), results obtained with radical hysterectomy were appreciably improved. However, the overall results did not change. Moreover, a lot of actinic complications were observed in patients treated by radiotherapy after a positive staging laparotomy. In order to reduce the rate of such complications the extraperitoneal approach was proposed. The Gynecologic Oncology Group (GOG) trial demonstrated that there were less radiation-induced bowel complications with the extraperitoneal approach [4], but the reduction was not significant enough and staging is no longer considered in most centres. Laparoscopic lymphadenectomy can, in same ways, be considered as a way of renewing the staging concept.

If laparoscopic staging is used as a method for selecting patients to be managed by radiation therapy and those who are candidates for abdominal surgery, the benefit is far from clear. Staging can be performed with a minimal scar, and this advantage should not be underestimated in patients who will be treated by radiation therapy. Peritoneal adhesions are a source of radiation enteritis observed in patients irradiated after surgery, and they are minimal after laparoscopic dissections. However, for those patients who will be managed by radical hysterectomy, the vast majority in the stage I and early stage II population, the benefit is more than questionable: the hazards of laparoscopy are just added to the risks and drawbacks of laparotomy. Moreover, as when staging laparotomy was performed, we can hope for an improvement in the results obtained in the subpopulation of patients treated by radical hysterectomy, but no improvement in the overall results can be expected.

It is a mistake to expect an improvement in oncological results when selecting high-risk patients for a therapy (radiotherapy) with well-known limits. The only hope lies in the future with the new therapies: chemotherapy, chemoradiotherapy and gene therapy. As there is no immediate chance of improvement for high-risk patients, the only thing we can do is to make surgery for low-risk patients safer and more patient-friendly.

Herein lies the philosophy of laparoscopy: improving the cost effectiveness of surgery, which remains the best tool in the management of node-negative early cervical cancer. This result cannot be obtained if laparoscopy is combined with abdominal surgery, but it can be fully accomplished if vaginal surgery is used. Vaginal surgery is usually better accepted by patients. In addition, it is safer because the mortality rate after vaginal hysterectomy is three times less than after abdominal hysterectomy [5] including radical hysterectomy [6]. That is the rationale for laparoscopically assisted vaginal radical hysterectomy, to which we have given the name 'coelio-Schauta', after the French 'coelioscopie' (meaning laparoscopy) and the name Schauta.

General principles

Radical vaginal hysterectomy is not conceptually different from radical abdominal hysterectomy. It differs from simple vaginal hysterectomy by the addition of removal of the upper part of the vagina and the pelvic cellular tissue (paracervix) surrounding the cervico-vaginal junction. Depending on the extent of the additional resection, many classes of vaginal radical hysterectomy can be defined. The Piver and Rutledge classification [7] could be extrapolated to the vaginal radical hysterectomy. However, this classification does appear excessively sophisticated for the abdominal operations and is even more inappropriate for the vaginal operations. A classification distinguishing — besides the simple extrafascial colpohysterectomy which is not a radical hysterectomy — the proximal (modified) and the distal (classic) types is enough. The basic anatomosurgical difference between the two operations has been explained in Chapter 7. The proximal vaginal hysterectomy corresponds to the Stoeckel variant of the Schauta operation. The distal vaginal hysterectomy corresponds to the Amreich variant of the Schauta operation. In this chapter the role of laparoscopic assistance in the Amreich radical-type operation will be described.

Laparoscopy in the Schauta–Amreich procedure can be limited to the completion of lymphadenectomy. The two operations are performed in two separate steps, either within an interval of a couple of days or in the same surgical session. We performed this two-step procedure (see below) during our first 5 years' clinical experience.

Laparoscopic assistance can be pushed further and used for the preparation of the extended hysterectomy. This preparation can be carried even further, and used for full laparoscopic radical hysterectomy in which the vaginal route is used only to take out the specimen. Our concept is different, as laparoscopy is used as preparation for an operation which remains essentially vaginal. Experience of the classic Schauta procedure has shown that laparoscopy can help with the two most difficult steps of the classical vaginal operation: identification and development of the paravesical and pararectal spaces and division of the paracervix at the pelvic side wall. The other steps of the classical operation can be quickly and safely performed through the vaginal approach: there is no need to perform them under laparoscopic guidance.

Identification of the paravisceral spaces is the key to success in radical hysterectomy. Doing this through the vaginal route requires a lot of experience. Moreover, when a distal radical hysterectomy which requires a large opening of those spaces has to be performed, a paravaginal Schuchardt's incision is mandatory, and this is not 'patient-friendly'. On the other hand, identifying and developing the paravesical and pararectal spaces is very simple through the abdominal route using either laparotomy or laparoscopy. In the laparoscopic-vaginal procedure the two spaces are prepared under laparoscopic guidance. The spaces are developed down to the levator muscle. Then the vaginal fascia will have to be perforated (at the right place) to find again the spaces during the

vaginal step of the procedure. Moreover, laparoscopic separation of the areolar tissue of the paravisceral spaces improves the mobility of the uterus, making the vaginal operation easier.

Division of the paracervix at the pelvic side wall is performed only in the distal type of laparoscopically assisted radical vaginal hysterectomy. The anatomy of this structure means that it should be managed differently in the proximal and the distal variants of radical hysterectomy. The paracervix is a condensation of the pelvic cellular tissue around arteries and veins going from the hypogastric vessels to the uterus and vagina. The uterine vessels are arranged pyramidally. They are numerous and occupy a large space at the point of contact of the vagina and cervix. More laterally (from the centropelvic area to the pelvic wall) they become less numerous and bunch together. For this reason, it is quite easy to divide laparoscopically the paracervix at the level of the pelvic wall (i.e. by performing a distal radical hysterectomy) using a stapler or any other tool. Moreover, the obliquity of the pelvic wall facilitates clamping from above—while it is difficult to clamp from below.

Conversely, management of the paracervix at an intermediate level (i.e. by performing a proximal radical hysterectomy) cannot be easily carried out from above using either the EndoGIA (the opening of which is too small) or bipolar coagulation or clips (the vessels are too numerous), but it is easy to carry out from below using classic clamps. That is the reason why Querleu and myself have chosen to clamp the paracervix from below for the radical proximal hysterectomy and to clamp it from above for the distal radical hysterectomy.

Techniques

The two techniques for distal laparoscopically assisted vaginal radical hysterectomy defined above will be described.

Laparoscopic lymphadenectomy combined with Schauta–Amreich hysterectomy

The two-step operation is described here for two reasons. First it is necessary to master the classic Schauta technique before any attempt is made at the coelio-Schauta procedure. Second, evidence that the new coelio-Schauta procedure is superior to this simple combination of two well-defined operations is still lacking. As a consequence, the classic Schauta–Amreich procedure will be described in detail, as good knowledge of this is mandatory to comfortably perform the laparoscopically assisted vaginal radical hysterectomy or coelio-Schauta procedure.

LAPAROSCOPIC STEP

The laparoscopic step of the two-step operation is described in Chapters 3 and 4. I favour the extraperitoneal approach, while not omitting assessment of the peritoneal cavity before performing the retroperitoneal operation. In France, assessment of the retroperitoneal lymph nodes is usually limited to the interiliac area. In cases where the interiliac lymph nodes are not involved the risk of missing metastasis in the common iliac or para-aortic area is low.

VAGINAL STEP

Vaginal radical hysterectomy performed after laparoscopic lymphadenectomy does not differ from the classical procedure, except that it is easier to perform immediately or early following laparoscopy. It would be harder to perform if the interval is more than 10 days after postoperative oedema and relaxation of the pelvic cellular tissue is replaced by fibrosis and sclerosis.

Schuchardt's incision

Schuchardt's incision is a mediolateral episiotomy performed for two reasons: it makes the operative field wider and it opens the paravisceral spaces. The incision is made on the left side of the patient (for the right-handed surgeon). The puborectal muscle is divided and, cranially to it, the pararectal space is entered. Then, turning around the caudal edge of the paracervix with a blunt instrument moving from the dorsal side to the ventral side of the cardinal ligament, the paravesical space is entered.

Making the vaginal cuff

Making the vaginal cuff is initiated while putting a series of Kocher's forceps at the level of the junction between the upper third and the median third of the vagina. While pulling on these forceps a sort of internal prolapse of the vagina is created. The outer layer of the prolapsed cylinder is incised, taking care to divide the three layers of the vagina (skin, muscle and fascia) but preserving the inner layer of the prolapsed cylinder. Making the incision properly is easy to do on the ventral face and also on the dorsal face of the vagina, but it is rather difficult to perform on the lateral faces. It is very important to perform the lateral incision properly: if the incision is too ventral and too shallow, the opening of the lateral spaces will be impossible; if the incision is too dorsal and too deep, the vaginal cuff will be separated from its connection with the paracervix which will become difficult to reach. To make the lateral incision easier, it is recommended to first make the ventral and dorsal parts of the incision, and then to move to the lateral parts where the incision has to be made at the appropriate length and depth to join the ventral and dorsal incisions.

Opening the vesicovaginal space

After separating the vaginal cuff from the rest of the vagina, the cuff over the cervix is closed with a series of Chrobak forceps placed on a frontal line. Using these forceps the cuff is pulled dorsally. At the same time the peripheral vaginal flap is grasped at 12 o'clock and pulled ventrally. The two opposing actions expose an artificial anatomical structure designated by Amreich as the 'supravaginal septum'. This structure is nothing other than a condensation of the connective fibres located between the inferior pole of the bladder and the anterior face of the vagina—the endopelvic fascia.

At this point in the operation it is essential to keep in mind the details of the anatomy of this area, as the anatomy is significantly modified by surgical preparation. First remember that the bladder floor is in direct connection with the upper part of the anterior vaginal wall. The connective fibres interposed joining the two organs are dense, especially at the level of the ureteral orifices and at the level of the bladder neck. Traction on the cervix before vaginal incision makes visible (for the experienced surgeon) three little depressions which limit the Pavlic triangle which is the 'vaginal mirror' of the bladder trigone. Anatomical connections between the vagina and the bladder floor explain why a traction exerted on the vaginal cuff attracts the bladder base directly into the operative field, along with the terminal part of the ureters.

The supravaginal septum, which has to be perforated in order to enter the vesicovaginal space, has a triangular shape. It has to be opened on the middle line close to its basis. This is the point at which the connections between the bladder and vagina are less tight (at an equal distance from the three landmarks of the Pavlic triangle). The scissors must be handled perpendicular to the vagina, tangential to the inferior pole of the bladder. Once the septum is opened the finger enters and develops the vesicovaginal space. A speculum is put in place. The remaining lateral fibres are divided with scissors. The finger is introduced again, and then the speculum . . . and so on until reaching the space located on the ventral face of the vesicouterine peritoneal cul-de-sac. Identification of the bladder with a probe introduced through the urethra may help.

Managing the bladder pillar on the left side

Now that the paravesical space on the left side is free (by

Schuchardt's incision) and the vesicouterine space has been developed, the next step in the operation is to manage the structures lying between the two spaces—the bladder pillar. This structure is composed of two parts: the lateral part is the ventrolateral expansion of the paracervix (the anterior parametrium); the medial part is the condensation of the vesicouterine connective fibres at the level of the ureteral orifice. As a result of traction exerted on this medial bladder pillar, the ureter is attracted into the operative field but it is hidden by the lateral bladder pillar. The pillar can be managed by cutting its medial part first. However, we prefer, as recommended by Amreich, to start with division of the lateral part. This division makes the ureter visible and makes the following step of the operation safer.

The first step in the management of the bladder pillar is to identify the contours of the ureter. This is done by palpation. The forefinger of the left hand is introduced into the vesicouterine space and exerts on the pillar a pressure from inside to outside. The forefinger of the right hand is introduced into the paravesical space. The pillar is palpated between the two fingers. A characteristic 'pop' makes the contours of the ureter perceptible. The forefinger of the right hand is taken away and the scalpel is introduced. The fibres of the lateral bladder pillar are cut. The ureter is seen. Be very careful while doing this incision: make a shallow incision, then palpate, then a shallow incision and so on. Having seen the ureter, the remaining management of the bladder pillar is easy.

With the ureter's 'knee' under direct visual control, the bladder pillar can be divided without any risk. The division of the lateral part of the pillar can be extended more dorsally (the more dorsal the division is extended, the larger the paracervical resection will be): the inferior vesical artery or branches of it are frequently divided during this complementary incision. Haemostasis is achieved after section when necessary. Division of the medial part of the pillar is carried out while moving upwards to the knee of the ureter. This division frees the anterior (ventral) face of the paracervix at the level of its insertion on the cervicovaginal junction. A little depression can then be identified by palpation at the superior edge of the paracervix. We call it the 'paraisthmic window': the arch of the uterine artery lies at this level. Once the arch of the artery has been identified the descending branch is dissected from inside to outside: it reaches the operating field in the concavity of the knee of the ureter. 'Unroofing' of the ureter is carried out in the opposite way to that used in abdominal surgery, and it ends with cutting the uterine artery as close as possible to its origin.

Managing the bladder pillar on the right side

Managing the bladder pillar on the side opposite to the paravaginal incision requires the pararectal and the paravesical spaces on the opposite side to be opened directly.

To open the paravesical space, two forceps are placed at the edge of the peripheral vaginal incision line: one at the 9 o'clock and the other one at the 11 o'clock positions. Traction is exerted on them divergently and at the same time traction is exerted in the opposite direction on the vaginal cuff. A triangular depression appears. Its base is constituted by the line joining the two forceps. The bottom of this depression corresponds to the entry to the paravesical space. The tip of the scissors is put at the contact of this landmark and the scissors are pushed in a ventrolateral direction. Once the paravesical space is opened with the instrument, a finger is introduced into it and the space is widened. In order to open the pararectal space, the forceps put at 11 o'clock is moved to 7 o'clock. The pararectal space is opened in the same way as on the ventral face.

Once the paravesical and pararectal spaces are opened, the preparation is completed by dividing a transverse structure attaching the peripheral vaginal flap to the paracervix and separating the two spaces: this lateral ligament is the inferior extension of the paracervix, the paracolpos. This lateral ligament is not identified on the left side because it is attached to the ventral flap of the paravaginal incision, namely to the anterior parametrium—the lateral part of the bladder pillar.

Opening the pouch of Douglas and dividing the rectum pillar

The preparation of the dorsal face of the specimen is much easier than the preparation of the ventral face. It starts with opening the rectovaginal space on the midline. This opening frees the posterior peritoneal cul-de-sac, but care must be taken not to work too close to the vagina and not to get lost in the fascia. The pouch of Douglas is entered. The rectal pillar—the rectovaginal ligament—is stretched while moving the rectum dorsally and the vagina ventrally using appropriate speculums. This ligament is divided by sharp dissection, which frees the posterior (dorsal) face and the inferior (caudal) edge of the paracervix.

Division of the paracervix

Once the two faces of the left paracervix are free the ligament can be clamped and divided. A right-angle curved dissector is pushed from behind through the broad ligament while guiding its tip with the forefinger of the other hand put at the contact of the 'paraisthmic window' we have described before, and which is the landmark of the superior edge of the paracervix. The dissector is opened; the superior (cephalic) edge of the ligament becomes free. A first clamp is placed on this ligament. Traction is exerted medially in order to put a second clamp at a distance from the first one, as close as possible to the pelvic insertion of the ligament. Then the ligament is divided and a suture is placed on the parietal stump. The knee of the ureter should be kept under permanent control throughout this step of the operation. The lowest point of the knee is located very close to the tip of the clamp. The same action is repeated on the right side. After division of the two paracervices, the posterior fold of the broad ligament is incised. Again care must be taken not to injure the ureter, which is still attached to the peritoneal fold. The section of the laterouterine peritoneum leads to the uterine horn. The uterus can be extracted after retroversion of the uterine fundus. The utero-ovarian ligament, tube and round ligament are clamped and cut at the contact of the myometrium then, depending on the age of the patient, a salpingo-oophorectomy may be performed.

Peritonization and closure of the vagina are carried out as they would be after a simple vaginal hysterectomy. The paravaginal incision is closed layer after layer.

Distal coelio-Schauta procedure

The distal coelio-Schauta procedure differs from the two-step operation only in details. However, those details make the operation much easier.

LAPAROSCOPIC STEP

This step starts with the pelvic dissection. The transumbilical transperitoneal route can be used for the laparoscopic step of the distal coelio-Schauta. The retroperitoneal approach can be used as well, but it is mandatory to act through an infraumbilical port as the aim of laparoscopic preparation is not only to assess the interiliac lymph nodes. Preparation of the radical vaginal hysterectomy cannot be carried out without a panoramic view of the pelvic cavity.

Preparation for vaginal radical hysterectomy involves dividing the paracervix at the level of its insertion on the pelvic side wall. To do this we have to develop the paravisceral spaces. This is not difficult because the paravesical space has already been opened during the lymphadenectomy. It only has to be developed down to the level of the levator muscle. The only possible danger when developing this space is injury to the veins coming from the vagina and going convergently to the internal iliac vein. Remember that in the standing position the vagina is located in a horizontal plane and the cervix in a vertical plane. In the supine position the paracervix

appears located in a frontal plane whose obliquity is the same as that of the umbilicococcygeal axis: work can be carried out easily and safely along the ventral face of the paracervix. Conversely, the caudal expansion of the paracervix—the paracolpos—appears almost parallel to the plane of the levator muscle, and the paravaginal veins may be at risk at this point.

To open and develop the pararectal space proceed in the same way as for the paravesical space. The pararectal space is deeper and more narrow. To enter this space the crossing point of the ureter and the uterine artery has to be identified. The entrance to the pararectal space is found dorsal and lateral to this crossing point. The development of the space is made by blunt dissection using two forceps (or one forceps and the suction device), the first pushing the rectum medially and the second running along the dorsal face of the paracervix. At this level there is a risk of injury to the hypogastric vein or to the rectal veins emptying into the hypogastric vein at a right angle.

Once the two paravisceral spaces have been developed, the paracervix can be managed. The ligament is stretched by pushing medially the bladder and the rectum using two forceps placed in the paravesical and in the pararectal spaces respectively, the tip of the two instruments being at the contact of the levator muscle. The vessels which represent the skeleton of the ligament can be managed in different ways. They may be electively divided after preventive haemostasis using bipolar cautery or after having put clips on them (two on the parietal side, one on the visceral one). We favour use of the EndoGIA (Autosuture®) stapler, or an equivalent, introduced through an ipsilateral iliac port. Two shots are needed; the first shot is placed on the anterior trunk of the hypogastric artery (Fig. 8.1) and the second shot on the vessels located caudally to the artery (Fig. 8.2). This step is not difficult: the space is large, the vessels to be treated are few and the axis that is worked along is correct. The anteroposterior obliquity of this axis is of the utmost importance; the lateral obliquity is also very important. To cut the visceral branches of the hypogastric artery, the stapler has to be introduced parallel to the pelvic wall, which means that the lateral iliac port has to be used. If the median port is used, the contact with the pelvic wall is at the wrong angle and there is a risk of cutting the parietal branches of the hypogastric artery. Consequently, the lateral iliac ports need to have 10–12-mm doors.

After dividing the paracervix, move directly to the vaginal step of the operation.

VAGINAL STEP

The main technical difference between the distal coelio-Schauta and the classic Amreich operation is the absence

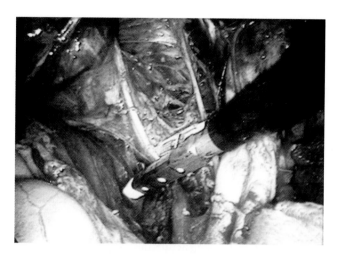

Fig. 8.1 Distal coelio-Schauta procedure, management of the paracervical ligament on the right side of the patient. The ligament lies obliquely between the paravesical space (upper right part of the figure) and the pararectal space (lower left part of the figure). The EndoGIA stapler is dividing the cranial part of the ligament, i.e. the common trunk of the inferior vesical artery and the uterine artery.

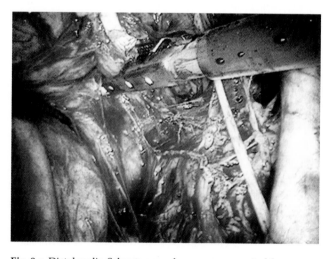

Fig. 8.2 Distal coelio-Schauta procedure, management of the paracervical ligament on the right side of the patient. The cranial and caudal parts of the paracervical ligament have been divided, and the paravesical and pararectal spaces communicate freely. The two sets of staples are visible where the stapler touches the pelvic wall.

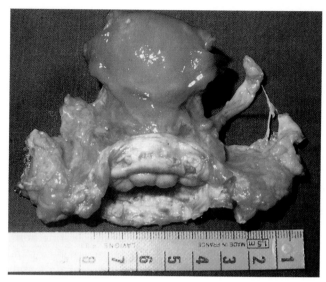

Fig. 8.3 The operative specimen from the distal coelio-Schauta procedure.

of the paravaginal Schuchardt incision. The vaginal cuff is made directly. The vesicovaginal and the rectovaginal spaces are opened as described on the side opposite to the paravaginal incision in the classic Schauta–Amreich operation, using two forceps placed at the edge of the vaginal incision to identify the opening of the paravesical space on both sides. The opening for the pararectal space is made while dividing the most caudal part of the uterosacral ligament. The job is very easy because the spaces have been previously prepared under laparoscopic guidance. In addition, division of the lateral ligament that is separating the part of the paracolpos related to the vaginal cuff from the part related to the remaining vagina is very easy.

For the following steps of the operation no haemostasis is necessary. The bladder pillar is managed in the same way as in the classic Schauta–Amreich procedure. The arch of the uterine artery is identified and the descending branch of the arch is dissected from inside to outside and finally divided at its origin (i.e. separated from the inferior vesical artery). Finally, the cephalic part of the uterosacral ligament and the posterior fold of the broad ligament are divided. Again the ureter is at risk and care must be taken. This part of the operation is bloodless because of the haemostasis provided by the control of the vessels in the paracervix, which is a very significant advantage of the laparoscopically assisted procedure.

After the extirpation of the operative specimen (Fig. 8.3) the question of peritoneal repair has to be discussed. Avoiding repair is, at the moment, popular. There are advantages in leaving open the lateropelvic spaces, enabling the prophylaxis of lymphocysts. However, the risk of incarceration of an intestinal loop into this latero-pelvic space does exist, especially after an operation as radical as the distal coelio-Schauta procedure. Having experienced such a complication, we recommend performing peritonization while leaving an opened linear peritoneal wound along the pelvic brim.

In cases where the laparoscopic preparation has been performed using a retroperitoneal approach, peritonization can be performed easily through the vaginal route. Where the transperitoneal approach has been used, the peritonization cannot be performed through the vaginal route. The bladder peritoneum and the rectal peritoneum can only be approximated transversally in the centro-pelvic area. The lateral parts of the peritonization are performed laparoscopically using straight needles (Vicryl no. 000) and separate cross stitches with extracorporeal knots.

Conclusion

Radical vaginal hysterectomy is a valuable addition to the armamentarium of oncological gynaecologists. Extra effort must be taken in training to learn the vaginal techniques. However, this effort is rewarded, as many patients with early cervical cancer will be able to avoid laparotomy. Laparoscopic preparation makes the operation relatively easy to learn and also provides a chance to determine the lymph-node status before going ahead with surgery.

References

1 Dargent D, Salvat J (1989). *L'Envahissement Ganglionnaire Pelvien.* Paris: McGraw-Hill.

2 Fuller AJ Jr, Elliott N, Kosloff C, Lewis JL (1982). Lymph node metastases from carcinoma of the cervix stages IB and IIA: implications for prognosis and treatment. *Gynecol Oncol* **13**:165–174.

3 Nelson JH, Macasaet MA, Lu T *et al* (1974). The incidence and significance of paraaortic lymph nodes metastasis in late invasive carcinoma of the cervix. *Am J Obstet Gynecol* **118**:749–756.

4 Weiser EB, Bundy BN, Hoskins WJ *et al* (1989). Extraperitoneal versus transperitoneal selective para aortic lymphadenectomy in the pretreatment surgical staging of advanced cervical carcinoma (a Gynecologic Oncologic Group study). *Gynecol Oncol* **33**:283–289.

5 Wingo PA, Huezo CM, Rubin GL *et al* (1992). The mortality risk associated with hysterectomy. *Am J Obstet Gynecol* **67**:756–757.

6 Dargent D, Kouakou F, Adeleine P (1991). L'opération de Schauta 90 ans après. *Lyon Chir* **87**:324–328.

7 Piver MS, Rutledge F, Smith JP (1974). Five classes of extended hysterectomy for women with cervical cancer. *Obstet Gynecol* **44**:265–272.

9 Laparoscopic radical hysterectomy for cervical cancer

Michel Canis, Arnaud Wattiez, Gérard Mage,
Patrice Mille, Jean-Luc Pouly and
Maurice-Antoine Bruhat

Introduction

Laparoscopic hysterectomy and pelvic lymphadenectomy were first reported in 1989 and 1991, respectively [1,2]. Since then, several laparoscopic techniques of radical hysterectomy combined with a vaginal approach have been reported [3–9]. Our first case was carefully selected—a patient with stage IA2 squamous carcinoma of the cervix, who had received preoperative caesium radiotherapy. For such a controversial laparoscopic procedure this cautious approach was necessary [3]. In 1992, Dargent first performed proximal laparoscopic transection of the cardinal ligament with an EndoGIA [6]. Following this report, and with increased experience, our technique became more radical, enabling us to treat patients by surgery alone [10]. If all the previously reported advantages of laparoscopic surgery can be confirmed in patients operated on for cervical carcinoma, this approach will appear very attractive. Until now, however, the series published have included only a small number of cases with a short follow-up [11,12], and this procedure cannot be considered as a standard.

Patient set-up and initial steps

The preoperative work-up includes: (i) an intravenous pyelogram; (ii) a chest X-ray and MRI scan to measure the volume of the tumour and to assess the pelvic and para-aortic nodes; and (iii) a complete preanaesthetic examination. A mechanical bowel preparation is administered on the day before surgery, so that the bowel can be easily pushed away from the pelvis, thus minimizing the Trendelenburg to 10° or less, which is essential during long laparoscopic procedures.

Under general anaesthesia with endotracheal intubation, the procedure is performed in a low lithotomy position. To easily perform the vaginal steps of the operation, it should be possible to increase the flexion and the abduction of the thighs. A Foley catheter is placed. The uterus is mobilized with a Valtchev mobilizer, without cervical dilatation. Compared with the curette, which we used at the beginning of our experience, this device improves uterine anteversion, thus facilitating the exposure for the posterior steps of the operation. It also allows a better exposure of the cervicovaginal area because of the direct mobilization of the cervix, which previously was only mobilized by the pressure applied on the uterine fundus. Vaginal and rectal probes may be necessary to facilitate the dissection of the rectovaginal space. A complete set of laparoscopic instruments should be available, including three curved laparoscopic scissors, three 3-mm large bipolar forceps, three atraumatic grasping forceps, two atraumatic haemostatic forceps, endoclips, two needle holders, one Clark knot pusher, a high-flow electronic insufflator (9l/mm) and a powerful suction-irrigation apparatus [13]. A second operating table with all the instruments required for a laparotomy is prepared to allow an immediate repair of a large vessel injury. Vaginal retractors and Chrobak forceps are necessary to carry out the vaginal step [14].

A 10-mm, 0° laparoscope is inserted intraumbilically. According to the uterine size and mobility, the ancillary trocars are inserted high enough to ensure that all the instruments can be used during every step of the operation. Whenever possible, the trocar entry sites are chosen to ensure that the instruments will be perpendicular to the tissue during key steps of the operation, such as the haemostasis of the cardinal ligaments and the dissection of the ureters. Usually two 5.5-mm trocars are inserted lateral to the rectus muscle, thus avoiding the episgastric vessels. A 10-mm trocar is placed on the midline or lateral to the umbilicus in small patients. This 10-mm trocar allows an immediate insertion of endoclips, and of sutures with curved needles. Moreover, this diameter is required for easy extraction of lymph nodes. In difficult cases, a fourth ancillary trocar may be necessary to dissect the distal part of the ureter.

The surgeon stands on the patient's left, usually operating with the instruments inserted in the left and the median suprapubic ports. The first assistant is on the patient's right, holding the video camera and working with the instruments inserted through the right trocar. The second assistant stands between the patient's legs, mobilizing the uterine cannula. One nurse stands on the patient's left making the instruments immediately available to the surgeon; occasionally she works as a third assistant, holding the left instrument when the surgeon is working with the median and the right instruments. One or two circulating nurses are in the room. The anaesthetist, who monitors the patient's pulse rate, blood pressure and capnia, should be used to working in extensive laparoscopic procedures.

Two video monitors are necessary. One is placed at the patient's right foot, for the surgeon, the second assistant and the nurse, one at the patient's left foot for the first assistant. Although we only work with two monitors, a third screen located over the patient's head would be useful for the second assistant and for the occasions when the surgeon stands between the patient's legs for para-aortic node dissection.

Whenever possible, three rules should be followed. First, the peritoneum is incised without previous coagulation while it is elevated with an atraumatic forceps. In this way the intra-abdominal pressure and the carbon dioxide enter the retroperitoneal space, thus facilitating the dissection. The opening of the retroperitoneal space is more difficult when both peritoneal leaves are stuck together by previous coagulation. Second, all bleeding, however minimal, should be stopped immediately to maintain optimal visibility. Indeed, a small amount of bleeding stains the retroperitoneal tissues, making the operation more difficult. To achieve this meticulous haemostasis, the retroperitoneal spaces are dissected with two instruments always including a bipolar forceps. As palpation is impossible, vision is essential for the endoscopic surgeon. Third, large vessels such as the uterine artery or the infundibulopelvic ligament should be skeletonized and stretched when applying bipolar coagulation. In this way the diameter of the vessels is decreased and the coagulation is more effective, because the electric current is applied on the vessel, not on the surrounding tissue.

Aspiration of the peritoneal fluid for cytological examination and inspection of the entire peritoneal cavity are performed first. This evaluation establishes if the laparoscopic approach is feasible. Poor local conditions, such as extensive adhesions or a very large uterus, may lead to conversion to laparotomy. To enable a satisfactory dissection of the left pelvic nodes, the sigmoid colon is mobilized. The round ligaments are coagulated and cut above the external iliac vein, allowing easy access to the pelvic lymph nodes and to the paravesical fossa. Then the lateral end of the round ligament is elevated and the peritoneum is incised above the external iliac vessels.

The adnexae are managed according to the patient's age, the volume of the tumour and the pathological diagnosis. In patients ≤40 years old with a ≤3-cm well-differentiated squamous cell carcinoma, the ovaries are preserved. The adnexal vessels are stretched, pushing the uterus toward the opposite pelvic side wall and pulling the adnexa laterally. In this way the adnexal vessels are easily coagulated with bipolar electrocautery and cut with scissors. Then the adnexa is elevated and pulled laterally; the medial peritoneum is incised parallel to the ovarian vessels, allowing free mobilization of the adnexa which will be sutured in the paracolic gutter with non-absorbable sutures. The right lateral peritoneal incision is extended up the paracolic gutter; this is not necessary on the left side where the sigmoid colon has been mobilized. Traction on the ovarian vessels is minimized, twisting should be carefully avoided.

When the ovaries are removed the approach is different. While pulling both the adnexa and the uterus towards the opposite pelvic side wall, the lateral peritoneal incision is extended up to the infundibulopelvic ligament. The ureter is identified by inspection or by dissection and the infundibulopelvic ligament is coagulated and cut.

Lymphadenectomy

The umbilical artery is identified and dissected up to the internal iliac artery to ensure complete dissection of the pelvic nodes and easier identification of the internal iliac artery, which will be the main landmark for the dissection of the pararectal fossa. Then, while pulling the umbilical artery medially, the paravesical fossa is opened bluntly using scissors and a bipolar forceps or an atraumatic probe such as the aspiration lavage cannula. At this moment, the dissection of the paravesical fossa can be stopped when the obturator nerve has been identified. The lymph nodes are separated from the external iliac vein, the obturator internus muscle, the iliopubic bone and the obturator nerve as previously described [15]. At the end of the dissection, to complete or to check the excision of the obturator nodes the external iliac vessels are separated from the lateral pelvic side wall. The lymph nodes are immediately removed from the abdomen. While extracting the nodes, the abdominal wall is protected using an endo-bag or the 10-mm trocar with a 5-mm forceps and a 5-mm external reducer.

When indicated, the para-aortic lymph nodes located below the inferior mesenteric artery are removed. This technique has been described by others [16–18]. To achieve a satisfactory dissection of the nodes located below the left renal vein, we have found that the ancillary trocars should be inserted closer to the umbilicus than to the pubic symphysis, higher than usual for pelvic procedures such as radical hysterectomy. However, the dissection of the nodes located below the level of the inferior mesenteric artery is much easier than the dissection of the upper para-aortic area below the left renal vein. When necessary, the laparoscope is introduced through the median 10-mm suprapubic trocar, or in the left suprapubic area to dissect the left side of the aorta as recommended by Pomel *et al.* [18].

Radical hysterectomy

Anatomy (Fig. 9.1)

The cardinal ligament should be represented as a parallelepiped oblique anteriorly and medially. The limits of this volume are:
1 the upper limit is the uterine artery;
2 the posterior surface is identified while dissecting the pararectal fossa;
3 the inferior surface is freed from the levator muscle;
4 the anterior surface is more complex—laterally it is identified when dissecting the paravesical space, medially it is connected to the bladder;
5 the lateral surface is the origin of this ligament and of the vessels along the pelvic side wall;
6 the medial surface is connected to the uterus.

The cardinal ligament is connected to the bladder by two vesicouterine ligaments, one is medial to the ureter and the second lateral to it [19]. To free the ureter, this external ligament will be coagulated and cut in two steps, one above and one below the ureter. It should be understood that the obliquity of the ureter is different to that of the cardinal ligament. Posteriorly the ureter enters in the

ligament just under its upper limit (i.e. the uterine artery), so that the ureter can be freed by cutting the uterine artery. Whereas in the anterior part of the parallelepiped the ureter enters the bladder, is located deeper and the dissection of this distal part requires several steps.

To excise the parametrium, five of the six surfaces of the parallelepiped should be dissected and cut, while freeing the ureter from the parametrium.

Dissection of the paravesical and pararectal spaces (Fig. 9.2)

This essential step which exposes the cardinal ligament is usually bloodless. However haemostasis, if necessary, should be meticulous. While pulling the umbilical artery, the paravesical space is easily identified. The loose connective tissue is dissected bluntly with scissors and a bipolar forceps. It is sometimes necessary to push the uterus towards the contralateral infundibulopelvic ligament and/or to pull the peritoneum medially. Once the space has been identified, the paravesical fossa is developed up to the levator muscle while moving the bipolar forceps and the scissors in opposite directions. When developing the posterior part of this space, which identifies the anterior surface of the parametrium, be cautious to avoid trauma to the uterine veins as their haemostasis would be difficult at this time.

To dissect the pararectal space, the posterior peritoneum is grasped and pulled medially. Thereafter, posterior to the internal iliac artery, the fossa is opened bluntly, accounting for the direction of the vessels of the cardinal ligament which are not perpendicular to the pelvic side wall, but oblique anteriorly and medially. To facilitate the dissection of the lower part of the fossa up to the levator

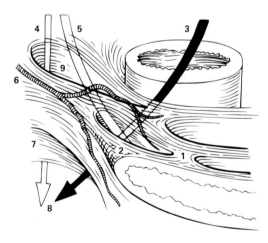

Fig. 9.1 Anatomy of the cardinal ligament. 1, Internal part of the vesicouterine ligament; 2, external part of the vesicouterine ligament; 3, space between the lateral and the anterior part (external part of the vesicouterine ligament) of the cardinal ligament; 4, space between the paravesical and the pararectal space; 5, ureter; 6, umbilicouterine artery; 7, cardinal ligament; 8, levator muscle; 9, pararectal fossa. (Adapted from Frobert [19].)

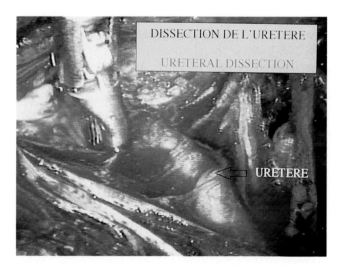

Fig. 9.2 Opening the pararectal fossa. The paravesical fossa has already been opened.

muscle, an aspiration lavage cannula is placed inside the fossa to retract the peritoneum and the ureter and to improve the view with short aspirations whenever the operating field is obscured by blood or lymph. Three working instruments are necessary to expose and to dissect this posterior fossa. At the bottom of this space the pelvic splanchnic nerve [20,21] is identified and preserved whenever possible.

As the treatment of bleeding is more difficult at laparoscopy, the technique used to open the pelvic fossae may differ from that used at laparotomy. Indeed, at laparotomy the fossae were always opened up to the levator muscle in one step, a more progressive approach may be preferred at laparoscopy, the deepest part of the fossae being dissected only after the section of the upper part of the lateral surface of the cardinal ligament (i.e. the uterine vessels). When these vessels are coagulated and cut, the retraction which can be achieved is improved, the deeper part of the fossae is more easily exposed and the bleeding encountered during the dissection is more easily controlled. A bleeding in the deeper part of the posterior fossa would be difficult to control when it occurs at the beginning of the dissection.

Rectovaginal space and the uterosacral ligaments

The posterior step should be one of the first steps of the procedure. The section of the posterior uterine ligaments allows easier mobilization of the uterus and facilitates the dissection of the parametrium and the ureters. Furthermore, these steps are easier when there is no bleeding from the anterior steps of the operation. When incising the posterior peritoneum, decide how large the excision of the peritoneum and the uterosacral ligaments will be, and where the ureter will be freed from the peritoneum and the periureteral plane opened. This point is essential, as the peritoneal vascular support to the ureter is important to prevent postoperative ureteral complications.

The posterior peritoneum is grasped under the infundibulopelvic ligament and pulled medially. Then the peritoneum is dissected from the underlying tissue and incised towards the uterosacral ligament. During this step, the ureter is identified and separated from the peritoneum. Extending this incision below the ureter up to the posterior cul-de-sac requires the coagulation of the upper part of the uterosacral ligament. Then the peritoneum, which will be excised, is pulled anteriorly and medially, to free the ureter from the peritoneum and from the uterosacral ligament. To dissect the rectovaginal space the uterus is anteverted and anteflexed, if possible according to the tumour anatomy. The rectum is elevated and pulled posteriorly. The rectovaginal space is developed with scissors and bipolar coagulation. A vaginal probe may be

used to identify the plane and to improve the exposure of the lower part of the dissection. This plane may be difficult to identify. However, an avascular space can be found in most patients. If many vessels are encountered, the correct plane has not been identified and it will almost always be found closer to the vagina. A similar technique is used to separate the rectum from the uterosacral ligaments.

The ureter is checked, and further separated from the uterosacral ligaments, which can then be safely coagulated as their lateral aspect has been identified when opening the pararectal fossa.

Section of the cardinal ligament

The haemostasis of the vessels along the pelvic side wall is the treatment of the lateral surface of the cardinal ligament. Several techniques including Endoclips and EndoGIA have been proposed for the haemostasis of these vessels [6]. In most cases we have used bipolar coagulation and found it to be safe—we have had no postoperative haemorrhage among 17 patients. Preventive haemostasis is the key to an effective and quick haemostasis. However, coagulation of bleeding areas induces carbonization, which prevents the efficacy of bipolar coagulation. The vessels of the cardinal ligament are dissected, coagulated and cut. Generally, four vessels are identified during this dissection. If the paravesical space is developed laterally to the umbilical artery, the umbilico-uterine artery is cut before its bifurcation, whereas when it has been dissected medially to the umbilical artery, this artery and its bladder branch will be preserved. This second technique should be preferred to prevent urological complications as much as possible.

Both cardinal ligaments should be coagulated and cut before the dissection of the ureters. Haemostasis of all the uterine vessels makes the dissection of the ureters much easier.

Dissection of the ureter and the vesicouterine ligaments (Fig. 9.3)

Dissection of the vesicovaginal plane is the first step. It should be large enough to allow the dissection of the vesicouterine ligaments and to identify the inferior margin of the vaginal cuff.

To dissect the bladder, the uterus is pushed medially and posteriorly toward the promontory [22]. The anterior peritoneum is elevated and incised, starting from the round ligament. The plane is developed with curved scissors and bipolar coagulation. To achieve this dissection several steps are often necessary, the lower part of the vesicovaginal plane is exposed only when grasping and

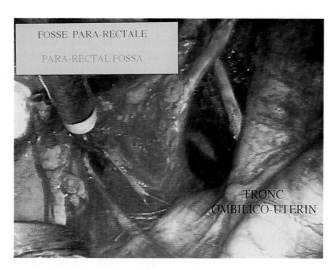

FOSSE PARA-RECTALE

PARA-RECTAL FOSSA

TRONC
OMBILICO-UTERIN

Fig. 9.3 Dissection of the right ureter.

carefully elevating the posterior surface of the bladder. This movement should be slow and careful to avoid bladder injuries, which may be easily induced by an atraumatic forceps, because the longer part of the forceps is outside the abdomen. When the dissection is difficult, follow this procedure: (i) avoid bleeding; (ii) improve the exposure, checking the uterine position and the bladder elevation; (iii) fill the bladder with methylene blue; (iv) elevate the bladder with two grasping forceps, thus exposing the space by pulling in two directions, the frontal and the sagittal planes; and (v) use a probe in the anterior vaginal cul-de-sac.

The dissection of the ureter includes two steps: the section of the uterine artery and the dissection of the internal part of the vesicouterine ligament.

The ureter is freed from the uterine artery with a dissector working on its medial side. Adequate exposure is obtained by pulling posteriorly the posterior peritoneum still adherent to the ureter. Coagulation of the uterine artery is achieved with bipolar coagulation; this haemostasis is easy as this vessel has already been cut laterally. This second section of the uterine artery is required only to free the ureter. Both parts of the uterine artery will be removed. The lateral part is excised when freeing the lateral part of the cardinal ligament from the pelvic floor, whereas the medial part is removed with the uterus.

Then the ureter is dissected up to its entry in the bladder. A perfect exposure of this distal part of the ureteric tunnel is often difficult to obtain. A fourth suprapubic instrument may be necessary. First, the uterus is pushed laterally and posteriorly towards the opposite pelvic side wall without any anteversion or anteflexion. Second, the bladder is elevated with an atraumatic forceps placed close to the estimated site of the ureteral extremity.

Third, the ureter is pulled back laterally to allow the dissection of its medial surface. Grasping the ureter is avoided whenever possible, either by pulling on the posterior peritoneum or using a Babcock forceps. The ureteric tunnel is developed using a 5-mm curved dissector. As in laparotomy, the correct plane is in contact with the ureter. Haemostasis and the section of the internal vesicouterine ligament should avoid ureteral trauma. When possible, haemostasis is achieved with Endoclips.

At this point, the cardinal ligament has to be freed from its lateral connections to the bladder. This is achieved in two steps, one above and one below the ureter, so that all the tissues located between the vesicovaginal and paravesical spaces will be coagulated and cut. The upper part is dissected with a curved forceps inserted through one lateral trocar and then coagulated and cut. Exposure is essential. The installation is similar to that described above, except for the ureter which is pulled medially.

The ureter is then freed from its inferior attachments to the cardinal ligament. The vesicovaginal space is further dissected, allowing the section of the lateral part of the vesicouterine ligament, which is essential for a radical excision of the cardinal ligament [19]. To expose this ligament, the bladder and the uterus are retracted as above. The ligament is sequentially coagulated with bipolar coagulation and cut. The dissection of the bladder is then completed. During all these steps, care should be taken to avoid dissection of the lateral surface of the distal end of the ureter from the bladder.

Finally, while elevating the cardinal ligament with an atraumatic grasping forceps, its fifth surface (i.e. inferior) is freed from the levator muscle. This step is stopped when the vagina is identified. A probe may facilitate the identification of the vagina.

Vaginal step

The procedure is finished vaginally. In this way an adequate vaginal resection, 3 cm from the tumour margins, is easier. As in a Schauta operation [23], several long Kocher claw forceps are used to identify the vaginal incision. Then the vagina is incised and dissected for 1 cm, which allows the anterior and posterior vaginal edges to be grouped together with three or four Chroback forceps. When necessary, the dissection of the vesicovaginal and rectovaginal spaces is completed up to the planes identified at laparoscopy. Similarly, the paravesical and pararectal spaces are identified. When a complete excision of the cardinal ligament has not been achieved laparoscopically, strong haemostatic forceps, such as angled Rodgers forceps, are used to grasp the lower part of the parametrium laterally and the uterosacral ligaments posteriorly. With increased experience in the laparoscopic

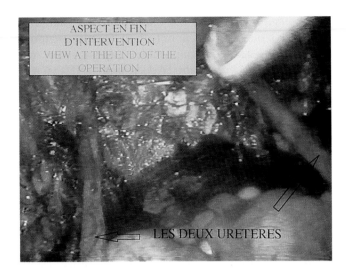

ASPECT EN FIN
D'INTERVENTION
VIEW AT THE END OF THE
OPERATION

LES DEUX URETERES

Fig. 9.4 Aspect of the ureters at the end of the operation.

approach, this vaginal step is shorter including the vaginal excision and suture. Frozen sections are needed to check the vaginal margins. Haemostasis is achieved with Vicryl no. 1, the vagina is closed with Vicryl no. 0.

The pneumoperitoneum is re-established, the haemostasis and ureteral peristalsism are checked (Fig. 9.4). A thorough peritoneal lavage is carried out. The pelvic peritoneum is left open.

Postoperative course

The bladder catheter, which we previously left in for 6 days, is now removed on the third day. Antibiotic therapy is initiated peroperatively and continued until the bladder catheter is removed. The patients are discharged 48 hours later, once satisfactory micturition has been achieved. An intravenous pyelogram is performed on the twelfth day.

Discussion

Our experience in laparoscopic radical hysterectomy seems promising. The operating time has become acceptable. No postoperative haemorrhage has been observed, confirming that bipolar coagulation is reliable in the treatment of large vessels [22]. The intraoperative complications have resolved with minimal sequelae and the postoperative complications are acceptable. The magnification provided by the laparoscope is an advantage as it minimizes trauma to the ureters and to the bladder. As meticulous haemostasis is required to avoid staining of the retroperitoneal tissue, the laparoscopic approach should be atraumatic and has even been described as a microsurgical approach [11]. Despite the longer operating time, most of the well-known advantages of laparoscopic

surgery, such as decreased stress and hospital stay, were confirmed in patients who underwent a laparoscopic radical hysterectomy, making the surgical treatment of cervical cancer more acceptable.

Others groups have reported their experience in the laparoscopic management of cervical cancer. A major step forward came from Dargent and Mathevet, who described a technique combining laparoscopic proximal haemostasis of the cardinal ligament and a Schauta operation. Knowledge of the Schauta operation is very useful when using a laparoscopic approach, because the dissection of the distal part of the ureter is the most difficult and the longest laparoscopic step. Several groups are using this technique. By contrast, we have developed a complete laparoscopic approach [24]. Spirtos *et al.* recently reported a similar technique [8]. A complete laparoscopic procedure is, in our opinion, less traumatic and allows for a more logical surgical technique, as it is not always easy to find the same planes and anatomical spaces using different surgical approaches to the pelvis. The longer operating time is the main disadvantage of the laparoscopic approach. Several years and prospective studies will be necessary to compare these two surgical techniques. Whatever the technique used, the vaginal approach is the best choice for incision of the vagina, as it allows visual control of the vaginal resection ensuring satisfactory tumour margins. By contrast, from our experience in laparoscopic hysterectomy, it is necessary to check the peritoneum by laparoscopy after the vaginal step. This allows for removal of the blood clots which are always found after the removal of the uterus, performance of a careful peritoneal lavage and checking the haemostasis using the magnification provided by the laparoscope. Meticulous haemostasis is a major advantage of laparoscopic surgery, it probably decreases the incidence of postoperative haematoma and postoperative *de novo* adhesion formation. Until now, we have never closed the peritoneum and have had no postoperative bowel occlusion. However, Dargent and Mathevet reported one case of bowel occlusion resulting from incarceration of a bowel loop in the pararectal fossa, and recommended careful closure of the peritoneum by a combined vaginal and laparoscopic approach. Our series include a case of vaginal vault evisceration, but this was caused by necrosis of the vagina not by the non-closure of the pelvic peritoneum.

Other instruments have been proposed for haemostasis of the cardinal ligament at the pelvic side wall. Dargent *et al.* and Spirtos *et al.* both used an Endostapler [8,9,14]. This instrument requires two lateral suprapubic trocars of 10 or 12 mm in diameter. However, from our experience of haemostasis of the adnexal vessels, this instrument is less reliable than bipolar coagulation, which is much slower.

Dargent reported postoperative bleeding in a patient whose vessels were treated with Endoclips [14], but we have used Endoclips to treat some vessels and found it to be safe. Before the application of an Endoclip, the vessel should be completely skeletonized, and this may be difficult. The thermal damage induced by the bipolar coagulation did not appear to be a major problem, and this technique is always our first choice. Endoclips are sometimes used to treat the proximal part of vessels, but they should not be used on the distal part, because they are generally removed by the grasping forceps during the following surgical steps.

Until now there has been no recurrence in our experience. However, the value of a new technique cannot be established from a limited number of selected cases with a short follow-up. Similar results have been reported by other groups [11–14], but much larger and longer series will be necessary to demonstrate that the laparoscopic technique is safe and can be proposed as a valuable alternative to the conventional approach by laparotomy. Also, the extent of the excision does not seem to be compromised by the laparoscopic approach, and is similar to that achieved previously by laparotomy. This result has been recently confirmed by Spirtos *et al.*, who routinely measured the parametrial width and the vaginal margin in 10 cases [8].

Laparoscopic radical hysterectomy is still at the investigational stage and should be reserved for gynaecological oncology surgeons trained in extensive laparoscopic procedures. These cautious conclusions are justified by the following arguments.

First, in our centre, many cases were performed by two senior surgeons with a large experience of laparoscopic surgery, in an environment where endoscopic surgery has been used extensively for many years [13]. Second, the surgical environment of laparoscopy and of laparotomy are different [25]. For instance, at laparoscopy the intra-abdominal pH is lower [26]. Following the report from Sahakian *et al.*, who demonstrated that peritoneal lavage with a buffered solution (Ringer's lactate) decreases postoperative adhesion formation after an endoscopic procedure performed with a pneumoperitoneum created with carbon dioxide [27], this difference seems important when considering postoperative healing. The intra-abdominal pressure minimizes small-vessel bleeding, but it may appear to be a disadvantage when considering intraoperative dissemination of malignant cells. This has been demonstrated by experimental and clinical studies about trocar-site metastasis [28–30]. One case occurred in a patient treated for a cervical cancer who had a laparoscopy before the treatment of the cancer. Interestingly this patient had a recurrence less than 6 months after the completion of the postoperative radio-therapy, suggesting that the tumour had unusual and very poor biological behaviour [30]. At laparoscopy intra-abdominal packing is impossible, implying that the trauma to the peritoneum is decreased, and that the protection of the upper abdomen is impossible. However, some data suggested that laparoscopy may also be beneficial for cancer patients. Allendorf *et al.* demonstrated in a murine model that intradermal tumours are more easily established and grow more aggressively after a laparotomy than after a laparoscopy [31]. In the same way, Mathew *et al.*, who reported in a rat model a significantly increased incidence of abdominal wall metastasis after laparoscopic manipulation of an intraperitoneal tumour, also noticed that the tumour growth was more important after a laparotomy than after a laparoscopy [29]. By contrast, Volz *et al.* clearly established in a nude mice model that tumour growth after intraperitoneal injection of cancer cells is significantly improved by a pneumoperitoneum [32]. Unfortunately there was no laparotomy control group in this study. When the results of clinical studies are so rare, and experimental data so conflicting, it seems logical to wait for more information before proposing a new technique as a gold standard.

From the technical point of view, the uterine cannulation appears to be the main disadvantage of the laparoscopic approach. The trauma to the tumour should be minimized: the instrument applied on the external cervical surface should be smooth, cervical dilatation should be avoided, uterine manipulations should be minimal and gentle. It has been noticed that many steps can be achieved without, or with only minimal, uterine retraction. As the vaginal excision is decided from below, palpation of the tumour is less common at laparoscopy than at laparotomy, so that surgical trauma to the tumour may not be much more important using this approach. During the preoperative evaluation we should decide, depending on the tumour anatomy, whether or not uterine cannulation and the laparoscopic approach are reasonable. Thereafter the technique will be adapted to these possibilities; anteflexion should be avoided when the posterior vaginal cul-de-sac is involved, so that the posterior steps are probably more safely achieved vaginally. Moreover, most patients who are operated on for a large tumour receive preoperative radiotherapy, so that the consequences of the uterine manipulation are minimized.

As stated before: '... any surgical procedure can be achieved endoscopically by experienced surgeons; therefore the main question is not to know whether or not the procedure is possible but if it is valuable and safe. These questions are to be answered using large prospective clinical trials, not wonderful pictures or beautiful videotapes' [33].

References

1 Reich H, De Caprio J, McGlynn F (1989). Laparoscopic hysterectomy. *J Gynecol Surg* **5**:213–216.
2 Querleu D, Leblanc E, Castelain B (1991). Laparoscopic lymphadenectomy in the staging of early carcinoma of the cervix. *Am J Obstet Gynecol* **164**:579–581.
3 Canis M, Mage G, Wattiez A, Pouly J-L, Manhes H, Bruhat M-A (1990). La chirurgie endoscopique a-t-elle une place dans la chirurgie radicale du cancer du col utérin? *J Gynecol Obstet Biol Reprod* **19**:921.
4 Querleu D (1991). Hystérectomies élargies de Schauta–Amreich et Schauta–Stoeckel assistées par coelioscopie. *J Gynecol Obstet Biol Reprod* **20**:747–748.
5 Nezhat CR, Burrell MO, Nezhat F, Benigno BB, Welander E (1992). Laparoscopic radical hysterectomy with paraaortic and pelvic node dissection. *Am J Obstet Gynecol* **166**:864–865.
6 Dargent D, Mathevet P (1992). Hystérectomie élargie laparoscopico-vaginale. *J Gynecol Obstet Biol Reprod* **21**:709–710.
7 Kadar N, Reich H (1993). Laparoscopically assisted radical Schauta hysterectomy and bilateral laparoscopic pelvic lymphadenectomy for the treatment of bulky stage IB carcinoma of the cervix. *Gynaecol Endosc* **2**:135–142.
8 Spirtos NM, Schlaerth JB, Kimball RE, Leiphart VM, Ballon SC (1996). Laparoscopic radical hysterectomy (type III) with aortic and pelvic lymphadenectomy. *Am J Obstet Gynecol* **174**:1763–1768.
9 Dargent D (1993). Laparoscopic surgery and gynecologic cancer. *Curr Opin Obstet Gynecol* **5**:294–300.
10 Piver MS, Rutledge F, Smith JP (1974). Five classes of extended hysterectomy for women with cervical cancer. *Obstet Gynecol* **44**:265–272.
11 Nezhat CR, Nezhat FR, Burrell MO *et al* (1993). Laparoscopic radical hysterectomy and laparoscopically assisted vaginal radical hysterectomy with pelvic and paraaortic node dissection. *J Gynecol Surg* **9**:105–120.
12 Querleu D (1993). Case report: laparoscopically assisted radical vaginal hysterectomy. *Gynecol Oncol* **51**:248–254.
13 Bruhat M-A, Mage G, Pouly J-L, Manhes H, Canis M, Wattiez A (1992). *Operative Laparoscopy*. New York: McGraw-Hill.
14 Dargent D, Mathevet P (1995) Schauta's vaginal hysterectomy combined with laparoscopic lymphadenectomy. *Baillieres Clin Obstet Gynaecol* **9**:691–705.
15 Wattiez A, Raymond F, Canis M *et al* (1993). Lymphadenectomie iliaque externe par coelioscopie. *Ann Chir* **47**:523–528.
16 Childers JM, Hatch KD, Tran AN, Surwit EA (1993). Laparoscopic para-aortic lymphadenectomy in gynecologic malignancies. *Obstet Gynecol* **82**:741–747.
17 Querleu D, Leblanc E (1994). Laparoscopic infrarenal paraaortic lymph node dissection for restaging of carcinoma of the ovary and of the tube. *Cancer* **73**:1467–1471.
18 Pomel C, Provencher D, Dauplat J *et al* (1995). Laparoscopic staging of early ovarian cancer. *Gynecol Oncol* **58**:301–306.
19 Frobert JL (1981). *L'hysterectomie élargie dans le traitement du cancer du col utérin*. MD thesis, University of Lyon.
20 Kobayashi T (1967). Presentation of the pelvic parasympathetic nerves in radical hysterectomy for cancer of the cervix. In: *Congress Edition of the 5th World Congress of Gynecology and Obstetrics, Scandinavia*, 32.
21 Sakamoto S (1986). Radical hysterectomy with pelvic lymphadenectomy. The Tokyo method. In: Coppleson M, ed. *Gynecologic Oncology*. Edinburgh: Churchill Livingstone, 877–886.
22 Masson F, Pouly J-L, Canis M *et al* (1996). Hysterectomie per-coelioscopique: une série continue de 318 cas. *J Gynecol Obstet Biol Reprod* **25**:340–352.
23 Schauta F (1908). *Die erweiterte Vaginale Totalexstirpation des Uterus beim Collumcarcinom*. Wien: J Safar.
24 Canis M, Mage G, Pomel C *et al* (1995). Laparoscopic radical hysterectomy for cervical cancer. *Baillieres Clin Obstet Gynaecol* **9**:675–689.
25 Canis M, Mage G, Wattiez A *et al* (1994). The role of laparoscopic surgery in gynecologic oncologic. *Curr Opin Obstet Gynecol* **6**:210–214.
26 Perry CP, Tombrello R (1993). Effect of fluid instillation on postlaparoscopy pain. *J Reprod Med* **38**:768–770.
27 Sahakian V, Rogers RG, Halme J, Hulka J (1993). Effect of carbon dioxide-saturated normal saline and ringer's lactate on post surgical adhesion formation in rabbits. *Obstet Gynecol* **82**:851–853.
28 Nduka CC, Monson JRT, Menzies-Gow N, Darzi A (1994). Abdominal wall metastases following laparoscopy. *Br J Surg* **81**:648–652.
29 Mathew G, Watson DI, Rofe AM, Baigrie CF, Ellis T, Jamieson GG (1996). Wound metastases following laparoscopic and open surgery for abdominal cancer in a rat model. *Br J Surg* **83**:1087–1090.
30 Pastner B, Damien M (1992). Umbilical metastases from a stage IB cervical cancer after laparoscopy: a case report. *Fertil Steril* **58**:1248–1249.
31 Allendorf JDF, Bessler M, Kayton MI *et al* (1995). Increased tumor establishment and growth after laparotomy vs laparoscopy in a murine model. *Arch Surg* **130**:649–653.
32 Volz J, Köster S, Weiss M *et al* (1996). Pathophysiology of a pneumoperitoneum in laparoscopy. A swine model. *Am J Obstet Gynecol* **174**:132–140.
33 Canis M, Mage G, Wattiez A, Pouly J-L, Manhes H, Bruhat M-A (1992). Vaginally assisted laparoscopic radical hysterectomy. *J Gynecol Surg* **8**:103–106.

10 Radical vaginal trachelectomy

Michel Roy and Marie Plante

Introduction

The concept of 'limited radical surgery' is now better accepted in all fields of oncology. In gynaecology, vulvar cancer is the best example of this new trend: hemivulvectomy and/or 'wide local excision' with unilateral inguinal lymphadenectomy are now considered acceptable for most stage I and II tumours [1]. Fertility-preserving surgery has been advocated in germ cell [2] and early epithelial ovarian cancers [3]. For microinvasive cervical cancer (International Federation of Gynecology and Obstetrics (FIGO) stage IA1), conization with negative margins is now widely used to preserve fertility [4]. This concept can be extended to stage IA2, IB (Fig. 10.1) and IIA cancers under certain conditions using Dargent's operation, the 'radical vaginal trachelectomy'. Dargent first performed this procedure in 1986 and published his results in 1994 [5]. At the same time the technique fulfills the needs for radicality, along with the possibility of preserving childbearing capacity.

The technique of this new operation will be described, its indications defined and the results available from three groups in France and Canada analysed below.

Technique

Radical vaginal trachelectomy is a modification of the Schauta–Stoeckel technique of vaginal radical hysterectomy [6]. The only difference is the preservation of the upper cervix and the uterine corpus. It is preceded by laparoscopic pelvic lymphadenectomy, which is described in Chapter 3. Laparoscopic para-aortic node biopsies are performed following the same indications as usual.

The initial steps of the radical trachelectomy are identical to the Schauta–Stoeckel procedure. In summary, the procedure is performed without a preliminary paravaginal (Schuchardt) incision. A good vaginal cuff is created by grasping circumferentially the vaginal mucosa with straight Kocher clamps, about 1 cm from the cervix. The vaginal mucosa is then incised above the clamps and used

to cover the cervix with four to six Chrobak forceps placed side by side. The dissection of the vesicouterine space is carried out in the midline using sharp and blunt dissection. The anterior peritoneum is kept intact. The paravesical and pararectal spaces are then opened. The cardinal ligaments are identified between the paravesical and the pararectal spaces at the same time as the bladder pillars, between the paravesical and the vesicouterine spaces. The ureter is located by palpation between two fingers and the bladder pillars are divided, so that the ureter is easily visualized, freed and pushed upwards.

From then on, the operation differs from the Schauta–Stoeckel procedure. The next step in the radical trachelectomy is to isolate the superior edge of the cardinal ligament: a clamp is pushed from behind through the parametrium close to the uterus, just below the cross of the uterine artery. The cardinal ligament is then clamped and divided at 1.5–2 cm from its insertion onto the cervix (Fig. 10.2).

After the division of the cardinal ligament, the cervicovaginal branch of the uterine artery is identified, dissected, cut and ligated (Fig. 10.3). Care must be taken not to ligate the uterine artery. The posterior cul-de-sac is opened and the inferior part of the uterosacral ligament is divided. The cervix is excised just below the isthmus (Fig. 10.4), attempting to leave about 8–10 mm of cervical tissue in place. A frozen section for pathological assessment of the endocervical margin of the specimen is obtained, during which time a cervical dilator is placed into the cervical canal to slowly distend it.

According to the results of the frozen section, one of three situations can occur:

1 If the endocervical margin is positive for tumour, a safe radical trachelectomy is not possible and the operation should be converted into a vaginal radical hysterectomy.

2 If tumour is found within 3–8 mm of the endocervical margin, more cervical tissue should be removed if possible.

3 If the tumour is at least 8–10 mm from the endocervical margin, the resection is satisfactory.

The peritoneum of the posterior cul-de-sac is closed

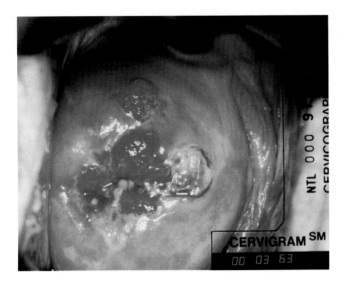

Fig. 10.1 Typical small exocervical cancer before surgery.

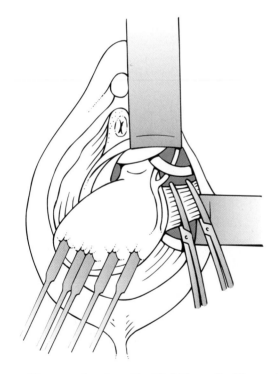

Fig. 10.2 The ureters have been identified. The cardinal ligaments are clamped below the level of the uterine arteries. (Courtesy of Hélène Roy MD.)

with a purse-string suture. A prophylactic cerclage is placed using a non-absorbable suture, at the level of the internal os (Fig. 10.5). Finally, after having removed the cervical dilator, closure is performed by suturing the vaginal mucosa to the stroma of the residual cervix with interrupted sutures, taking care not to invert the vaginal

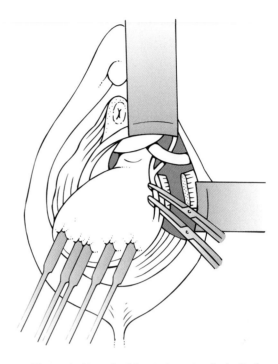

Fig. 10.3 The cervical branch of the uterine artery is electively controlled. (Courtesy of Hélène Roy MD.)

mucosa into the endocervical canal (Fig. 10.6). Drains are left in the lateral fornices when indicated.

The abdomen is reinsufflated and laparoscopic evaluation of the retroperitoneum is done to verify haemostasis.

Postoperative follow-up

The patient should be evaluated 4 weeks after surgery to look for vaginal adhesion formation, cervical granulation tissue that can cause contact bleeding and cervical stenosis. Cervical dilatation can be carried out if indicated. Further follow-up consists of a colposcopic evaluation of the new transformation zone, cytology and pelvic examination every 3–4 months for 2 years and 6 months thereafter. Endocervical curettage may have to be performed for the following indications: unsatisfactory colposcopic examination, abnormal cytology and contact bleeding.

Complete healing usually occurs about 3–4 months after the procedure. The transformation zone is then evaluable by colposcopy (Fig. 10.7).

Indications

Radical vaginal trachelectomy is usually offered to women who wish to retain their childbearing capacity. The selection criteria for this procedure include:
1 Desire to preserve fertility.
2 No clinical evidence of impaired fertility.

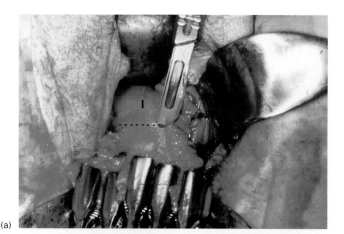

(a)

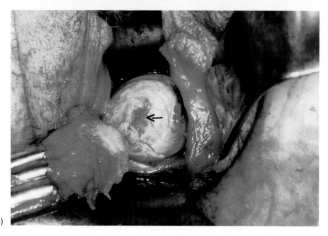

(b)

Fig. 10.4 (a) The cervix is removed immediately below the isthmus, leaving a 10-mm upper cervix. I, level of the internal os; dashed line, level of the section of the cervix. (b) Portion of the cervix being removed. Arrow, cervical canal.

3 FIGO stage IA2–IB and exophytic IIA.
4 Lesion size ≤2.5 cm.
5 Limited endocervical involvement at colposcopic and/or MRI evaluation, confirmed intraoperatively by frozen section.
6 No evidence of pelvic lymph-node metastasis, confirmed by laparoscopic lymphadenectomy.

However, patients with endophytic lesions, lesions measuring more than 3 cm and those showing widespread capillary-like space invasion on biopsy and/or conization should probably not be offered the procedure.

Results

Three groups have reported data on the radical vaginal trachelectomy procedure so far: Dargent and Mathevet in Lyon, France reported 47 cases (D. Dargent & P. Mathevet, personal communication), Roy and Plante in Québec City, Canada [7] 30 cases and Covens in Toronto, Canada [8] 25

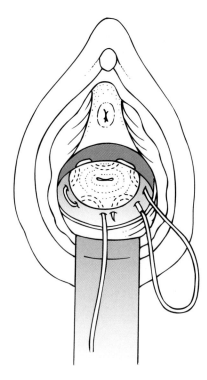

Fig. 10.5 A permanent cerclage is placed around the isthmus. (Courtesy of Hélène Roy MD.)

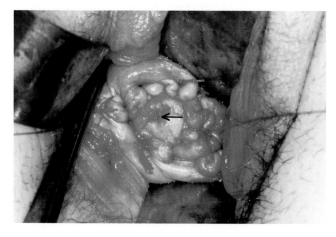

Fig. 10.6 The vagina is sutured to the upper endocervix. Arrow, cervical canal.

cases. The majority of patients had cervical lesions measuring between 3 mm and 2 cm and were FIGO stage IB. Adenocarcinoma accounted for over 25% of the cases in the series (Table 10.1).

Table 10.2 shows that the operating time is comparable to abdominal or vaginal radical hysterectomy performed with laparoscopic lymphadenectomy, but the blood loss is less [9]. The time spent in hospital is the same. The intra-

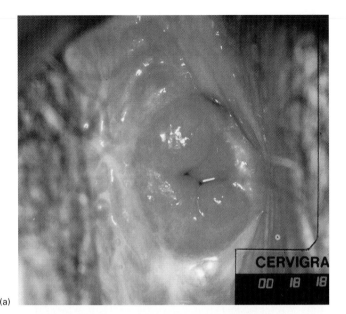

(a)

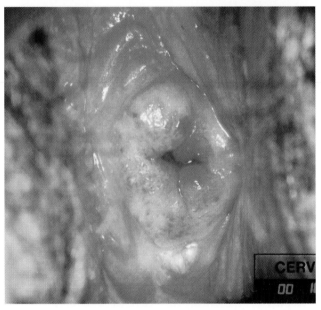

(b)

Fig. 10.7 Postoperative status. The glandular tissue and a new squamocolumnar junction is available for colposcopic follow-up: (a) before and (b) after acetic acid application. Note the new transformation zone.

Table 10.1 Patients' characteristics.

	Study		
	Dargent*	Roy [7]	Covens [8]
Age (years)		32 (22–42)	31 (25–38)
Histology			
Adenocarcinoma	8†	12†	9
Squamous cell carcinoma	39	18	16
Tumour size (mm)		3–30	3–20
Capillary-like space involvement		4	13
FIGO stage			
IA1	4	1	
IA2	14	7	
IB	27	20	25‡
IIA	2	2	
Total patients	47	30	25

* Personal communication.
† Including two patients with neuroendocrine tumour.
‡ Stage IB or less.

Table 10.2 Operative results.

	Study		
	Dargent*	Roy [7]	Covens [8]
Operative time	2 h†	4 h 45 min	3 h
Blood loss (ml)	250	200	500
Complications	6‡	4‡	5‡

* Personal communication.
† Not all patients had lymphadenectomies at the same time.
‡ A total of six patients required laparotomy.

and postoperative complications listed in Table 10.2 consisted of one immediate laparotomy for intractable bleeding, one laparotomy and one colpotomy for postoperative pelvic haematomata and six cystotomies. Three vascular injuries requiring laparotomy occurred during the laparoscopic lymphadenectomy. In all cases, the planned trachelectomy was performed. Cervical stenosis was noted in the follow-up of three patients, one of these cases required multiple cervical dilatations. The long-term complication rate is unevaluable, because the follow-up for most patients is too short.

The follow-up times range from 6 months to 12 years. So far, recurrences have been documented in four of the 100 patients (4%; excluding the two patients with neuroendocrine tumours diagnosed on the final pathology report). Dargent reported two recurrences; one patient developed para-aortic lymph-node metastasis and died with pulmonary metastasis despite radio-chemotherapy. She had an adenocarcinoma of the cervix with capillary-like space involvement on the specimen but negative pelvic nodes. The second patient developed pelvic lymph-node metastasis 7 years after her trachelectomy. She also had capillary-like space involvement on the specimen. One of Coven's patients recurred in the parametrium 13 months postsurgery. She had a 4.1-mm deep adenocarcinoma with vascular-like space involvement on the trachelectomy specimen. In the Quebec series, one patient presented a recurrence in the parametrium 16 months after surgery, progressed while receiving radiation therapy and died of metastatic disease.

Recurrence rates suggest that the radical trachelectomy as described by Dargent seems to be radical enough for the treatment of selected patients with invasive cancer of the cervix. The finding of proximal parametrial node invasion in two patients by Dargent and the recurrences in the parametrium in the other cases indicate that a significant parametrial length has to be removed along with the specimen. The fact that three recurrences occurred among patients with capillary-like space involvement indicates this should be seriously considered to be a contraindication for trachelectomy. The extent of capillary-like space involvement must be carefully evaluated and the risk associated with it clearly explained to the patients.

Reproductive outcome

Table 10.3 shows the reproductive outcome of patients in the three series cited above. Among a total of 102 patients, 40 patients have attempted pregnancy: 24 succeeded and had a total of 18 live births; three patients are currently expecting their first baby. Six abortions occurred (one abortion was induced because of a Down's syndrome). The infertility and abortion rates though do not seem to be higher than the normal population.

When a patient becomes pregnant, routine obstetric care is followed until 20 weeks, from then antenatal visits should be made every 2 weeks instead of 4 weekly. Weekly visits after 28 weeks are important in order to check for cervical incompetence. In the first 13 patients of Dargent's

series where prophylactic cerclage was not carried out routinely, two late abortions and two early labours occurred. Since the routine addition of a permanent suture to avoid cervical incompetence, the rate of prematurity is lower. However, the efficacy of the prophylactic cerclage has not been fully studied. Caesarean section is indicated for delivery.

Conclusion

Radical trachelectomy appears to be a safe procedure for selected cases of early cervical cancer: fertility seems to be preserved in most patients. However, patients must be carefully selected. Because of the limited follow-up in most cases, the criteria for indications and contraindications are not yet well defined. At the present time, we should be conservative and offer the procedure to patients with lesions measuring more than 2.5 cm in size, lesions with endocervical extension or with widespread capillary-like space involvement in exceptional cases. Further studies should help to define those parameters in the future.

References

1 Di Saia P (1985). Management of superficially invasive vulvar carcinoma. *Clin Obstet Gynecol* **28**:196–203.
2 Williams SD, Gershenson DM, Horowitz CJ, Scully RE (1992). Ovarian germ cell and stromal tumors. In: Hoskins WJ, Perez CA, Young RC, eds. *Principles and Practice of Gynecologic Oncology.* Philadelphia: JB Lippincott, 715–730.
3 Guthrie D, Davy NILJ, Phillips PR (1989). Study of 656 patients with 'early' ovarian cancer. *Gynecol Oncol* **17**:363.
4 Jones WB, Mercer GO, Lewis JL Jr, Rubins SC, Hoskins WJ (1993). Early invasive carcinoma of the cervix. *Gynecol Oncol* **51**:26.
5 Dargent D, Brun JC, Roy M, Mathevet P, Reny I (1994). La Trachélectomie élargie (T.E.), une alternative à l'hystérectomie radicale dans le traitement des cancers infiltrants développés sur la face externe du col utérin. *J Obstet Gynecol* **2**:285–292.
6 Stoeckel W (1928). Die Vaginale Radical Operation des collum Karzinoms. *Zentralbl Gynakol* **52**:39–63.
7 Roy M, Plante M (1998). Pregnancies following vaginal radical trachelectomy for early-stage cervical cancer. *Am J Obstet Gynecol* **179**(6):1491–1496.
8 Covens A (1998). Prospective study of fertility-preserving surgery for invasive cancer of the cervix. Presented at the meeting of the Society of Obstetricians and Gynecologists of Canada (SOGC), Victoria BC.
9 Roy M, Plante M (1996). Vaginal radical hysterectomy (VRH) versus abdominal radical hysterectomy (ARH) in the treatment of early stage cervical cancer. *Gynecol Oncol* **62**:336–339.

Table 10.3 Obstetric results.

	Study			
	Dargent*	Roy [7]	Covens [8]	Total
Patients attempting pregnancy	22	6	10	38
Patients becoming pregnant	13	6	5	24
Live births	10	5	3	18
Spontaneous abortions	3	1	2	6
Total patients	47	30	25	102

* Personal communication.

11   Laparoscopic ovarian transposition

Eric Leblanc and Denis Querleu

Introduction

Gynaecological malignancies are often managed by radiotherapy alone or combined with surgery. The ovaries are very sensitive to radiation. A dose of less than 3 Gy usually causes little harm, but a dose over 6 Gy regularly leads to ovarian failure. Between these two limits, the ability of the ovaries to restore a normal function is mainly related to the woman's age.

The adverse effects of castration are well known. Hormonal privation is associated with a higher incidence of osteoporosis and cerebrovascular or cardiovascular accidents. Moreover, vasomotor dysfunction, urogenital and sexual disturbances, may affect the quality of life.

Therefore, unless contraindicated, particularly in young women, both ovaries should be transposed out of the future irradiation field in order to preserve the hormonal function and, if possible, fertility. Nevertheless, several questions must be answered to ensure the safety and the effectiveness of the procedure. The risk of transposing a metastatic ovary, the occurrence of benign pathology or recurrent malignancy on the retained ovary and the assessment of hormonal function will be discussed below.

History

McCall *et al.* demonstrated in 1957 that *in situ* preservation of ovarian tissue at the time of surgery for cervical malignancy is technically feasible and can preserve the hormonal function of the ovaries [1].

Technically, numerous surgical methods of varying interest have been described. Cyclic ovarian fluid secretion precludes subcutaneous [2] or extraperitoneal placements [3]. Other studies have advocated intraperitoneal ovarian positioning upon or laterally to the psoas muscle [1], in the paracolic gutters [4] or behind the uterine isthmus in cases undergoing pelvic lymph-node irradiation [5].

Larue-Charlus *et al.* published the first use of laparoscopy for ovarian transposition in cervical cancer treatment [6]. The operation consisted of a temporary suspension of the adnexa to the anterior abdominal wall, leaving a significant amount of irradiation to the ovaries.

Technique

Two methods of laparoscopic transposition are described below, which mimic the standard laparotomy procedures: the laterocolic and median retrouterine transpositions. The indications for both techniques depend on the method of irradiation to be employed.

Laterocolic ovarian transposition

Usually laterocolic ovarian transposition is performed during a laparoscopic lymphadenectomy. As an elective procedure, it can be carried out as a day case. The patient is placed in the Trendelenburg position. After completion of the pneumoperitoneum, the trocars are displayed. Four ports are necessary: two 10-mm ports for the umbilical optical device and the median suprapubic clip-applier and two operative lateropelvic 5-mm ports.

The operation begins with a thorough exploration of the abdominal and pelvic cavities. The adnexae are thoroughly inspected. Any suspicious aspect on their surface must be biopsied and submitted for frozen-section examination.

In cases undergoing conservative surgery, the fallopian tube is severed from the ovary with preservation of its vasculature. Otherwise a complete adnexal transposition will be performed. The adnexa is grasped and both leaves of the broad ligament are incised below the ovary, in the avascular area. The fallopian tube and the utero-ovarian pedicle are then divided without any risk to the uterine vessels or the underlying ureter. Haemostasis is provided either by clips, suture, bipolar cautery or stapling devices. Clips are not safe enough and we do not use them any more. Suturing is effective but time consuming. Stapling devices are quick, safe but expensive. We use them only when the utero-ovarian pedicle is thick. Bipolar coagulation is our method of choice because it is simple, cheap and effective.

The next step in the procedure is the pediculization of the ovary or adnexa on its infundibulopelvic vessels. The initial peritoneal incision of the broad ligament is extended upwards with scissors, just beneath the ovary and the infundibulopelvic ligament. Special attention must be paid to the ureter, particularly when it crosses the external iliac vessels.

The dissection of the infundibulopelvic pedicle is carried out as high as possible under the caecum or the sigmoid colon. The ovary or adnexa is then anchored with a transparietal suture, high in the laterocolic gutter, above the level of the anterior iliac spine. Its vessels must not be twisted.

A tunnel can also be created under the peritoneum of the laterocolic gutter, through which the ovary will be introduced and brought out into the abdominal cavity a few centimetres higher. This manoeuvre will retain the ovary intraperitoneally and its vessels extraperitoneally and prevent the risk of bowel strangulation around the ovarian vessels as suggested by Belinson *et al.* [7]. We favour this technique (Fig. 11.1).

Finally, clips are applied to the utero-ovarian ligament stump for later radiological localization in order to obtain a precise dosimetry (Figs 11.2 & 11.3). The peritoneum is left open. The procedure is usually performed on each side.

Medial ovarian transposition

In cases of lateropelvic irradiation for Hodgkin's disease or lymphoma, some authors advocate laparoscopically moving the ovaries from the pelvic node area to the posterior part of the uterus [8]. They can be protected during the irradiation with a median lead shield. Without any dissection, the ovaries are approximated on the midline by a suture that ties both utero-ovarian ligaments and the posterior serosal surface of the isthmus. Again, they are marked with clips.

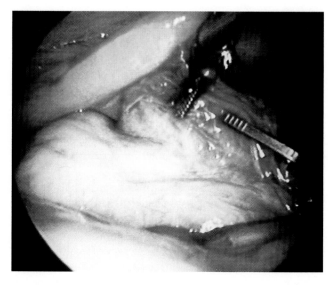

Fig. 11.2 A laparoscopic view of the transposed ovary. Clips are placed for radiological identification.

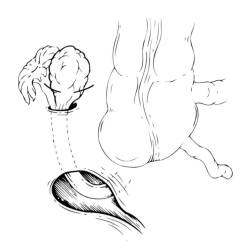

Fig. 11.1 The right adnexa is transposed as high and lateral as possible. The ovarian pedicle is passed in a peritoneal tunnel. (Redrawn from Querleu [39] with permission.)

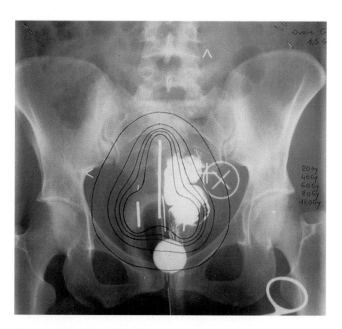

Fig. 11.3 Film showing the location of the transposed ovaries (top right and top left), receiving 1.5 and 1.4 Gy, respectively. The 120, 80, 60, 40 and 20 Gy isodoses are drawn.

Materials

From March 1989 to March 1996, our centre performed 36 laparoscopic ovarian transpositions: one for perineal sarcoma in an 11-year-old girl, two for Hodgkin's disease and 33 for cervical carcinoma. In these cases laterocolic ovarian transposition was performed only in patients under 40, with early-stage epidermoid carcinoma (stage 1A to 2B). A laparoscopic pelvic lymphadenectomy was carried out before treatment. If there was no lymph-node involvement, the management combined brachytherapy on the tumour and radical surgery 6 weeks later. Otherwise, cervical cancer was treated by irradiation alone. Laterocolic ovarian transposition was achieved during this operation if frozen section of the lymph node was negative.

There was no morbidity related to the operation. The operating time averaged 10–15 minutes per side. Three symptomatic functional cysts occurred 15 and 10 months after the procedure. Two of them were treated by ultrasound-guided needle aspiration; the last spontaneously disappeared. The maximal dose of irradiation received by the ovaries was <300 cGy (mean 220) in all cases for a total dose of 6000 cGy to the cervical tumour.

There were no clinical or biological signs of castration (FSH-LH and oestradiol levels) in 26 out of 36 patients (72%) after more than 6 months of follow-up.

Complications

Intraoperative complications

BLEEDING

Bleeding is the most frequent complication. It can come from the utero-ovarian vessels, the ovary itself, the peritoneum or the ovarian vessels. It is usually managed by bipolar coagulation. In some cases, the ovary or adnexa may have to be removed to control bleeding.

TORSION OF THE VASCULAR PEDICLE

This problem results in an infarction of the ovary that can lead to oophorectomy [9] or to loss of the ovary.

URETERAL INJURY

Ureteral injury is another potential complication. It can occur during section of the utero-ovarian pedicle (especially when using staplers) or incision of the broad ligament. It is therefore very important to locate it before any dissection and to keep it in sight during incision of the broad ligament.

Postoperative complications

FUNCTIONAL OVARIAN CYSTS

The incidence of symptomatic ovarian cyst in retained ovaries is low. The estimated rate is 1.8–5.2% [10] in cases of standard hysterectomy and 4.9% [11] to 7.6% [12] after radical hysterectomy. The diagnosis can be true ovarian cysts or peritoneal inclusion cysts.

The effect of transposition on the incidence of benign cysts has been established retrospectively by Chambers *et al.* [13]; in the absence of radiotherapy, laterocolic ovarian transposition leads to 24% of symptomatic cysts requiring reoperation vs 7% if there is preservation without transposition. Postoperative irradiation does not significantly alter these results [14].

Clinically, large symptomatic cysts are detectable by abdominal rather than pelvic examination. Ultrasound or CT scan are of help but, in this context, their interpretation is sometimes difficult. If the aspect is compatible with a functional cyst, expectant management or ultrasound-guided fine-needle aspiration are the mainstay of management. Surgery or laparoscopy may be indicated if there is a suspicious ultrasound pattern of diagnostic doubt (e.g. appendicitis), or an increase, recurrence or persistence of the abnormalities after a few weeks.

There is no prophylaxis for such cysts. Preventive suppressive hormonal treatment has no effect and, anyway, is illogical because the aim of ovarian transposition is to avoid taking drugs.

OVARIAN CARCINOMA

Radiation-induced ovarian tumours

There is no cause for concern because the dose is very low. A study reported by Darby *et al.* evaluated the risk of ovarian cancer in patients treated, some decades earlier, by low-dose radiation therapy for metropathia haemorrhagica [15].

Primary ovarian cancer

Simultaneous primary ovarian and cervical carcinoma is an extremely rare circumstance that is observed in women with Peutz–Jeghers syndrome [16]. Following hysterectomy, the overall incidence of ovarian cancer has been estimated to be 0.2% [17].

Ovarian metastases

Metastases are very infrequent in cases of early cervical carcinoma. A Gynecologic Oncology Group (GOG) study of 770 stage I patients reported an overall incidence of 0.6% [18]. This rate is higher in advanced stage carcinomata (18.7%) [18].

The histological type may play a role. Ovarian metastases are quite exceptional in epidermoid carcinoma. In 1981, Baltzer reported four cases of metastasis in a series of 749 epidermoid cervical cancers (0.5%). In three out of four, there was an infiltration of the uterine corpus [19]. In a series of 278 patients with stage 1–3 epidermoid carcinoma, Tabata did not find any ovarian metastases, although 21.6% of patients presented with lymph-node metastases [20].

The incidence of metastasis seems to be slightly higher in stage I adenocarcinoma: 2/150 (1.3%) in Kjorstad's study [21], 2/121 (1.7%) in a Gynecologic Oncology Group report and 2/26 (7.7%) of Tabata's cases. In all reports, infiltration of the uterine corpus was significantly associated with the presence of ovarian metastasis. The correlation with lymph-node involvement is more controversial: it has been noted in both of Tabata's patients, in three out of five patients in Brown's review of the literature [22], but in no cases reported by Kjorstad *et al.* [21] and Sutton *et al.* [18].

Subsequent recurrence on transposed ovaries

Michel *et al.* reported the first case of epidermoid ovarian metastasis occurring on a transposed ovary [23]. The patient had been treated by a radiosurgical combination for an early-stage node-negative epidermoid tumour invading the uterine isthmus. The cystic ovarian epidermoid recurrence occurred 3 years later without any other localization.

Parham *et al.* recently reported a case of metastasis occurring 6 months after radiosurgical treatment of a bulky adenocarcinoma of the uterine cervix with involvement of the endocervix [24]. A cystic recurrence occurred 6 months after the initial treatment and the patient died 1 year later.

Ultrasound or CT scan monitoring of transposed ovaries is required at least yearly to check for cyst development and/or sometimes occult cancerization.

OVARIAN FAILURE

This is the most worrying issue of this procedure. It is suspected by the loss of menses in non-hysterectomized patients, the presence of specific symptoms such as hot flushes, a decrease in the oestrogen status of the vaginal epithelium and a modification of hormonal serum levels—an increase in the gonadotropins FSH and LH and a drop in ovarian hormone levels. As the spontaneous incidence of ovarian failure is as low as 1% [25], almost all losses of ovarian function may be attributed to the ovarian transposition.

There are different explanations for the failure, and these are described below.

Weakness of ovarian blood supply

After ovarian preservation, 85% of patients following simple hysterectomy and 80% following radical hysterectomy retain hormonal function [26] until the expected time of menopause. From an anatomical point of view, it is known that in older patients, ovarian vascularization is mainly provided by the uterine artery, particularly after 45 years [27]; therefore, the division of the utero-ovarian vessels could result in a loss of blood supply in some patients. Chambers states that laterocolic transposition does not increase the incidence of early menopause compared with preservation without transposition [13].

Chemotherapy can alter ovarian function

Platinum-based chemotherapies are less toxic than other regimens, such as MOPP (methchlormethamine-vincristine-procarbazine-prednisone), for Hodgkin's disease [28].

Failure to protect against radiation

The results are very different according to the institutions. In cervical cancer patients treated by radical surgery plus laterocolic ovarian transposition and subsequent external beam pelvic irradiation, Husseinzadeh reported, in 1984, a preserved hormonal function rate of 83% in a series of 14 patients [9]. In 1991, Chambers *et al.* reported a 71% success rate in another series of 14 patients with a median follow-up of 35 months [14]. Bidzinski *et al.* observed a 100% success rate in a series of 24 transposed women with cervical cancer treated by radical surgery with postoperative brachytherapy and an 80% success rate in 15 patients treated by adjunctive postoperative teletherapy [29]. Comparing retrospectively two series of patients with cervical cancer treated by surgery and laterocolic ovarian transposition, Feeney *et al.* [17] stated that postoperative radiotherapy reduces the effectiveness of the procedure: 3/104 (2.9%) without postoperative radiotherapy experienced menopausal symptoms vs 14/28 (50%) in the group with postoperative irradiation at 24 months and 83% at 60 months. Anderson *et al.* reported the worst results with an 83% failure in a series of 24 patients, and therefore concluded that ovarian transposition was not useful in patients likely to need radiation therapy [26].

Age and radiation dose are the most important prognostic factors of ovarian castration after radiotherapy treatment. The two factors cannot be considered separately. As suggested by Lushbaugh and Casarett [30] in women over 40, the total dose that induces menopause was 600 cGy, while it could reach 2000 cGy fractioned in impubescent girls. When considering the lower limit of tolerance, Chambers *et al*. [14] and Husseinzadeh *et al*. [9], demonstrated that under 300 cGy, the likelihood of maintaining ovarian function will be approximately 90%. A steep dose–response effect on the induction of menopause was observed for irradiation over 300 cGy.

Other factors that may affect the dose delivered to the ovaries

1 The technique of irradiation therapy. When brachytherapy alone is used after transposition, ovarian failure occurs in 24%; if external irradiation is added this rate rises to 37% [26].
2 The geometry of the irradiation fields (AP/PA or four-field box). A four-field box is more toxic than a two-field AP/PA technique. The addition of a para-aortic irradiation field in spite of shields increases the dose to the ovaries, and Husseinzadeh feels this should result in this procedure being abandoned [31].
3 The distance between the ovary and the source. The radiation effects decrease exponentially as soon as the ovary is moved away from the source. The higher and more lateral the dissection, the more effective the protection [28], but possibly with an increased risk of cyst [14].
4 The use of ovarian shields during irradiation. In the study reported by Haie-Meder *et al*., the measured dose to the transposed ovaries was 10.5% of the delivered dose when ovaries were located under shielding blocks, and 4.4% if ovaries were outside the irradiation field [32].

Finally, it is probably the combination of these different factors, at different degrees, that results in the variable failure rates of the procedure. To prevent ovarian failure, our policy is not to transpose beyond the age of 40. To increase the chances of success, bilateral transposition appears to be more effective than unilateral transposition. Adnexa have to be widely mobilized on their pedicle to allow the most high and lateral fixation, especially in cases of lymph-node irradiation. In hysterectomized patients, hormonal monitoring by serum FSH and oestradiol sampling once a year, or if the patient is symptomatic, is advised. This exploration can be coupled with morphological monitoring. In cases of hormonal menopause, the patient will be prescribed a hormone replacement therapy.

Indications

Laparoscopic ovarian transposition can be relevant in young women every time pelvic radiation therapy is indicated alone or associated with surgery.

Carcinoma of the uterine cervix

This was the first indication for the procedure, since it has been demonstrated that preservation of ovarian function does not adversely alter the course of cervical cancer [1,12]. However, if there is a risk of ovarian metastasis, transposition should be avoided in the following stuations.
1 In any suspicious ovarian lesion (biopsy with a frozen section may help to rule out malignancy).
2 In advanced stage or bulky early cervical carcinoma, involving the endocervix or the uterine isthmus, and (for some authors) when lymph nodes are positive.
3 In non-bulky adenocarcinoma, in which transposition is acceptable only in very young women [33].

When preoperative brachytherapy is indicated, laterocolic ovarian transposition is performed during laparoscopic lymphadenectomy. The early division of uteroadnexal pedicles and the temporary storage of the adnexa in the paracolic gutter will help the posterior dissection of the interiliac area.

If two applications of brachytherapy are scheduled, the adnexae are dissected and fixed in the paracolic gutter, positioning their pedicle extraperitoneally as previously described. At the time of the radical surgery the adnexae are left in the high paracolic situation. If only one immediate application is planned, it is simpler to anchor the ovary in the paracolic gutter with a transparietal suture that will be cut at the end of the radiation treatment in order to let the ovaries fall back in the Douglas cul-de-sac.

When considering the geometry of the radiation fields, ovaries must be as high laterally and anteriorly as possible. When external beam irradiation is associated, block shields are indicated.

Vaginal carcinoma

There are very few indications for laterocolic ovarian transposition in vaginal epidermoid carcinoma, primarily because patients are usually beyond 50 years old. Clear cell vaginal adenocarcinomata in patients exposed in their intrauterine life to diethylstilboestrol have a very different epidemiology and management. They occur in very young women (median age 19 years). They are not hormone dependent and are often detected at an early stage. They can be effectively managed conservatively [34]: wide local excision followed by local irradiation or even brachytherapy alone. In this situation, the ovaries alone are transposed at the time of pelvic lymphadenectomy to preserve not only hormonal function but also fertility [35].

Pelvic and gynaecological non-uterine sarcoma

Laterocolic ovarian transposition can be indicated in some rare tumours, such as vaginal, perineal or other soft-tissue pelvic sarcoma, that afflict predominantly children and are often treated by a combination of chemotherapy, irradiation and more limited surgery.

Ovarian dysgerminoma

According to the patient's age, childbearing status and intraoperative staging, the treatment can consist of unilateral oophorectomy with radiation therapy of pelvic and para-aortic areas. Contralateral ovarian transposition (if not dysgenetic) will preserve hormonal function and fertility [35]. However, chemotherapy is becoming the treatment of choice in advanced dysgerminoma in younger patients.

Pelvic Hodgkin's disease or other lymphoma

Although they are not gynaecological tumours, they are treated by a combination of chemotherapy and lymphnode irradiation, including the pelvic channels. The technique of medial transposition, advocated by some authors [8], is easier to perform than the laterocolic transposition, but it seems to be less effective [36]. Therefore, even in these indications, we recommed laterocolic ovarian transposition.

As a conclusion to this section, it is important to underline another advantage of this technique, which not only spares young women the effects of an early menopause, but also, in some cases, allows childbearing. In the series reported by Haie-Meder *et al.*, the incidence of birth was 19%, with no childhood abnormalities. Although some authors insist there is a risk of fetal abnormality from radiochemotherapy treatment [37], the outcome in children born from cancer patients is generally considered to be standard. Other workers have pointed out an increased risk of low birth weight or prematurity as a result of the irradiation effect on the uterine muscle [38].

Conclusion

The risk of developing an ovarian metastasis or a primary neoplasm in a transposed ovary is real, especially in cases with a large tumour volume, but rare. On the other hand, hormone replacement therapies are becoming better tolerated and easy to use, but they are relatively expensive. Long-term patient compliance may be a problem and, at the present time, the late adverse effects are not known.

Finally, the success rate of 60–80%, with few adverse effects from laterocolic ovarian transposition, means that young women under 40 with non-hormone-dependent pelvic tumours can be offered this option. This ovarian protection spares them an early menopause, well before their physiological menopause, and preserves their fertility potential.

References

1 McCall M, Keaty EC, Thompson JD (1958). Conservation of ovarian tissue in treatment of carcinoma. *Am J Obstet Gynecol* **75**:590–605.

2 Kovacev KE (1968). Exteriorization of the ovaries under the skin of young women operated upon for cancer of the cervix. *Am J Obstet Gynecol* **101**:756–759.

3 Bieler EU, Schnabel T, Knobel J (1976). Persisting cyclic ovarian activity in cervical cancer after surgical transposition of the ovaries and pelvic irradiation. *Br J Radiol* **49**:875–879.

4 Hodel K, Rich WM, Austin P, DiSaia PJ (1982). The role of ovarian transposition in conservation of ovarian function in radical hysterectomy followed by pelvic irradiation. *Gynecol Oncol* **13**:195–202.

5 Trueblood HW, Enright LP, Ray GR (1970). Preservation of ovarian function in pelvic radiation for Hodgkin's disease. *Arch Surg* **100**:236–237.

6 Larue-Charlus S, Pigneux J, Audebert A, Papras Y, Emperaire JC (1987). Transposition ovarienne temporaire au cours des curiethérapies utéro-vaginales. Description d'une technique originale. *Contracept Fertil Sex* **15**:595–596.

7 Belinson JL, Doherty M, McDay JB (1984). A new technique for ovarian transposition. *Surg Gynecol Obstet* **159**:157–160.

8 Willams RS, Mendenhall N (1992). Laparoscopic oophoropexy for preservation of ovarian function before pelvic node irradiation. *Obstet Gynecol* **80**:541–543.

9 Husseinzadeh N, Nahnas WA, Velkley DE, Whitney CW, Mortel R (1984). The preservation of ovarian function in young women undergoing pelvic radiation therapy. *Gynecol Oncol* **18**:373–379.

10 Bukovsky I, Liftshitz Y, Langer R, Weintraub Z, Sadovsky G, Caspi E (1988). Ovarian residual syndrome. *Surg Gynecol Obstet* **167**:132–134.

11 Ellsworth LR, Allen HH, Nisker JA (1983). Ovarian function after radical hysterectomy and pelvic node dissection. *Gynecol Oncol* **145**:185–188.

12 Webb GA (1979). The role of ovarian conservation in the treatment of carcinoma of the cervix with radical surgery. *Am J Obstet Gynecol* **122**:476–484.

13 Chambers SK, Chambers JT, Holm C, Peschel RE, Schwarz PE (1990). Sequelae of lateral ovarian transposition in unirradiated cervical cancer. *Gynecol Oncol* **39**:155–159.

14 Chambers SK, Chambers JT, Kier PDR, Peschel RE (1991). Sequelae of lateral ovarian transposition in irradiated cervical cancer patients. *Int J Radiat Oncol* **20**:1305–1308.

15 Darby SC, Reeves G, Key T, Doll R, Stovall M (1994). Mortality in a cohort of women given X-ray therapy for metropathia haemorrhagica. *Int J Cancer* **56**:793–801.

16 Eisner RF, Neiberg RK, Berek JS (1989). Synchronous primary neoplasms of the female reproductive tract. *Gynecol Oncol* **33**:335–339.

17 Feeney DD, Moore DH, Look KY, Stehman FB, Sutton GP (1995).

The fate of the ovaries after radical hysterectomy and ovarian transposition. *Gynecol Oncol* **56**:3–7.

18 Sutton GP, Bundy BN, Delgado G *et al* (1992). Ovarian metastases in stage 1b carcinoma of the cervix. *Am J Obstet Gynecol* **166**:50–53.

19 Baltzer J, Lohe KJ, Hopke W, Zander J (1981). Metastatischer Befall der Ovarien beim Operierten Plattenepithel Karzinom der Cervix. *Geburtshilfe Frauenheilkd* **173**:857–860.

20 Tabata M, Ichinoe K, Sakuragi N, Shina Y, Yamaguchi T, Mabuchi Y (1987). Incidence of ovarian metastasis in patients with cancer of the uterine cervix. *Gynecol Oncol* **28**:255–261.

21 Kjorstad KE, Bond B (1984). Stage 1B adenocarcinoma of the cervix: metastatic potential and patterns of dissemination. *Am J Obstet Gynecol* **150**:297–299.

22 Brown JV, Fu YS, Berek JS (1990). Ovarian metastasis are rare in Stage 1 adenocarcinoma of the cervix. *Obstet Gynecol* **76**:623–626.

23 Michel G, Zarca D, Guettier X, Castaigne D, Charpentier P (1989). Une observation de métastase sur ovaire transposé, après traitement radiochirurgical d'un épithélioma épidermoide du col utérin. Comment minimiser le risque? *Cah Cancer* **1**:121–123.

24 Parham G, Heppard MCS, DiSaia P (1994). Metastasis from a stage 1B cervical adenocarcinoma in a transposed ovary: a case report and review of the literature, *Gynecol Oncol* **55**:469–472.

25 Coulam CB, Adamson SC, Annegers JF (1986). Incidence of premature ovarian failure. *Obstet Gynecol* **67**:604–606.

26 Anderson B, La Polla J, Turner D, Chapman G, Buller R (1993). Ovarian transposition in cervical cancer. *Gynecol Oncol* **49**:206–214.

27 Prouvost MA, Canis M, Le Bouëdec G, Achard JL, Mage G, Dauplat J (1991). Transposition ovarienne percoelioscopique avant curiethérapie dans les cancers du col stade 1A et 1B. *J Gynecol Obstet Biol Reprod* **20**:361–365.

28 Dein A, Menutti MT, Kovach P, Gabbe SG (1984). The reproductive potential of young men and women with Hodgkin's disease. *Obstet Gynecol Surv* **39**:474–482.

29 Bidzinski M, Lemieszczuk B, Zielinski J (1993). Evaluation of the hormonal function and features of the ultrasound picture of transposed ovary in cervical cancer patients after surgery and pelvic irradiation. *Eur J Gynaecol Oncol* **14**:77–80.

30 Lushbaugh CC, Casarett GW (1976). The effects of gonadal irradiation in clinical radiation therapy: a review. *Cancer* **37**:1111–1120.

31 Husseinzadeh N, Van Haken ML, Aron B (1994). Ovarian transposition in young patients with invasive cervical cancer receiving radiation therapy. *Int J Gynecol Cancer* **4**:61–65.

32 Haie-Meder C, Milka-Cabanne N, Michel G *et al* (1993). Radiotherapy after ovarian transposition: ovarian function and fertility preservation. *Int J Radiat Oncol Biol Phys* **25**:419–424.

33 Querleu D, Castelain B (1992). Le devenir de l'ovaire transposé dans le traitement des cancers du col utérin chez la femme jeune. *Cah Oncol* **1**:235–238.

34 Herbst A, Anderson D (1990). Clear cell adenocarcinoma of the vagina and cervix secondary to intrauterine exposure to diethylstilbestrol. *Semin Surg Oncol* **6**:343–346.

35 Michel G, Castaigne D, Gerbaulet A, Lhommé C, Prade M (1992). Transposition ovarienne dans les cancers gynécologiques. *Cah Oncol* **1**:27–29.

36 Hadar H, Loven D, Herskovitz P, Bairey O, Yagoda A (1994). An evaluation of lateral and medial transposition of the ovaries out of radiation fields. *Cancer* **74**:774–779.

37 Holmes G, Holmes F (1978). Pregnancy outcome of patients treated for Hodgkin's disease. *Cancer* **41**:1317–1322.

38 Mulvilhill JJ, McKeen EA, Rosner F, Zarrabi MH (1987). Pregnancy outcome in cancer patients. Experience in a large cooperative group. *Cancer* **60**:1143–1150.

39 Querleu D (1995). *Techniques chirurgicales en gynécologie.* Paris: Masson.

12 Laparoscopic colorectal surgical techniques

Camran Nezhat, Daniel S. Seidman,
Fariba Nasserbakht, Farr Nezhat and
Ceana H. Nezhat

Introduction

Major intestinal operations are performed routinely by experienced gynaecological oncology surgeons as part of their primary therapy for a specific gynaecological malignancy, the management of complications related to cancer or its therapy or the treatment of recurrent tumour [1]. These surgical procedures include repair of simple enterotomies, colostomies and ileostomies, colostomy closures, bowel resection with reanastomosis, intestinal bypass procedures and urinary conduits [1–22].

The revolution in laparoscopic surgery over the last decade includes bowel surgery. To a large extent, this progress was pioneered by gynaecologists. The first procedure, appendectomy, was developed by gynaecologists over a decade ago [23] and was adopted in routine care [24,25]. Surgical tools were gradually developed, including improved insufflation devices, powerful suction-irrigation probes to facilitate hydrodissection, stapling devices, and non-crushing bowel clamps and graspers suitable for handling bowel. The growing experience and skill with laparoscopic surgery, combined with the availability of new instruments, led to more complex laparoscopic bowel operations. These procedures were developed by gynaecologists [24,26–32] and general surgeons [33–51], and included appendectomy, colostomy, ileostomy, partial and total rectosigmoid colon resection with reanastomosis, hemicolectomy and abdomino-perineal resection.

Advantages of laparoscopic bowel surgery

The benefits of laparoscopic intestinal surgery are similar to those of other laparoscopic procedures, including less postoperative pain, a lower risk of wound dehiscence, early ambulation and, generally, a more rapid convalescence. Laparoscopy for intestinal surgery may mean a quicker return of bowel function and a decreased use of analgesics. These benefits are especially important for patients with malignant disease who may be prone to cardiovascular and pulmonary complications, and who have a higher risk of surgical scar dehiscence. More rapid recovery may permit earlier initiation of chemotherapy or radiotherapy. The risk of adhesion formation is reduced with laparoscopic surgery [52,53]. In a recent study involving porcine models, it was suggested that adhesion formation following lymphadenectomy may be less than that following laparotomy [54]. The laparoscope magnifies pelvic and abdominal anatomy, and may improve observation and identification of metastatic lesions on the upper abdomen, the surfaces of the liver and diaphragm, the posterior cul-de-sac and the posterior aspect of the broad ligaments. Other possible benefits are less blood loss, decreased fluid requirements and less immunosuppression, resulting from reduced stress and fewer blood transfusions [55].

Disadvantages of laparoscopic bowel surgery

Basic surgical principles must always be observed, regardless of whether the intestinal operation is performed by laparoscopy or laparotomy. These principles include excellent exposure of the operating field, avoiding spillage of enteric contents in the peritoneal cavity and retrieving the specimen intact for complete pathological analysis [44]. The anastomosis must be well vascularized, free of tension and circumferentially intact [44]. At laparoscopy, optimal retraction of the adjacent organs may be difficult, and the surgeon's depth perception may be challenged by the two-dimensional vision of video.

A significant restriction of laparoscopic bowel surgery is poor tactile feedback because direct palpation is not possible. The use of a colonoscope during surgery can reduce this shortcoming by improving the operator's ability to locate and assess bowel lesions. Laparoscopic sonography, using specially designed probes, may help to identify structures beneath the visualized surface, and it is an important intraoperative diagnostic tool.

Concerns about laparoscopic bowel surgery for malignancy

The major objections to laparoscopic surgery for cancer patients are inadequate tumour clearance and possible metastasis to trocar port sites.

Preliminary data suggest that resected tumour specimens have acceptable distal and proximal resection margins [43]. The efficacy of laparoscopic lymphadenectomy has also been questioned [56]. The amount of residual lymph-node tissue is directly related to the surgeon's experience [57,58]. The yield of laparoscopic lymphadenectomy has been shown to be satisfactory [43,48,49]. Abdominal wall tumour implantation has been reported following laparoscopy for cancer of the ovary [59,60], stomach [61], gallbladder [62], pancreas [63] and colon [64]. However, these are anecdotal case reports. Preliminary surveys of laparoscopy for gynaecological [65] and colon cancer [66] suggest that port-site recurrence is infrequent. Further, gynaecologists [67] and general surgeons [68] have advocated placing all specimens in a laparoscopic pouch for transanal or transabdominal removal to reduce the risk of inadvertent metastasis.

Indications

The role of laparoscopic surgery for gynaecological operations is rapidly expanding [69–71]. The most frequent indication for laparoscopic bowel surgery is probably adhesiolysis. This approach is successful in managing incomplete bowel obstruction due to adhesions, but the operator must be experienced. The indications for laparoscopic bowel resection include colonic segmental resection for colonic metastasis with intra- or extra-corporeal anastomosis. Traumatic bowel injury can be repaired with laparoscopic primary repair or segmental resection. Closure of ileostomy or colostomy can be performed laparoscopically.

Improved survival following intensified cytoreduction has been suggested [72] and this may be a role for laparoscopic surgery. The carbon dioxide laser has long been used to ablate endometriotic implants on the peritoneum and other intra-abdominal organs [73,74]. The carbon dioxide laser has also been used to vaporize and excise metastases of ovarian cancer in the abdomen [75,76] and ovarian intestinal metastases [77,78]. Observation and accessibility to the upper abdomen, including the diaphragm, and deep pelvis are better at laparoscopy. This improved access and observation, combined with magnification, may facilitate identification and treatment of metastatic lesions, and allow intensified cytoreduction with the carbon dioxide laser.

Contraindications

Contraindications to laparoscopic colon surgery include diffuse faecal peritonitis, unprepared bowel, extensive multiple adhesions and large bulky tumours. Other less common contraindications include large phlegmon, acute inflammatory bowel disease, liver cirrhosis and large abdominal aortic aneurysm.

The importance of careful patient selection for laparoscopic bowel surgery has been emphasized [44,68], although absolute contraindications have not been formally defined [51]. By respecting the contraindications noted above and the skill of the operator, complications associated with the procedure can be decreased. The more experienced laparoscopist may regard some of the previously described contraindications to be support for performing, rather than avoiding, laparoscopic surgery. Additionally, improved instrumentation and operative techniques may increase the margin of safety for operative laparoscopy.

Laparoscopic intestinal surgery for endometriosis

While most of our experience with laparoscopic intestinal surgery involve treating endometriosis [24,26–31], there are similarities between deeply infiltrating endometriosis and malignant metastasis to the bowel. Although endometriosis is a benign disease, severe cases may involve widespread implants that penetrate deep into the peritoneal surface and affect every organ in the abdominal cavity, from the urinary bladder to the diaphragm. The radical laparoscopic procedures that were developed to treat intestinal endometriosis may be applicable to typical secondary cancer involvement of the bowel.

This section is primarily based on our experience with laparoscopic intestinal procedures performed for severe endometriosis. Recent achievements by general surgeons in intestinal laparoscopic operations will also be discussed.

Preoperative bowel preparation

All patients should undergo outpatient mechanical and antibiotic bowel preparation. Two days before the operation, the patient consumes only clear liquids. The day before surgery, the patient drinks a gallon of oral solutions containing polyethylene glycol 3350, sodium chloride, bicarbonate, and potassium chloride. The night before surgery, the patient should undergo a Fleet enema and take 1 g of metronidazole orally. Two grams of cefoxitin sodium (Mefoxin) are administered intravenously 30 minutes before the scheduled procedure.

Laparoscopic operative set-up

Laparoscopy is performed under general endotracheal anaesthesia. A 10-mm trocar is directly inserted infraumbilically. An operating laparoscope is inserted and a camera is attached to the laparoscope. After visual verification that the trocar has been properly placed in the peritoneal cavity, pneumoperitoneum is induced. Under direct guidance, three 5-mm suprapubic trocars are placed, one each in the lower left and right quadrants, and one in the midline, 5–6 cm above the pubic symphysis (Fig. 12.1). The number, size and location of the trocars may be modified depending on the procedure. One of the 5-mm trocars may be exchanged for a 10–12 mm one if a large instrument will need to be used. The grasping forceps are inserted through the lower right sleeve, the bipolar electrocoagulator through the midline and the suction irrigator probe through the lower left port. Then, using the video laparoscope system through the umbilical

channel, the pelvic and abdominal organs are examined. If the carbon dioxide laser is used, a direct lens–laser coupler is attached to the laparoscope. The laser is placed through the operating channel of the laparoscope or through one of the ancillary 5-mm trocars, and may be used for cutting and coagulating small blood vessels (Fig. 12.1). Electrosurgery, harmonic scalpel, sharp scissors or any other cutting modality can replace the carbon dioxide laser. The power of the laser is set between 40 and 80 W. Haemostasis is accomplished with the laser, bipolar electrocoagulation or surgical clips.

Laparoscopic appendectomy

Technique

The appendix is examined and mobilized after lysis of periappendiceal or pericaecal adhesions. This is done carefully because there may be attachment to the lateral

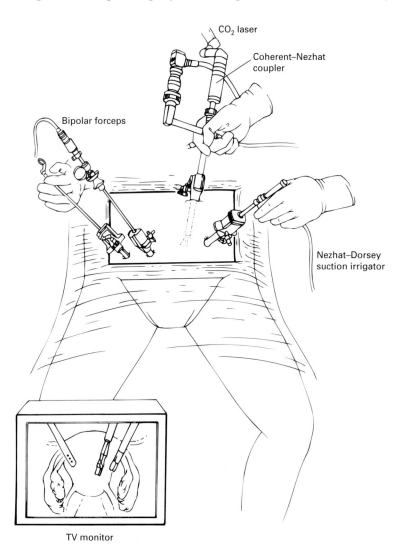

Fig. 12.1 Instrument placement for appendectomy by operative laparoscopy. (© C. Boyter 1994.)

pelvic wall or a retrocaecal appendix. Next, the bipolar electrocoagulator and carbon dioxide laser are used sequentially to desiccate and cut the mesoappendix close to the ileocaecal area.

At this point the bipolar forceps is withdrawn and the Endoloop applicator is inserted through the suprapubic midline puncture. Two chromic or polydioxanone Endoloop sutures are passed to the base of the appendix, 3–5 mm from the caecum, and tied one on top of the other. Both suture ends are cut. A third Endoloop suture is applied (Fig. 12.2), 1 cm distal to the other sutures, and cut, leaving a 15-cm tail to facilitate retrieval should the appendix inadvertently fall into the pelvic well. The appendix is cut between the second and third sutures. Luminal portions of the appendiceal stump and the removed appendix are seared with the carbon dioxide laser or sterilized with Betadine solution (Fig. 12.3). The abdomen is irrigated copiously with lactated Ringer's. Recently, we have omitted the third Endoloop, thoroughly coagulating the distal part of the appendix using bipolar forceps and are not using Betadine solution.

The appendix is removed from the abdomen with a long grasping forceps passed through the operating channel of the laparoscope, a suprapubic port or inside a pouch, and submitted for pathology. If appropriate, an appendix extractor is used through the central port after replacing the central 5-mm trocar with a 10-mm one. Instruments, possibly contaminated, are removed from the surgical field. No adjunctive therapy is used. Finally,

the appendiceal and other operative sites are inspected for haemostasis by completely emptying the abdominal cavity of carbon dioxide gas, and then reinflating it. Finally, the cavity is irrigated with lactated Ringer's.

Experience

In our first 100 cases, appendectomies were accomplished in 4–21 minutes [24]. No major intraoperative complications occurred. All patients were discharged from the hospital within 24 hours of surgery. Seven remained overnight because of patient preference or surgery performed late in the day. The average hospital stay was 14 hours. All patients resumed a regular diet the day after surgery. Except for mild periumbilical ecchymosis, no apparent postoperative complications were noted in the study group.

Comment

A number of techniques are employed for laparoscopic appendectomy, and the procedure is common [25]. Although this operation has a favourable cost–benefit ratio, complications including stump blowout, wound infection, haemorrhage and postoperative ileus have been described [79,80].

Laparoscopic repair of enterotomies of the small bowel, colon and rectum

Technique

Intentional or inadvertent enterotomies created during diagnostic or therapeutic laparoscopy can be corrected

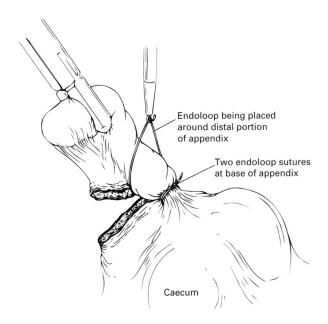

Endoloop being placed around distal portion of appendix

Two endoloop sutures at base of appendix

Caecum

Fig. 12.2 Endoloop sutures are placed around the base of the appendix. (Redrawn from Nezhat *et al* [85] with permission of the McGraw-Hill Companies.)

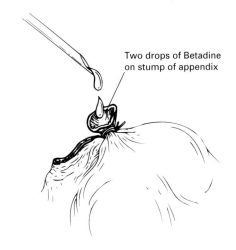

Two drops of Betadine on stump of appendix

Fig. 12.3 Luminal portions of the appendiceal stump are seared with the carbon dioxide laser. (Redrawn from Nezhat *et al* [85] with permission of the McGraw-Hill Companies.)

successfully using the laparoscopic approach. The pelvic and abdominal cavity is thoroughly irrigated and any bowel contents are removed. The location of the enterotomy is evaluated and any necrotic tissue is removed. We usually perform repairs with a single-layer closure incorporating mucosa, submucosa, and serosa using 0 Dexon or Vicryl on a curved or straight needle, and intracorporeal or extracorporeal knot tying. The repair can be vertical or transverse, depending on the size of the enterotomy (Fig. 12.4). Care should be taken to avoid bowel stricture. If the laceration is extensive, it is safer to resect the injured portion of the bowel. The bowel is mobilized laparoscopically, and resection and reanastomosis may be completed through a minilaparotomy incision or completely laparoscopically.

The repair is evaluated using one of the following methods. To assess the integrity of small bowel and colon closures, the abdominal and pelvic cavities are filled with lactated Ringer's. The bowel is observed under the fluid for the presence of air bubbles, indicating that the closure is not airtight. To evaluate rectum and rectosigmoid colon repairs, the posterior cul-de-sac is filled with lactated

Ringer's, sigmoidoscopy is performed and the rectum is inflated with air, again observing for air bubbles. Postoperatively, patients receive 1 g cefoxitin for three doses every 8 hours. They are given clear liquids orally after their bowel function resumes and their postoperative course is closely monitored.

Experience

In a published series [34] the indications for surgery were endometriosis in 18 cases, pelvic adhesions in seven and adhesions with Crohn's disease in one. All women had preoperative antibiotic and mechanical bowel preparation as described.

The enterotomies were secondary to carbon dioxide laser vaporization or excision of endometriosis and/or lysis of adhesions adjacent to or involving the bowel wall in 23 patients, and trocar insertion in three. The three enterotomies related to trocar insertion occurred in women who had prior abdominal surgery. The injuries included nine small bowel, four colonic and 13 rectal enterotomies.

The enterotomies were repaired without laparotomy. All patients tolerated solid low residual diets within 72 hours of surgery. Twenty-three patients were discharged from the hospital within 24 hours of surgery. No clinical complications related to the laparoscopic bowel repair were noted, and no patients developed infection or obstruction. No fistulae occurred and all repairs healed without clinical evidence of infection.

Comment

It is possible to repair laparoscopically enterotomies of the small bowel, colon and rectum that occur during laparoscopic procedures in patients who have had preoperative bowel preparation. The results of repair in unprepared bowel, as might occur with penetrating trauma, have not yet been determined.

Laparoscopic treatment of infiltrative endometriosis involving the rectosigmoid colon and the rectovaginal septum*

Severe endometriosis commonly involves the uterosacral ligaments, rectovaginal septum and the rectosigmoid

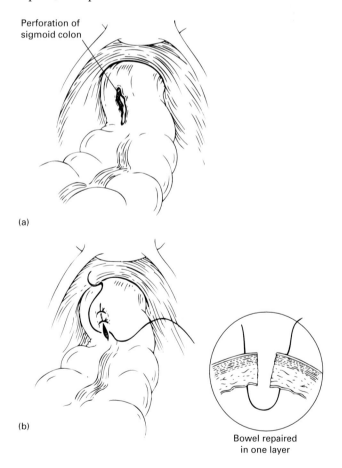

(a)

(b)

Bowel repaired in one layer

Fig. 12.4 (a) Perforation of sigmoid colon. (b) The enterotomy is repaired in one layer using a 0 polyglactin suture.

---

* *Editor's note*: This section is not directly related to cancer surgery. It has, however, been included to: (i) emphasize the technical possibilities of laparoscopic surgery; (ii) inform gynaecological oncologists, who may be consulted in cases of rectal endometriosis; (iii) show that reconstructive bowel surgery may be performed with the assistance of laparoscopic techniques; and (iv) inspire new ideas on surgical strategy in exenterative surgery of central disease, in combination with vaginal surgery.

colon with partial or complete obliteration of the posterior cul-de-sac. Medical management is generally unsatisfactory. We have successfully treated deep colorectal endometriosis with laparoscopic techniques. This procedure may be applied to the management of gynaecological malignancies involving the rectosigmoid colon.

Technique

The procedures are performed under general anaesthesia in the modified dorsolithotomy position. The assistant should stand between the patient's legs and perform rectovaginal examination with one hand. With the other hand, the assistant holds the uterus up with a rigid uterine elevator while both the assistant and the surgeon observe the monitor. For rectovaginal septum and uterosacral ligament endometriosis, 5–8 ml of dilute vasopressin (10 units in 60–100 ml of lactated Ringer's) are injected into an uninvolved area with a 16-gauge laparoscopic needle. The peritoneum is opened and, using hydrodissection, a plane is created in the rectovaginal septum.

Locating and assessing the ureters before proceeding with this procedure is of paramount importance. Any alteration in the direction of the ureters should be identified in advance. Because ureters are lateral to the uterosacral ligaments, we try to stay between the ligaments as much as possible. Using hydrodissection and making a relaxing incision lateral to the uterosacral ligament allows the ureters to retract laterally. This affords increased protection of the ureters. Different degrees of ureterolysis often are necessary to free the ureters from the surrounding fibrotic diseased tissue and from ovarian tumours. Hydrodissection with the carbon dioxide laser and blunt dissection can be used for ureterolysis, enterolysis and ovarian resection. Sharp scissors, fibre lasers, harmonic scalpel, unipolar electrode or hot scissors are rarely used for these dissections.

While the assistant examines the rectum, the involved area is completely excised or vaporized until the loose areolar tissue of the rectovaginal space and the normal muscularis layers of the rectum are reached. In women whose rectum is pulled up and attached to the back of the cervix between the uterosacral ligaments, the uterus is anteflexed sharply and an incision is made at the right or left pararectal area, then extended to the junction of the cervix and the rectum. If the involvement of the rectum is more extensive and the assistant's finger is not long enough, a sigmoidoscope, a sponge on forceps or a rectal probe is used. Two advantages of using the sigmoidoscope are that it helps the surgeon to identify the rectum and it aids in identifying or ruling out bowel perforation because air bubbles can be seen passing from the air-inflated rectum into the posterior cul-de-sac, the latter being filled with irrigation fluid. While the assistant guides the surgeon by rectovaginal examination, the rectum is completely freed from the back of the cervix. Generalized oozing and bleeding may occur and can be controlled with an injection of 3–5 ml dilute vasopressin (1 ampoule in 100 ml), laser or bipolar electrocoagulation. Occasional bleeding from the stalk vessels, caused by dissection or vaporization of the fibrotic uterosacral ligaments and pararectal areas, is controlled with bipolar electrocoagulator or surgical clips.

Endometriosis rarely penetrates the mucosa of the colon, but commonly involves the serosa, subserosa and muscularis. This is probably true for most metastatic lesions to the colon. When significant portions of both serosal and muscularis layers have been excised or vaporized and the mucosa is reached, the bowel wall may be reinforced by 0 to 000 polydioxanone or polyglactin sutures. The involved areas can be excised or vaporized thoroughly by an experienced videolaparoscopist. The procedure is demanding and requires maximum cooperation between the assistant and surgeon.

The rectum is thoroughly evaluated, and small perforations can be repaired laparoscopically as described. Consultation with a colorectal surgeon is always recommended.

Experience

From January 1985 to January 1990, a total of 185 patients, ages 25–41, were managed [31]. They had endometriosis of the lower colon, rectum, uterosacral ligaments or rectovaginal septum. All were referred for treatment because previous surgical or hormonal management failed to relieve their discomfort. Excluding nine patients with bowel perforation and one with a partial bowel resection, all were discharged within 24 hours. The surgical procedures (from initial laparoscopy to termination) lasted from 55 to 245 minutes. All patients had benign disease, but a large number underwent additional surgical procedures including uterolysis, presacral neurectomy, hysterectomy with unilateral or bilateral oophorectomy, myomectomy and appendectomy. The patients were instructed to have nothing by mouth for 24 hours postoperatively except for sips of water, and if no complications were noted the diet was gradually increased. Patients with bowel perforation or resection were allowed nothing by mouth until they had passed flatus and, otherwise, were instructed to avoid constipation by eating a high-fibre diet. Minor complications were shoulder pain, abdominal wall ecchymosis, urine retention and dyschezia for 1–2 weeks.

Comment

Although laparoscopic procedures for cancer are not necessarily the same as those for endometriosis, the two disease processes have common characteristics, including invasion and obliteration of the posterior cul-de-sac. The benefits of the laparoscopic approach, demonstrated for endometriosis, may be similar for some cases of malignancy involving the rectosigmoid colon and rectovaginal septum.

Severe rectal involvement may result in attachment of the rectum to the posterior aspect of the vagina and cervix, and the lower portions of the ureters. Laparoscopic surgery provides better magnification and visualization, improving the chance of detection and resection of the involved areas deep in the pelvis.

Dilute vasopressin adequately controls oozing during laparoscopic dissection, while the laser and bipolar forceps control active bleeding in these patients. Careful and meticulous dissection of severe fibrosis and infiltrating disease will ensure complete removal of the tumour down to the normal areolar tissue of the pararectal area or the bowel muscularis. Constant irrigation removes debris and charcoal, and hydrodissection will help differentiate between fibrosis and normal areolar tissue. A thorough understanding of the pelvic anatomy is critical, to avoid damage to the ureters or rectum.

Laparoscopically assisted anterior rectal wall resection and reanastomosis using a multifire stapler

Technique

For small isolated lesions in the lower rectum near the anus, the following technique can be used. The rectovaginal septum is delineated by the assistant who performs simultaneous vaginal and rectal examination. The rectum is mobilized along the rectovaginal septum anteriorly to within 2 cm of the anus, using scissors and blunt dissection or the carbon dioxide laser and hydrodissection. Mobilization is continued along the left and right pararectal spaces by coagulating and dividing branches of the haemorrhoidal artery, if necessary.

When the rectum is sufficiently mobilized, the lesion is prolapsed to the level of the anus, the perineal body is retracted and an RL30 multifire stapler is applied across the segment of the anterior rectal wall containing the nodule. Two staple applications usually are required to traverse the width of the involved mucosa. The tumour is then excised and two additional interrupted 2-0 polyglactin sutures are inserted along the staple line.

The rectum is returned to the pelvis under direct observation through the laparoscope and video monitor. The integrity of the anastomosis is verified by insufflation of air into the rectum while the cul-de-sac is filled with lactated Ringer's.

When there are multiple lesions or a larger portion of the bowel is involved, an entire segment of bowel is resected. The technique used depends on the location of the lesion. If the lesion is in the rectum or lower rectosigmoid colon and a hysterectomy is performed at the same surgery, the bowel is mobilized laparoscopically and the resection and reanastomosis are completed transvaginally or transanally using a circular stapler as described below. If the lesion is high in the sigmoid colon or other part of the colon, after laparoscopic mobilization of the bowel, the resection and reanastomosis are performed through a minilaparotomy at the left or right lower abdominal quadrant. Lesions involving the small bowel can be resected similarly by extending the umbilical incision and delivering the loop of bowel for anastomosis. This minilaparotomy approach has been successfully performed to repair bowel injury.

Experience

Our first procedure lasted 160 minutes [26]. The patient tolerated clear liquids on the first postoperative day and was discharged on the second day. Her recovery was uneventful, and at 8 weeks following surgery she was doing well, with no constipation, rectal pain or bleeding [26].

In a subsequent series [28], endometriosis invading deep into or through the muscularis propria of the rectum was present in 16 patients, with invasion deep into the anterior rectal wall in five. Using laparoscopic techniques, the entire rectum was mobilized, lesions in the rectovaginal septum were vaporized or excised, the lateral rectal pedicles were desiccated, and the presacral space was entered to the level of the levator ani muscles. In the patients with anterior rectal lesions, the rectum was prolapsed via the anal or vaginal canal, transected using two applications of an RL30 or RL60 stapler and reinforced using interrupted 2-0 polyglactin sutures. Resection can be performed without the stapler, instead using primary resection and suturing for repair. In women with circumferential lesions, the rectum was transected proximal to the lesion using Babcock clamps, and the proximal limb was prolapsed through the anorectum or vagina (Fig. 12.5). The anvil of the ILS 33 stapler was detached and secured in the proximal limb with a 0 polypropylene suture placed around the circumference of the bowel. The proximal limb was then returned to the abdominal cavity (Fig. 12.6). The rectal segment with the lesion was prolapsed out the anus or vagina and stapled closed with the RL60 (Fig. 12.7). The segment of rectum containing the lesion above the staple line was transected. The rectum was then returned to its normal position by reducing the prolapse transanally or transvaginally. The ILS 33 was placed into the rectum and the trocar was opened to pass through the stapled end of the rectal stump. Using the laparoscope, the anvil in the proximal limb was reattached to the trocar shaft (Fig. 12.6). Next, the bowel ends were approximated and the stapler fired to create a double-stapled end-to-end anastomosis. 'Donought' margins were inspected to be sure the rings were complete.

A proctoscope was used to inspect each anastomosis for structural integrity and haemostasis. The pelvic cavity was filled with lactated Ringer's and the rectum was insufflated with air to check for leakage. In two patients, air leaks were detected and further reinforcement was performed using three transanally placed polyglactin sutures. In the first 16 cases [28], one patient had partial proctectomy, but laparotomy was necessary for anastomosis as a result of an unsuccessful attempt to place a purse-string suture around the patulous rectal ampulla. Excluding the latter case, the average operating time was 190 minutes (range 90–420 minutes). The average blood loss was 77 ml (range 30–300 ml). The average time spent in hospital was 3.4 days (range 2–5 days). No visceral injuries, anastomotic leaks or pelvic sepsis occurred. Patients were discharged following spontaneous passing of flatus or after having a bowel movement, and when they could tolerate a full liquid diet.

Comment

Transperineal proctectomy with reanastomosis is an accepted, safe procedure. However, fixation of the rectum by rectal mesentery, lateral stalks and rectovaginal adherence means that this procedure is more applicable in selected cases of idiopathic rectal prolapse. In these cases, the points of fixation have weakened, allowing the rectum to spontaneously prolapse through the anal canal. At laparoscopy, the pelvic endometriosis is excised or vaporized, and the rectum is fully mobilized from its fascial and vascular attachments, allowing rectal prolapse. Extracorporeal transanal or transvaginal resection of the diseased segment is performed, followed by double-stapled reanastomosis of the bowel. While this double-staple technique is an accepted procedure for low colorectal anastomosis, it should be applied cautiously for malignancy [81–84].

Laparoscopic hysterectomy with partial proctectomy

Technique

After completing laparoscopic hysterectomy, the rectosigmoid colon is mobilized, as described, and prolapsed via the vaginal cuff. The prolapsed segment is extracorporeally transected proximal to the lesion and a 2-0 polypropylene purse-string suture is placed around the proximal limb of the bowel. The anvil of an ILS 33 stapler is placed through the purse-string into the proximal bowel and the proximal limb of bowel is replaced into the pelvis. Using Babcock clamps, the distal rectal segment is further prolapsed through the vagina. The bowel is resected, distal to the lesion and proximal to the anal canal, using the RL60 stapler.

The rectal stump is replaced through the vaginal cuff in the pelvis. A wet lap pack is placed in the vagina to prevent escape of pneumoperitoneum. The anastomosis is completed and inspected as described previously. The vaginal pack is removed and the vaginal cuff closed with intracorporeal sutures.

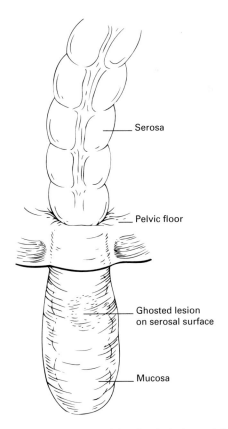

Fig. 12.5 The rectum is transected distal to the lesion and the proximal limb is prolapsed into the distal limb.

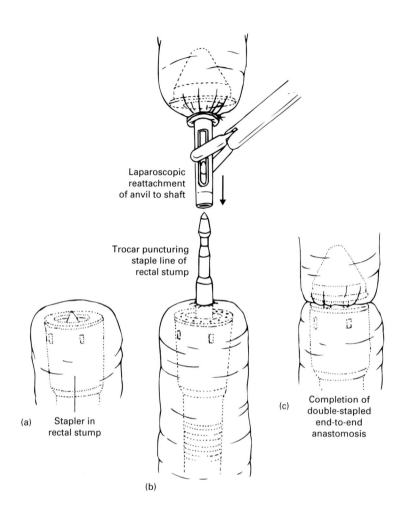

Laparoscopic
reattachment
of anvil to shaft

Trocar puncturing
staple line of
rectal stump

(a)   Stapler in
rectal stump

(b)

(c)   Completion of
double-stapled
end-to-end
anastomosis

Fig. 12.6 A 2-0 polypropylene purse-string suture is placed around the circumference of the proximal limb of the bowel. (a) The ILS stapler is placed into the rectum, and the anvil trocar within the proximal bowel is inserted into the stapling device using the laparoscope. The device is fired (b), creating an end-to-end anastomosis (c).

Laparoscopic disc excision and primary repair of the anterior rectal wall without a stapling device

The following technique for total laparoscopic resection of part of the colon wall and repair of the defect eliminates stapling devices and much of the complex and time-consuming dissection. It is used to treat selected cases of infiltrative symptomatic intestinal endometriosis.

Technique

The extent of bowel involvement is evaluated and the need for full-thickness disc excision is determined. We use a sigmoidoscope to completely clean the rectum, to further delineate the lesion, and to guide the surgeon. If the lesion is low enough, an assistant can identify it by performing a rectal examination. After the ureters are identified in each side, the lower colon is mobilized. Depending on the location of the lesion, the right and/or

left pararectal area(s) are separated from adjacent organs. Any bleeding which is not controlled with the carbon dioxide laser is managed with bipolar electrocoagulation or surgical clips.

Full-thickness excision begins above the area of visible disease. After identifying normal tissue, the lesion is held at its proximal end with grasping forceps inserted through the right lower quadrant trocar. An incision is made through the bowel serosa and muscularis, and the lumen is entered (Fig. 12.8). The lesion is completely excised from the anterior rectal wall (Fig. 12.9). Following complete excision of the lesion, the pelvic cavity is thoroughly irrigated and suctioned. The lesion is removed from the abdomen through the operative channel of the laparoscope using a long grasping forceps, or from the anus using polyp forceps, and submitted for pathology.

The bowel is repaired transversely in one layer. Two traction sutures are applied to each side of the bowel defect, transforming it into a transverse opening (Fig. 12.10). The stay sutures are brought out via the right

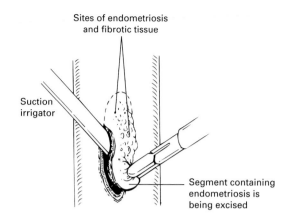

Fig. 12.8 An incision is made through the bowel serosa and muscularis, and the lumen is entered.

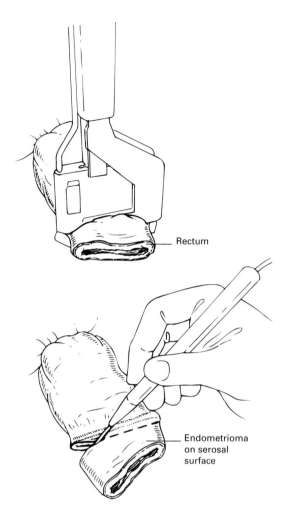

Fig. 12.7 The rectal stump is transected proximal to the lesion using an RL60 linear stapler.

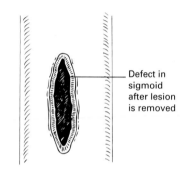

Fig. 12.9 The lesion is completely excised from the anterior rectal wall.

and 4, when they are able to tolerate clear liquids well. A low-residual diet is begun after the patient has a bowel movement.

Experience

Eight women, from 29 to 38 years old, who suffered from extensive symptomatic lower colon endometriosis associated with gastrointestinal symptoms were diagnosed with severe bowel endometriosis and had not responded to previous conservative surgical and hormonal therapy [30]. The subjects were evaluated preoperatively and intraoperatively by a colorectal surgeon; barium enema and sigmoidoscopy were performed as necessary. In addition, a rectovaginal examination confirmed severe lower colon endometriosis in all patients. Intravenous pyelograms, when performed, were normal in all but one woman, who had ureteral obstruction.

Patients underwent preoperative mechanical and antibiotic bowel preparation as described above. The duration of the operations (measured from the induction of anaesthesia until the procedure was terminated)

and left lower quadrant trocar sleeves. The sleeves are removed, then replaced in the peritoneal cavity next to the stay sutures, and the sutures are secured outside the abdomen. The bowel is then repaired by placing several interrupted through-and-through sutures in 0.3–0.6-cm increments until it is completely repaired (Figs 12.11 & 12.12). We use 0 polyglactin laparoscopic sutures and a straight or curved needle with extracorporeal or intracorporeal knot tying.

At the end of the procedure, the rectosigmoid colon is carefully examined using the sigmoidoscope as described earlier, to confirm that the closure is airtight and to ensure that there is no bowel stricture. Neither a Jackson–Pratt drain nor a nasogastric tube are used routinely. The Foley catheter is removed on the day of surgery. Oral feeding is resumed after the spontaneous release of flatus, usually on the first or second postoperative day. All patients are released from the hospital between postoperative days 2

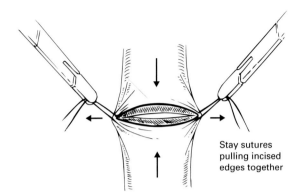

Fig. 12.10 Two traction sutures are applied to each side of the bowel defect, transforming it into a transverse opening.

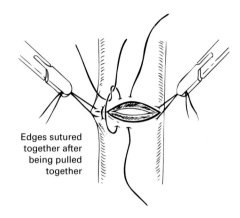

Fig. 12.11 The bowel is repaired by placing several interrupted through-and-through sutures in 0.3–0.6-cm increments.

ranged from 120 to 270 minutes [30]. The estimated blood loss was 150–350 ml. No patients required transfusion. Sigmoidoscopy was performed at 6 weeks and 6 months postoperatively. All anastomotic sites have healed well with no sign of stricture or fistula.

Comment

The laparoscopic procedure was similar to laparotomy. The only drawback to this procedure is the time necessary for laparoscopic suturing—our average was 2.5 minutes per suture. There are patient benefits from smaller incisions, a faster recovery time and a lower postoperative morbidity. A randomized trial has not been performed to compare this technique with laparotomy. However, our results with this technique in a large series were positive, and in the hands of experienced laparoscopists and carefully selected patients, this technique may prove useful in treating disease involving the anterior rectal wall with minimal complications.

Summary of cases treated

In a series of 356 women who underwent laparoscopic treatment of bowel endometriosis using the different techniques presented above, two cases were converted to laparotomy early in our experience. The first patient underwent laparotomy for repair of an enterotomy after the treatment of infiltrative rectal endometriosis. The second patient required laparotomy for anastomosis following an unsuccessful attempt to place a purse-string suture around a patulous rectal ampulla.

Significant postoperative complications occurred in 1.7% of patients. Two women developed leaks and pelvic infections. One woman required, laparoscopically, a temporary colostomy with subsequent take down and repair by laparotomy, whereas another woman was managed by

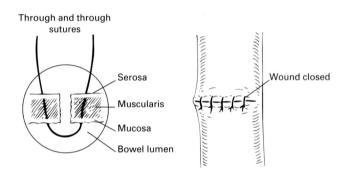

Fig. 12.12 The bowel is completely repaired.

prolonged drainage. A bowel stricture was a complication in one women, and thus required resection and reanastomosis by laparotomy. One women developed a pelvic abscess which did not respond to drainage; she underwent laparoscopic right salpingo-oophorectomy. Following wedge resection of the rectum, another woman had an immediate rectal prolapse which was reduced without surgical management. Her bowel symptoms persisted, and she finally had a colectomy.

Minor complications included skin ecchymosis, temporary urinary retention, temporary diarrhoea or constipation, and dyschezia.

At present, we treat bowel endometriosis by vaporizing and excising the lesions using the carbon dioxide laser, providing they are isolated and involve only serosa, subserosa or muscularis without mucosal penetration. The bowel is repaired and reinforced whenever there is a deep defect. For deeply infiltrative lesions, wedge resection of the anterior colon or rectum is performed. Depending on the size of the defect, the bowel is repaired transversely or vertically. If the lesion is low in the rectum, close to the anus, the rectovaginal septum is entered and completely dissected. The lower portion of the rectum is mobilized, and the nodule is brought out through the anus and resected. For multiple and extensive lesions, and those which affect a large portion of the rectum or rectosigmoid colon, the bowel is mobilized laparoscopically. Resection and reanastomosis are performed through a minilaparotomy incision, vaginally or transanally, depending upon the location of the disease. For the small bowel and ileocaecum, after the bowel is mobilized laparoscopically, the resection and reanastomosis are performed through a minilaparotomy. Appendiceal endometriosis is managed by appendectomy.

Conclusion

Laparoscopic procedures can be used for practically all types of intestinal surgery performed by the gynaecological surgeon. Numerous techniques have been proposed for laparoscopic colon surgery, and modifications are constantly devised [68,81]. The application of laparoscopic bowel surgery for oncology patients has been challenged [82]. Although some authorities believe that it should be an accepted surgical procedure [83], there is general agreement regarding the urgent need for randomized trials comparing laparoscopic and open colorectal surgery [84].

The benefits of laparoscopic surgery, including early ambulation and a decreased risk of surgical scar dehiscence and ventral hernia, are especially important for patients with malignancy. The laparoscopic approach may allow more intensive cytoreduction by utilizing the carbon dioxide laser for the ablation of metastatic implants on the intestine. However, it must be remembered that laparoscopic bowel operations require a high degree of skill and knowledge of instrumentation and techniques, and should be attempted only by experienced laparoscopists. Long-term data will be available soon about the outcome of these procedures in managing malignancy. The role of laparoscopic intestinal surgery will be determined only when follow-up results and survival analyses are available.

References

1 Barnhill D, Doering D, Remmenga S, Bosscher J, Nash J, Park R (1991). Intestinal surgery performed on gynecologic cancer patients. *Gynecol Oncol* **40**:38–41.

2 Photopulos GJ, Delgado G, Fowler WC, Walton LA (1979). Intestinal anastomosis after radiation therapy by surgical stapling instruments. *Obstet Gynecol* **54**:515–518.

3 Wheeless CR Jr (1979). Avoidance of a permanent colostomy in pelvic malignancy using the surgical stapler. *Obstet Gynecol* **54**:501–505.

4 Delgado G (1980). Use of the automatic stapler in urinary conduit diversions and pelvic exenterations. *Gynecol Oncol* **10**:93–97.

5 Castaldo TW, Petrilli ES, Ballon SC, Lagasse LD (1981). Rectosigmoid colectomy and reanastomosis to facilitate resection of primary and recurrent gynecologic cancer. *Obstet Gynecol* **139**:80–84.

6 Wheeless CR, Dorsey JH (1981). Use of the automatic surgical stapler for intestinal anastomosis associated with gynecologic malignancy. Review of 283 procedures. *Gynecol Oncol* **11**:1–7.

7 Krebs HB, Goplerud DR (1983). Surgical management of bowel obstruction in advanced ovarian carcinoma. *Obstet Gynecol* **61**:327–330.

8 Berek JS, Hacker NF, Lagasse LD (1984). Rectosigmoid colectomy and reanastomosis to facilitate resection in primary and recurrent gynecologic cancer. *Obstet Gynecol* **64**:715–720.

9 Burke TW, Weiser EB, Hoskins WJ, Heller PB, Nash JD, Park RC (1987). End colostomy using an end-to-end anastomosis instrument. *Obstet Gynecol* **69**:156–159.

10 Wheeless CR Jr (1987). Incidence of fecal incontinence after coloproctostomy below five centimeters in the rectum. *Gynecol Oncol* **27**:373–379.

11 Clarke-Pearson DL, Chin NP, DeLong ER, Rice R, Creasman WT (1987). Surgical management of intestinal obstruction in ovarian cancer. *Gynecol Oncol* **26**:11–18.

12 Hoskins WJ, Burke TW, Weiser EB, Heller PB, Grayson J, Park RC (1987). Right hemicolectomy and ileal resection with primary reanastomosis for irradiation injury of terminal ileum. *Gynecol Oncol* **26**:215–224.

13 Penalver M, Averette H, Sevin B, Lichtinger M, Girtanner R (1987). Gastrointestinal surgery in gynecologic oncology: evaluation of surgical techniques. *Gynecol Oncol* **28**:74–82.

14 Hatch KD, Shingleton HM, Potter ME, Baker VV (1987). Low rectal resection and anastomosis at the time of pelvic exenteration. *Gynecol Oncol* **32**:262–267.

15 Rubin SC, Hoskins WJ, Benjamin I, Lewis JL (1989). Palliative surgery for intestinal obstruction in advanced ovarian cancer. *Gynecol Oncol* **34**:16–19.

16 Wheeless CR Jr, Hempling RE (1989). Rectal J-pouch reservoir to decrease the frequency of tenesmus and defecation in low coloproctostomy. *Gynecol Oncol* **34**:379–382.

17 Lewis JL (1989). Intestinal surgery in gynecologic oncology. *Gynecol Oncol* **34**:30–33.

18 Kadivar TF, Nahhas WA (1989). 'Nongynecologic' surgical procedures performed on a gynecologic oncology service. *Gynecol Oncol* **35**:78–83.

19 Hatch KD, Gelder MS, Soong SJ, Baker VV, Shingleton HM (1990). Pelvic exenteration with low rectal anastomosis: survival, complication, and prognostic factors. *Gynecol Oncol* **38**:462–467.

20 Barnhill D, Doering D, Remmenga S, Bosscher J, Nash J, Park R (1991). Intestinal surgery performed on gynecologic cancer patients. *Gynecol Oncol* **40**:38–41.

21 Wheeless CR (1993). Low colorectal anstomosis and reconstruction after gynecologic cancer. *Cancer Suppl* **71**:1664–1666.

22 Hoffman MS, Gleeson N, Diebel D, Roberts WS, Fiorica JV, Cavanagh D (1993). Colostomy closure on a gynecologic oncology service. *Gynecol Oncol* **49**:299–301.

23 Semm K (1983). Kie endoskopische appendektomie. *Gynakol Prax* **7**:26–30.

24 Nezhat C, Nezhat F (1991). Incidental appendectomy during videolaseroscopy. *Am J Obstet Gynecol* **165**:559–564.

25 McAnena OJ, Willson PD (1993). Laparoscopic appendectomy:

diagnosis and resection of acute and perforated appendices. *Baillieres Clin Gastroenterol* **7**:851–866.
26 Nezhat C, Pennington E, Nezhat F, Silfen SL (1991). Laparoscopically assisted anterior rectal wall resection and reanastomosis for deeply infiltrating endometriosis. *Surg Laparosc Endosc* **1**:106–108.
27 Nezhat F, Nezhat C, Pennington E (1992). Laparoscopic proctectomy for infiltrating endometriosis of the rectum. *Fertil Steril* **57**:1129–1132.
28 Nezhat F, Nezhat C, Pennington E, Ambroze W (1992). Laparoscopic segmental resection for infiltrating endometriosis of the rectosigmoid colon: a preliminary report. *Surg Laparosc Endosc* **2**:212–216.
29 Sharpe DR, Redwine DB (1992). Laparoscopic segmental resection of the sigmoid and rectosigmoid colon for endometriosis. *Surg Laparosc Endosc* **2**:120–124.
30 Nezhat C, Nezhat F, Pennington E, Nezhat CH *et al* (1994). Laparoscopic disk excision and primary repair of the anterior rectal wall for the treatment of full-thickness bowel endometriosis. *Surg Endosc* **8**:682–685.
31 Nezhat C, Nezhat F, Pennington E (1992). Laparoscopic treatment of lower colorectal and infiltrative rectovaginal septum endometriosis by the technique of videolaseroscopy. *Br J Obstet Gynaecol* **99**:664–667.
32 Fowler D, White S (1991). Laparoscopy-assisted sigmoid resection. *Surg Laparosc Endosc* **1**:183–188.
33 Jacobs M, Verdeja J, Goldsetin H (1991). Minimally invasive colon resection (laparoscopic colectomy). *Surg Laparosc Endosc* **1**:144–150.
34 Nezhat C, Nezhat F, Ambroze W, Pennington E (1993). Laparoscopic repair of small bowel, colon, and rectal endometriosis: a report of twenty-six cases. *Surg Endosc* **7**:88–89.
35 Lange V, Meyer G, Schardey HM, Scildberg FW (1991). Laparoscopic creation of a loop colostomy. *J Laparoendosc Surg* **1**:307–312.
36 Schlinkert RT (1991). Laparoscopic-assisted right hemicolectomy. *Dis Colon Rectum* **34**:1030–1031.
37 Saclarides TJ, Ko ST, Airan M, Dillon C, Franklin J (1991). Laparoscopic removal of a large colonic lipoma: report of a case. *Dis Colon Rectum* **34**:1027–1029.
38 Phillips EH, Franklin M, Carroll BJ, Fallas MJ, Ramos R, Rosenthal D (1993). Laparoscopic colectomy. *Ann Surg* **216**:703–707.
39 Ballantyne GH (1992). Laparoscopically assisted anterior resection for rectal prolapse. *Surg Laparosc Endosc* **2**:230–236.
40 Scoggin S, Frazee R (1992). Laparoscopically assisted resection of a colonic lipoma. *J Laparoendoscop Surg* **2**:185–189.
41 Peters WR (1992). Laparoscopic total proctocolectomy with creation of ileostomy for ulcerative colitis: Report of two cases. *J Laparoendoscop Surg* **2**:175–178.
42 Wexner SD, Johansen OB, Nogueras JJ, Jagelman DG (1992). Laparoscopic total abdominal colectomy. *Dis Colon Rectum* **356**:651–655.
43 Monson J, Darzi A, Carey P, Gillou P (1992). Prospective evaluation of laparoscopic-assisted colectomy in an unselected group of patients. *Lancet* **340**:831–833.
44 Wexner SD, Johansen OB (1992). Laparoscopic bowel resection: advantages and limitations. *Ann Med* **4**:105–110.
45 Ambroze WL, Orangio GR, Tucker JG *et al* (1993). Laparoscopic assisted proctosigmoidectomy with extracorporeal transanal anastomosis: a pilot study. *Surg Endosc* **7**:29–32.
46 Quattelbaum JK, Flanders D, Usher CH (1993). Laparoscopically assisted colectomy. *Surg Laparosc Endosc* **3**:81–87.
47 Senagore AJ, Luchtefeld MA, Mackeigan JM, Mazier WP (1993). Open colectomy vs laparoscopic colectomy: are there differences? *Ann Surg* **59**:549–553.
48 Falk PM, Beart RW, Wexner SD *et al* (1993). Laparoscopic colectomy: a critical appraisal. *Dis Colon Rectum* **36**:28–34.
49 Peters WR, Bartels TL (1993). Minimally invasive colectomy: are potential benefits realized? *Dis Colon Rectum* **36**:751–756.
50 Vara-Thorbeck C, Carcia-Caballero M, Salvi M *et al* (1994). Indication and advantages of laparoscopy-assisted colon resection for carcinoma in elderly patients. *Surg Laparosc Endosc* **4**:110–118.
51 Ambroze WL, Orangio GR, Armstrong D, Schertzer M, Lucas G (1994). Laparoscopic surgery for colorectal neoplasms. *Sem Surg Oncol* **10**:398–403.
52 Nezhat C, Nezhat F, Metzger DA, Luciano AA (1990). Adhesion reformation after reproductive surgery by videolaseroscopy. *Fertil Steril* **53**:1008–1011.
53 Luciano AA, Moufauino-Oliva M (1994). Comparison of postoperative adhesion formation—laparoscopy versus laparotomy. *Infert Reprod Med Clin North Am* **5**:437.
54 Fowler JM, Hartenbach EM, Reynolds HT *et al* (1994). Pelvic adhesion formation after pelvic lymphadenectomy: comparison between transperitoneal laparoscopy and extraperitoneal laparotomy in a porcine model. *Gynecol Oncol* **55**:25–28.
55 Beart RW (1994). Laparoscopic colectomy: status of the art. *Dis Colon Rectum* **37**:547–549.
56 Johnson N (1994). Laparoscopic versus conventional pelvic lymphadenectomy for gynecologic malignancy in humans. *Br J Obstet Gynaecol* **101**:902–904.
57 Guazzoni G, Montorsi F, Bergmaschi F *et al* (1994). Open surgical revision of laparoscopic pelvic lymphadenectomy for staging of prostate cancer: the impact of laparoscopic learning curve. *J Urol* **151**:930–933.
58 Fowler JM, Carter JR, Carlson JW *et al* (1993). Lymph node yield from laparoscopic lymphadenectomy on cervical cancer: a comparative study. *Gynecol Oncol* **51**:187–192.
59 Gleeson NC, Nicosia SV, Mark JE, Hoffman MS, Cavanagh D (1993). Abdominal-wall metastases from ovarian carcinoma after laparoscopy. *Am J Obstet Gynecol* **169**:522–523.
60 Shepherd JG, Carter PG, Lowe DG (1994). Wound recurrence by implantation of a borderline ovarian tumor following laparoscopic removal. *Br J Obstet Gynaecol* **101**:265–266.
61 Cava A, Roman J, Quintela G, Martin F, Arambro P (1990). Subcutaneous metastases following laparoscopy in gastric adenocarcinoma. *Eur J Surg Oncol* **16**:63–67.
62 Pezet D, Fondrinier E, Rotman N *et al* (1992). Parietal seeding of carcinoma of the gallbladder after laparoscopic cholecystectomy. *Br J Surg* **79**:230.
63 Siriwarden A, Samarji W (1993). Cutaneous tumor seeding from a previously undiagnosed pancreatic carcinoma after laparoscopic cholecystectomy. *Ann R Coll Surg Eng* **75**:199–200.
64 Walsh DC, Wattchow DA, Wilson TG (1993). Subcutaneous metastases after laparoscopic resection of malignancy. *Aust NZ J Surg* **63**:563–565.
65 Childers JM, Aqua KA, Surwit EA, Hallum AV, Hatch KD (1994).

Abdominal-wall tumor implantation after laparoscopy for malignant conditions. *Obstet Gynecol* **84**:765–769.

66 Ramos JM, Gupta S, Anthone GJ, Ortega AE, Simons AJ, Beart RW Jr (1994). Laparoscopy and colon cancer: is the port site at risk? A preliminary report. *Arch Surg* **129**:897–899.

67 Amos NN, Broadbent JAM, Hill NCW, Magos AL (1992). Laparoscopic 'oophorectomy-in-a-bag' for removal of ovarian tumors of uncertain origin. *Gynecol Endoscopy* **1**:85–89.

68 Franklin ME Jr, Ramos R, Rosenthal D, Schuessler W (1993). Laparoscopic colonic procedures. *World J Surg* **17**:51–56.

69 Tadir Y, Fisch B (1993). Operative laparoscopy: a challenge for general gynecology? *Am J Obstet Gynecol* **169**:7–12.

70 Rock JA, Warshaw JR (1994). The history and future of operative laparoscopy. *Am J Obstet Gynecol* **170**:7–11.

71 Garry R (1992). Laparoscopic alternatives to laparotomy: a new approach to gynecologic surgery. *Br J Obstet Gynaecol* **99**:629–632.

72 Elsenkop SM, Nalick RH, Wang H *et al* (1993). Peritoneal implant elimination during cytoreductive surgery for ovarian cancer: impact on survival. *Gynecol Oncol* **51**:224.

73 Nezhat C, Crowgey S, Nezhat F (1989). Videolaseroscopy for the treatment of endometriosis associated with infertility. *Fertil Steril* **51**:237–240.

74 Nezhat C, Nezhat F, Silfen SL (1991). Videolaseroscopy: the CO_2 laser for advanced operative laparoscopy. *Obstet Gynecol Clin North Am* **18**:585–604.

75 Patsner B (1990). Carbon dioxide laser vaporization of diaphragmatic metastases for cytoreduction of ovarian epithelial cancer. *Obstet Gynecol* **76**:724–727.

76 Chevinsky AH, Minton JP (1990). Ablation of recurrent and metastatic intraabdominal tumor with the CO_2 laser. *Lasers Surg Med* **10**:5–11.

77 Fanning J, Hilgers RD, Richards PK *et al* (1994). Carbon dioxide laser vaporization of intestinal metastasis of epithelial ovarian cancer. *Int J Gynecol Oncol* **4**:324–327.

78 Amara DD, Nezhat C, Teng V, Nezhat F, Nezhat C, Rosati M (1995). Operative laparoscopy and management of ovarian cancer. *Surg Laparosc Endosc* **6**(1):38–45.

79 Fisher KS, Ross DS (1990). Guidelines for therapeutic decision in incidental appendectomy. *Surg Gynecol Obstet* **171**:95.

80 Nezhat C, Nezhat F, Nezhat CH (1992). Operative laparoscopy (minimally invasive surgery): state of the art. *J Gynecol Surg* **8**:111–141.

81 Velez PM (1993). Laparoscopic colonic and rectal resection. *Baillieres Clin Gastroenterol* **7**:867–869.

82 Cirocco WC, Schwartzman A, Golub RW (1994). Abdominal wall recurrence after laparoscopic colectomy for colon cancer. *Surgery* **116**:842–846.

83 Jensen A (1994). Laparoscopic-assisted colon resection. Evolution from an experimental technique to a standardized surgical procedure. *Ann Chir Gynaecol* **83**:86–91.

84 Slim K, Pezet D, Stencl J Jr *et al* (1994). Prospective analysis of 70 initial laparoscopic colorectal resections: a plea for a randomized trial. *J Laparoendoscop Surg* **4**:241–245.

85 Nezhat CR, Nezhat FR, Luciano AA, Siegler AM, Metzger DA, Nezhat CH (1995). *Operative Gynecologic Laparoscopy: Principles and Techniques*. New York: McGraw-Hill.

13   Appendectomy and omentectomy

Eric Leblanc and Denis Querleu

Appendectomy

Introduction

Appendectomy is currently one of the most frequent indications for laparoscopy in general surgery. The technique is now well codified. However, if an appendectomy is required every time an appendicitis is suspected, it can also be indicated in other circumstances. For example, since the 1980s, appendectomy has been included as part of the staging procedure for debulking adnexal tumours. Nevertheless, there has been little documentation of its true role in the literature.

Technique

Appendectomy is usually the last step in a staging operation. Thus, the patient's position should not be changed or additional ports placed. Only the two lateropelvic 5-mm and 10-mm suprapubic ports are used. One grasping forceps, a bipolar forceps and monopolar scissors are required.

After the caecoappendicular area and the position of the appendix have been checked, we perform a fully intraperitoneal appendectomy. The extremity of the appendix is grasped to expose the mesoappendix containing the appendicular vessels. These vessels are progressively desiccated with the bipolar forceps, 0.5–1 cm from the ileocaecal junction, and divided. The skeletonized appendicular base is then double ligated with Endoloops. The appendix is transected between these two sutures and removed through the 10-mm suprapubic port. The appendiceal stump is swabbed with iodine and left in the iliac fossa. This area is washed as soon as the procedure is completed.

VARIANTS

According to preferences or circumstances, the mesoappendix and/or the appendix can be managed either with extra- or intracorporeal sutures, clips or even EndoGIA. The appendix can also be exteriorized through the right-sided port orifice and ligated and cut outside the abdominal cavity; this is called the 'out' technique or the laparoscopically assisted appendectomy. Finally, the appendiceal stump is buried in the caecum with a circular purse-string suture.

For a heterotopic appendix, the adjuvant techniques described below can be helpful [1].

RETROCAECAL APPENDIX

The appendix is not immediately visible because it lays over the paracolic gutter, joined to the caecum by a short mesoappendix. A small tilt of the table to the left will facilitate rotation of the caecum and provide a better exposure of its posterior aspect and appendix. Sometimes, a retrograde operation must be performed when the appendiceal extremity is not visible. A primary transection of the base is performed with progressive withdrawal of the extremity. Haemostasis of the mesoappendix is performed close to the appendix along the dissection.

In the case of a true retrocaecal appendix which, for access, will need mobilization of the ascending colon, the risk of involvement is by definition nil and appendectomy is useless.

SUBHEPATIC APPENDIX

To facilitate the exposure and further dissections, the introduction of an accessory trocar under the right subcostal margin can be helpful. A reverse Trendelenburg with a slight left tilt of the table is recommended. As soon as the organ is correctly exposed, follow the same steps as given above for an orthotopic appendectomy.

Authors' series

Appendectomy was performed in 12 out of 22 patients with presumed stage I adnexal tumours. All appendiceal specimens were free of involvement. One complication occurred in the series: an abscess of the Douglas cul-de-sac that required surgical drainage.

Discussion

Laparoscopic appendectomy is one of the most frequently performed operations. In appendicitis, the role of laparoscopy vs laparotomy, which was initially controversial, has been established by randomized studies [2,3]. The complication rate is very low: 0–4% of complications in a large series, where the appendix had a normal appearance [4]. Most of the complications reported consisted of wound infections or intra-abdominal abcesses; but these results were from cases undergoing appendectomy for appendicitis. Other complications, such as enterocutaneous fistulae, injuries to other organs, wound herniation or trocar-site bleeding, have been reported as well but are quite rare [4].

In gynaecological oncology, appendiceal involvement has only been studied in ovarian and endometrial tumours.

OVARIAN CARCINOMA

The overall incidence of appendiceal involvement is about 30%. It is more frequent in the advanced stages (range 43–83%) and its systematic removal is justified for debulking purposes [5], especially since 20% of the appendix containing tumour appeared grossly normal in one reported study [6].

In the early stage, the indication for appendectomy is more controversial. A few studies report low rates of involvement: 4.3% in clinical stages I and II for Rose *et al.* [7] and 8.8% in stage I for Ayhan *et al.* [8]. Therefore, these authors advocate systematic appendectomy in the staging of early stage carcinoma. Another argument favouring routine appendectomy is the possibility of appendicitis associated with the carcinoma, which is kown to cause significant morbidity, particularly in elderly patients [8,9].

By contrast, appendectomy was thought to be useless for staging by other workers [5,9,10], because they did not find any involvement in their pooled series of 152 cases of stage I or II ovarian tumours.

The discovery of appendiceal involvement is important because it moves the diagnosis to a stage III, consequently implying a modification of the management, especially in stages IA or IB. Unfortunately, the appendiceal involvement is seldom isolated: in the series reported by Rose, patients who presented with appendiceal metastases always had an omental involvement (stage IIIA). This association was not pointed out by Ayhan.

In Fontanelli's study, the incidence of appendiceal involvement in the more advanced stage did not differ appreciably according to the side of the primary ovarian tumour. Appendiceal metastasis is thus one site of a general peritoneal dissemination, rather than a preferential spreading pathway.

The incidence of ovarian tumour histology has been studied by Fontanelli *et al.* [5], who reported a higher incidence of appendiceal involvement in cases of serous adenocarcinoma than in the mucinous types. This difference is considered to be due to a greater incidence of the serous tumours. Nevertheless, in cases of mucinous cystadenocarcinoma, Malfetano advocates a routine appendectomy, because these tumours are frequently metastatic from the gastrointestinal tract and the appendix can harbour the primary lesion [9].

Ayhan *et al.* [8] reported an incidence of appendiceal involvement in 6/38 non-epithelial tumours (2/15 stage I) compared with 37/94 in epithelial tumours (1/19 stage I). The difference was not statistically significant.

In second-look operations, appendiceal involvement is associated with multiple other microscopic or gross bulk tumour implants [5,7]. It has been the only site of recurrence in only one patient in Westerman's series [11].

FALLOPIAN TUBE CARCINOMA

The incidence of appendiceal metastasis in fallopian tube carcinoma has not been reported. The indication for appendectomy is the same as that in epithelial ovarian tumours.

ENDOMETRIAL CARCINOMA

In endometrial carcinoma, the appendiceal involvement is rarely isolated. In 1986 Westerman *et al.* reported a study of routine appendectomy in 233 patients who had undergone extensive gynaecological operations [11]. Among this group, 57 had an endometrial carcinoma; six appendices were metastasic (10.5%). In three cases, the appendix was macroscopically normal. In every case, appendiceal metastases were associated with other abdominal or extra-abdominal metastases. Routine appendectomy is not advocated at the time of laparoscopic management of an early endometrial carcinoma, because it does not influence the stage, the prognosis or the treatment. Conversely, if debulking surgery is carried out, appendectomy can be associated with the other procedures.

To our knowledge, appendiceal metastases have not been reported in other gynaecological malignancies.

Conclusion

Most authors reported above agree with the idea of a systematic appendectomy in advance-stage adnexal tumours as part of a maximal debulking procedure. These operations are generally performed through a laparotomy.

In earlier-stage tumours, the role of appendectomy as part of a standard laparoscopic staging procedure, which already includes multiple random peritoneal biopsies, omentectomy and comprehensive pelvic and para-aortic lymphadenectomies, is not established. However, most series are limited and the true incidence of the appendix as the sole site of extraovarian involvement is unknown. Because the morbidity is low, and the consequences of positive staging are important for patients, routine laparoscopic appendectomy may be indicated in early-stage ovarian carcinoma, especially within the framework of prospective studies.

In other gynaecological malignancies, appendectomy is indicated as part of a diagnostic laparoscopy only in cases with macroscopic abnormalities.

Omentectomy

Introduction

The great omentum is a frequent site of metastasis in gynaecological tumours, especially in adnexal carcinomata. Its involvement provides evidence of the extent of tumour outside the pelvis, worsens the prognosis and generally indicates the need for additional therapy.

As a staging procedure, laparoscopic removal of the omentum is usually an easy procedure. Conversely, as part of debulking surgery, laparoscopy is no longer indicated, because of the technical difficulties of managing huge tumour masses.

Anatomy [12]

The great omentum is a peritoneal bag that links the great curvature of the stomach to the transverse colon and falls down as an apron on the bowel loops. In infants it is thin and almost transparent; over the years it becomes fatty and can become very bulky in obese people. It is grossly square or crescent shaped. The anterior surface is fixed on the great curvature and continues to the two serosal leaves of the stomach, whereas the posterior surface is inserted on the transverse colon and close to the access to the lesser sac. Laterally, on the right side, the omentum joins the transverse mesocolon; on the left side, it reaches the left colon angulus and makes up the phrenocolic ligament, or sustentaculum lienis, on which lays the inferior pole of the spleen. Below the colon both surfaces are joined and make up the free part, or the apron, of the great omentum. The part between stomach and colon is called the gastrocolic ligament.

The great omentum has blood supplies from four or five epiploic arteries arising from both right and left gastroepiploic arteries. There is an anastomotic artery, in the posterior leaf between the right and left epiploic arteries, named Barkow's arch. This arch also gives ascending and descending branches. Omental veins are satellites of the arteries and join the portal system. Lymphatic channels are drained in the gastroepiploic nodes at the origin of the arteries, close to the pylorus for the right side and in the splenic hilus nodes for the left side. Lymphatic communications between the mesocolon and omentum can appear in cases of malignancy.

Technique

The patient is placed in the lithotomy position. As an elective procedure, four trocars are necessary: one 10-mm umbilical port for the laparoscope, two 5-mm ports laterally just above each anterior iliac spine and one 10-mm port with a 5-mm reducer under the left subcostal margin.

The instrumentation set consists of monopolar scissors, two grasping forceps and a bipolar forceps.

According to the extent of the omental resection, two techniques are described: the infracolic and the infragastric omentectomy.

INFRACOLIC OMENTECTOMY

The free part of the omentum is pushed into the upper abdomen to expose its posterior aspect. The Trendelenburg position can be slightly pronounced. Then, the omentum is grasped close to its insertion on the colon and is progressively separated from the large bowel using bipolar coagulation and sharp dissection (Fig. 13.1). This, almost bloodless, separation is performed from the left to

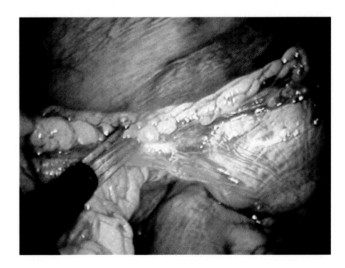

Fig. 13.1 The omentum is grabbed and stretched using Manhes forceps, then divided using monopolar cautery.

the right. Following this, the omentum is dividend from the gastrocolic ligament using the same instruments. The largest vessels are managed either with bipolar coagulation, clips or EndoGIA. When the omentum is too abundant, it is easier to divide it into two parts from the midline, before separating the two hemiomentums from the transverse colon (Fig. 13.2). If the omentum is small, it can be ligated on to the gastrocolic ligament using an Endoloop before division.

INFRAGASTRIC OMENTECTOMY

After separation from the transverse colon, the lesser sac (omental bursa) is entered (Fig. 13.3). The posterior aspect

of the stomach and the anterior part of the pancreas are clearly visible and can be checked. However, the entry into the lesser sac is not always evident. In case of difficulty, this dissection must be performed more on the left, close to the spleen. Then the dissection is carried on, up to and close to the great gastric curvature. The small vessels arising from the right gastroepiploic vessels on both sides of the stomach are desiccated with bipolar coagulation, or clipped and divided. This dissection is continued along the great curvature until the avascular area (between the right and left gastroepiploic vessels) is visible. Do not burn the stomach or injure the inferior pole of the spleen when pulling on the omentum. The frequent adhesions between the omentum and spleen can be managed with dessication-division.

On the right side, the dissection of the great curvature is completed as far as the origin of the right gastroepiploic vessels. They are divided, along with the remaining adhesions, with the gallbladder and the right colon. The whole omentum is now entirely mobilized and can be removed.

SPECIMEN REMOVAL

As soon as it is completely freed, the omentum is stored in an endoscopic bag before its removal through the abdominal wall or the vagina (Fig. 13.4).

Authors' series

Twenty-eight patients were staged for an apparent early adnexal (26 ovarian and two fallopian tube) carcinoma. The ovarian neoplasm series was composed of 13 epithelial tumours. Nine borderline tumours, three dysgermino-

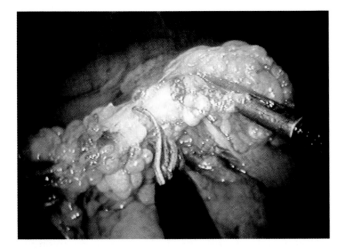

Fig. 13.2 The transverse colon is separated (infracolic omentectomy).

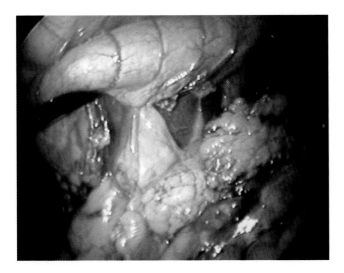

Fig. 13.3 The stomach is separated and the lesser sac is opened (infragastric omentectomy).

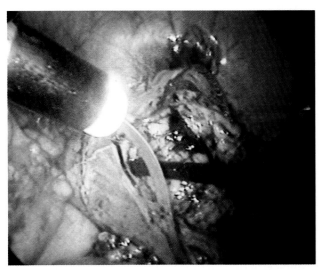

Fig. 13.4 The omentum is packed in a bag for later removal through an abdominal or vaginal minimal incision.

mata and one granulosa cell tumour. Nineteen patients were referred to our institution for a secondary laparoscopic staging, three patients were fully managed laparoscopically (two epithelial ovarian and one tubal cancer). The ages ranged from 21 to 68 years old.

Each patient had an omentectomy as part of their staging. An infracolic omentectomy was performed in 25 patients and an infragastric procedure in the other patient. In three cases the great omentum was found to be involved. Macroscopic disease was found in a borderline tumour and was associated with other positive peritoneal implants and cytology; no adjuvant treatment was administered. The second case occurred in a fallopian tube carcinoma and was the only site of metastasis. The last case was found in an invasive epithelial carcinoma. These patients were given six courses of platinum-based chemotherapy. Currently, with a median follow-up of 18 months (range 13–25 months), all 28 patients are alive with no evidence of disease.

No intraoperative or delayed complication occurred in that short series, which could be related either to omentectomy or to other steps in the staging. However, potential complications were observed, such as haemorrhages (especially in bulky fatty omentum), spleen injuries [13], and colon or gastric burns. In staging by laparotomy for early-stage ovarian carcinoma, Trimbos reported a 15% incidence of complications which were principally related to the retroperitoneal dissections [14]. Abdominal wall tumour implants seem to be a specific complication of laparoscopic management of ovarian tumours. Although the true incidence is unknown, it was estimated to be about 1% in a recent review [15], implying that endoscopic bags should be used for specimen removal.

Indications

OVARIAN CARCINOMA

Epithelial invasive carcinoma

In 1977, Green claimed that omentectomy should be associated with total abdominal hysterectomy and bilateral salpingo-oophorectomy (in [16]). Since the 1980s, the standard staging procedure has included random peritoneal biopsies, appendectomy and pelvic and infrarenal para-aortic lymphadenectomies. Reports of restaging procedures for presumed early-stage ovarian cancers revealed that 25–30% of the patients were moved up to stage III of the FIGO (International Federation of Gynecology and Obstetrics) classification [17,18]. This comprehensive staging is important in the early stages to decide whether an adjuvant treatment is indicated. Moreover, in young women with low-grade tumour in which this staging is

negative (true stage IA), conservative management can be considered to allow completion of pregnancies [19].

Technically, if no macroscopic tumour implant is visible on the free part or the gastrocolic ligament, an infracolic omentectomy seems to be adequate sampling [20].

The rates of positivity in apparent early stages ranged from 0 to 10.5%, with an average of 7.1% in a recent review of the literature [16,17,20,21]. The patient is moved to stage III of the FIGO classification. The positivity of the omentum is independent of the positivity of the other sites of spread, but is an indicator of positive para-aortic nodes [22]. Moreover, positivity of peritoneal sampling is not systematically correlated to positivity of the peritoneal cytology, because 61% of biopsy-proven peritoneal implants were found to be associated with negative cytology in Webb's series [23].

Borderline tumours

About 10% of epithelial tumours have a low malignant potential [24]. Surgery seems to be the optimal treatment in cases of borderline tumour in an apparent early stage [25,26]. The role of a staging procedure is only prognostic. Trope *et al.* reported the results of four consecutive randomized studies in 243 stage I–II borderline tumours [25]. The only recurrences occurred in four out of the 45 patients who did not undergo omentectomy. Hence, omentectomy is recommended to be routinely associated with total abdominal hysterectomy and bilateral salpingo-oophorectomy in most patients, or with unilateral adnexectomy in patients with stage I who desire to remain fertile [25]. In our series, except for two patients of more than 60 years who underwent total abdominal hysterectomy plus bilateral salpingo-oophorectomy, the others had conservative surgical therapy and staging. Laparoscopic management of borderline tumours has been reported in the literature. Darai *et al.* reported 25 cases of conservative therapy without omentectomy in the staging: four recurred, but in the pelvis only, and required additional surgery [27].

Germ cell tumours

Most of these tumours, such as dysgerminoma, immature teratoma and endodermal sinus tumour, are unilateral and occur in young women who wish to preserve their fertility. Because the prognosis is excellent in early stages, conservative management can be considered if the staging procedure is negative (this is what we did in our three cases reported above). The staging must be identical to that applied for an epithelial tumour [28]. Arakawa *et al.* reported two cases of lonely omental metastasis in dysgerminoma [29].

Sex cord tumours

The same indications can be used for the sex cord tumours, such as granulosa tumours or thecomata. Surgery is the gold standard of treatment. For metastatic tumours or poorly differentiated Sertoli–Leydig tumours, with or without heterologous elements, platinum-based chemotherapy is favoured but only modest activity can be expected [30].

FALLOPIAN TUBE CARCINOMA

There is no official FIGO staging system for the fallopian tube carcinoma and an adaptation of the staging system for ovarian carcinoma is currently used. Indeed, although tubal carcinomata are frequently diagnosed at an earlier stage than ovarian carcinomata two out of three are FIGO stage I or II, due to their development in a hollow viscus [31], their spread pattern is comparable to epithelial ovarian cancer. Therefore the surgical staging must be similar and include an omentectomy [32]. Moreover, it was the only site of dissemination in one of our two patients.

ENDOMETRIAL CARCINOMA

Positive omentum defines stage IVB in the FIGO staging system. Occult intraperitoneal spread is quite infrequent in apparent early-stage endometrial cancers. In 1987 Creasman *et al.* reported 35 cases out of 621 patients of the Gynecologic Oncology Groups (GOG) series (6%) [33], Grigsby *et al.* in 1992 reported four cases of stage 1 upstaged to IVB in 808 patients (0.4%) without detail [34], and Mangioni *et al.* reported five cases of upstaging in 1055 patients (0.5%) – two of these cases were due to positive omentum (0.2%) [35]. Thus, the role of omentectomy as a specific staging procedure in endometrial carcinoma is questionable.

Chen and Spiegel, in 1991 [36], reported a prospective study of routine omentectomy in 84 apparent stage 1 endometrial carcinoma. Omental metastases were found in seven (8.3%) of the cases; five were microscopic. Adnexal spread, papillary serous carcinoma, cul-de-sac implantation, node involvement and grade 3 tumour were the statistically significantly associated factors. The authors concluded that routine omental biopsy should be a part of the staging and, in the case of high-risk patients, an infragastric omentectomy should be considered. It could be performed as part of immediate or secondary laparoscopic staging.

Conclusion

Laparoscopic omentectomy is a safe and accurate procedure in peritoneal staging of early-stage adnexal malignancies or other gynaecological tumours which could possibly lead to occult abdominal spread. If microscopic involvement is looked for, resection of the free part is sufficient. In cases of macroscopic but apparently resectable involvement, total infragastric omentectomy is desirable. In cases of bulky tumour, laparotomy or neoadjuvant chemotherapy must be preferred. A secondary laparoscopic omentectomy can be performed in patients with apparent complete remission [37].

References

1 Pier A, Götz F (1994). Laparoscopic appendectomy, In: Cushieri A, Buess G, Pereissat J, eds. *Operative Manual of Endoscopic Surgery*. Berlin: Springer Verlag, 194–208.
2 Attwood S, Hill A, Murphy P *et al* (1992). A prospective randomized trial of laparoscopy versus open appendectomy. *Surgery* **112**:497–501.
3 Tate, J, Chung S, Lau W (1993). Laparoscopic versus open appendicectomy: prospective randomised trial. *Lancet* **342**:633–637.
4 Flowers JL (1995). Complications of appendectomy. In: Bailey RW, Flowers JL, eds. *Complications of Laparoscopic Surgery*. St Louis: Quality Medical Publishing, 161–184.
5 Fontanelli R, Paladini D, Raspagliesi F, Di Re E (1992). The role of appendectomy in surgical procedures for ovarian cancer. *Gynecol Oncol* **46**:42–44.
6 Sonnendecker E (1982). Is appendectomy mandatory in patients with ovarian carcinoma? *Am J Obstet Gynecol* **62**:978–979.
7 Rose P, Reale F, Fisher A, Hunter R (1991). Appendectomy in primary and secondary staging operations for ovarian malignancy. *Obstet Gynecol* **77**:116–118.
8 Ayhan A, Tuncer Z, Tuncer R, Yüce K, Ayhan A (1994). Is routine appendectomy beneficial in the management of ovarian cancer? *Eur J Obstet Gynecol* **57**:29–31.
9 Malfetano J (1987). The appendix and its metastatic potential in epithelial ovarian cancer. *Obstet Gynecol* **69**:396–398.
10 Bese T, Kosebay D, Kaleli S, Oz A *et al* (1996). Appendectomy in the surgical staging of ovarian carcinoma. *Int J Gynecol Obstet* **53**:249–252.
11 Westerman C, Mann W, Chumas J *et al* (1986). Routine appendectomy in extensive gynecologic operations. *Surg Gynecol Obstet* **162**:307–312.
12 Bouchet A, Cuilleret P (1991). *Anatomie topographique, descriptive et fonctionnelle*, Vol 4, 2nd edn. Paris: SIMEP.
13 Morris M, Gershenson DM, Burke TW, Wharton JT (1991). Splenectomy in gynecologic oncology, indications, complications and techniques. *Gynecol Oncol* **43**(Suppl. 2):118–122.
14 Trimbos JB (1990). Reasons for incomplete surgical staging in early ovarian carcinoma. *Gynecol Oncol* **37**:374–377.
15 Childers J, Aqua K, Surwitt E, Hallum A *et al* (1994). Abdominal-wall tumor implantation after laparoscopy for malignant conditions. *Obstet Gynecol* **84**:765–769.
16 Moore DH (1993). Primary management of early epithelial

ovarian carcinoma. In: Rubin SC, Sutton GH, eds. *Ovarian Cancer*. New York: McGraw-Hill, 498–507.

17 Young RC, Decker DG, Wharton JT *et al* (1983). Staging laparotomy in early ovarian cancer. *JAMA* **250**:3072–3076.

18 Helewa ME, Krepart GV, Lotocki R (1986). Staging laparotomy in early epithelial ovarian carcinoma. *Am J Obstet Gynecol* **154**:282.

19 Di Saia PJ, Creasman WT (1993). Epithelial ovarian cancer. In: Di Saia PJ, Creasman WT, eds. *Clinical Gynecologic Oncology*. St Louis: Mosby-Year Book, 333–425.

20 Bushbaum HJ, Brady MF, Delgado G (1989). Surgical staging of carcinoma of the ovaries. *Surg Gynecol Oncol* **169**:226–235.

21 Piver MST, Barlow JJ, Lele SB (1978). Incidence of subclinical metastasis in stage I and II ovarian carcinoma. *Obstet Gynecol* **52**:100–104.

22 Tsuruchi N, Kamura T *et al* (1993). Relationship between paraaortic lymph node involvement and intraperitoneal spread in patients with ovarian cancer—a multivariate analysis. *Gynecol Oncol* **49**:51.

23 Webb MJ (1983). The role of staging procedures in therapy. In: Grundmann E, ed. *Cancer Campaign*, Vol 7. Stuttgart: Fisher, 93–100.

24 Ozols RF, Rubin SC, Thomas G, Robboy S (1997). Epithelial ovarian cancer. In: Hoskins WJ, Perez CA, Young RC, eds. *Principles and Practice of Gynecologic Oncology*. Philadelphia: JB Lippincott: 919–986.

25 Trope C, Kaern J, Vergote I *et al* (1993). Are borderline tumors of the ovary overtreated both surgically and systematically? A review of four prospective randomized trials including 253 patients with borderline tumors. *Gynecol Oncol* **51**:236–240.

26 Kennedy AW, Hart WR (1996). Ovarian papillary serous tumor of low malignant potential. *Cancer* **78**:278–286.

27 Darai E, Teboul J, Walker F *et al* (1996). Epithelial ovarian carcinoma of low malignant potential. *Eur J Obstet Gynecol Reprod Biol* **66**:141–145.

28 Berek JS, Hacker NF (1987). Staging and second look operations in ovarian cancer. In: Piver MS, ed. *Ovarian Malignancies Diagnostic and Therapeutic Advances*. Edinburgh: Churchill Livingstone, 109–127.

29 Arakawa A, Kato N, Suzumori K, Yagami Y (1994). The two cases of the ovarian dysgerminomas. The cases with great omentum metastasis without tumor cells in ascites. *J Jpn Soc Cancer Ther* **29**:88–90.

30 Gershenson DM (1994). Management of early ovarian cancer: germ cell and sex cord – stromal tumors. *Gynecol Oncol* **55**(3 Pt 2):S62–72.

31 Markman M, Zaino R, Fleming P, Barakart R (1997). Carcinoma of the Fallopian tube. In: Hoskins WJ, Perez CA, Young RC, eds. *Principles and Practice of Gynecologic Oncology*. Philadelphia: JB Lippincott, 1025–1038.

32 Tulusan AH (1993). Cancer of the Fallopian tube. In: Burghardt E, ed. *Surgical Gynecologic Oncology*. Stuttgart: Georg Thiem Verlag 417–421.

33 Creasman WT, Morrow CP, Bundy BN *et al* (1987). Surgical pathologic spread patterns of endometrial cancer. *Cancer* **60**:2035–2041.

34 Grigsby P, Perez C, Kuten A *et al* (1992). Clinical stage 1 endometrial cancer: prognostic factors for local control and distant metastasis and implication of the new FIGO surgical staging system. *Int J Rad Oncol Biol Phys* **22**:905–911.

35 Mangioni C, De Palo G, Marubini E, Del Vecchio M (1993). Surgical pathologic staging in apparent stage 1 endometrial carcinoma. *Int J Gynecol Cancer* **3**:373–376.

36 Chen SS, Spiegel G (1991). Stage I endometrial carcinoma: role of omental biopsy and omentectomy. *J Reprod Med Obstet Gynecol* **36**:627–629.

37 Surwit E, Childers J, Atlas I, Nour K *et al* (1996). Neoadjuvant chemotherapy for advanced ovarian cancer. *Int J Gynecol Cancer* **6**:356–361.

Section 3
Adverse Effects of Laparoscopy in Gynaecological Oncology

14   Mismanagement of ovarian cancer by laparoscopy and laparotomy

Mitchell Maiman

Introduction

Ovarian carcinoma continues to be the leading cause of death from gynaecological malignancy in the USA, and the fourth most frequent cause of death from cancer in women in general. Epithelial ovarian carcinoma, which comprises about 70% of ovarian cancer, has its highest incidence in industrialized western countries. In these countries, approximately one in 70 women will develop ovarian cancer in her lifetime, and the majority will present with advanced disease. Approximately three-quarters of malignant ovarian tumours are detected only after disease has spread throughout the peritoneal cavity. Survival closely parallels the initial stage of the disease, with a favourable prognosis for women with localized cancer, but the survival rates for those with disease spread outside the pelvis are dismal. Early symptoms such as gastrointestinal disturbances, vaginal bleeding or urinary problems, while common, are very non-specific and rarely lead to early diagnosis. While routine pelvic examination of an asymptomatic adnexal mass may lead to the early diagnosis of ovarian cancer, only a small minority of neoplasms are detected by this method. Therefore, techniques that can potentially diagnose ovarian cancer in the pre-metastatic phase are likely to have a significant impact on subsequent outcome. Similarly, any delays in diagnosis or therapy or faulty application of oncological principles could have a potentially negative effect.

Patterns of spread

The surgical staging and management of ovarian carcinoma is based on our understanding of the natural history of the disease and its pattern of spread. In most cases, early growth is confined to the ovary, after which tumour penetration through the ovarian capsule occurs, allowing malignant cells to spread throughout the peritoneal cavity. In approximately 10% of patients, the ovarian lesion is not the primary event, and histological evidence of extraovarian disease is apparent with normal sized ovaries. Such cases of 'peritoneal cancer' are particularly unamenable to early diagnosis. As ovarian cancer progresses, cells follow the normal circulation of peritoneal fluid, and intra-abdominal implantation occurs in areas such as the paracolic gutters, the undersurface of the right diaphragm, the cul-de-sac, the pelvic and peritoneal surfaces, the serosa of the small intestine, the rectosigmoid and, most commonly, the omentum. While peritoneal involvement is the dominant mode of spread, retroperitoneal involvement via lymph nodes that drain the ovary is also quite common, and may occur early in the disease process. Para-aortic and paracaval lymph nodes up to the level of the renal vessels are the most commonly involved, but pelvic and inguinal node metastases are frequently encountered. Transdiaphragmatic spread to the lymph nodes on the thoracic surface of the diaphragm may lead to pleural effusions, and a right-sided malignant pleural effusion is frequently the first extraperitoneal manifestation. Haematogenous spread of ovarian cancer to the liver, bone and central nervous system is rare, and usually a late manifestation. Extrinsic compression of the small and large bowel and involvement of the myenteric plexus leads to impaired motility, and patients eventually die as a result of functional intestinal obstruction, increasing intraperitoneal tumour volume and progressive starvation.

Surgical staging

Ovarian carcinoma is surgically staged, and thorough evaluation of all areas at risk of neoplastic disease must be performed. It is critically important that correct and optimal surgery is executed during the initial surgical attempt, as an incomplete evaluation may adversely affect the patient's prognosis and contribute to future morbidity. A vertical abdominal incision, preferably supraumbilical, is recommended because of limited access to the upper abdomen through low transverse incisions. Upon entering the abdomen, aspiration of ascites or peritoneal lavage should be performed to obtain multiple cytological specimens of the pelvis, paracolic gutters and undersurface of the diaphragm before surgical manipulation is initiated.

Exploration of the entire abdomen and pelvis, including all intestinal surfaces, should next be performed to define the extent of disease. In patients with advanced disease, the goal of surgery is optimal cytoreduction and tumour debulking, while the emphasis in cases of apparent early disease is on careful surgical staging. Frozen section should be sent to confirm the diagnosis of cancer and define the histological type. Total abdominal hysterectomy and bilateral salpingo-oophorectomy is the procedure of choice, with intact tumour removal. In cases of bulky pelvic disease, a retroperitoneal approach can facilitate a safe and effective resection. Omentectomy, pelvic and para-aortic lymph-node sampling, and biopsies of the paracolic gutters, cul-de-sac, lateral pelvic walls, vesicouterine reflection, subdiaphragmatic area and any adhesions, as well as random peritoneal biopsies, should be performed.

The 1986 FIGO staging system is most commonly used in the assignment of surgical stage (Table 14.1). After proper staging, most ovarian cancer patients have advance-stage disease. Patients with disease confined to the ovaries are designated as stage I, while those with only pelvic spread are considered stage II. Stage III disease includes intraperitoneal disease or positive retroperitoneal or inguinal nodes. The substage is assigned based on the size of the largest tumour nodule. Stage IV disease involves liver parenchyma, or it may be diagnosed by documenting cytologically positive pleural fluid or supraclavicular adenopathy. The histological grade is assigned in all cases, and is a particularly important prognostic factor.

While, in general, the management of early-stage invasive epithelial ovarian carcinoma is total abdominal hysterectomy and bilateral salpingo-oophorectomy, omentectomy, pelvic and para-aortic lymph-node biopsies, multiple peritoneal biopsies, diaphragmatic evaluation and peritoneal washings, carefully selected patients with stage IA grade I tumours who wish to maintain their fertility may be considered for a unilateral ovarian procedure. There is never a role for partial ovarian excision or ovarian cystectomy, and capsular rupture is best avoided. In contrast to this approach, patients with germ cell tumours of the ovary rarely require bilateral salpingo-oophorectomy and hysterectomy, and the future reproductive capacity of these typically young patients can usually be maintained. The bilaterality rate of most malignant germ cell tumours is almost zero, except for the dysgerminoma where the opposite ovary may be involved in 15–20% of cases. This requires careful evaluation of the contralateral ovary with liberal biopsy. Therefore, conservative management, unilateral salpingo-oophorectomy and surgical staging is usually the procedure of choice. In patients with ovarian stromal tumours, most commonly granulosa cell tumours, unilateral conservative procedures and surgical staging may also be considered in instances of confined unilateral involvement in patients who wish to maintain their fertility. In peri- or postmenopausal patients, however, total abdominal hysterectomy and bilateral salpingo-oophorectomy is the procedure of choice. Ovarian cystectomy alone is contraindicated in stromal tumours. In addition, careful evaluation of the endometrium is required, as the high oestrogen levels associated with granulosa cell tumours often result in endometrial hyperplasia or carcinoma. Ovarian epithelial tumours of low malignant potential

Table 14.1 FIGO (International Federation of Gynecology and Obstetrics; 1986) staging system for ovarian cancer.

Stage	Characteristic
I	Growth limited to the ovaries
IA	Growth limited to one ovary; no ascites; no tumour on the external surfaces; capsule intact
IB	Growth limited to both ovaries; no ascites; no tumour on the external surfaces; capsule intact
IC	Tumour either stage IA or stage IB but with tumour on the surface of one or both ovaries, or with capsule ruptured, or with ascites containing malignant cells or with positive peritoneal washings
II	Growth involving one or both ovaries on pelvic extension
IIA	Extension or metastases to the uterus or tubes
IIB	Extension to other pelvic tissues
IIC	Tumour either stage IIA or stage IIB with tumour on the surface of one or both ovaries, or with capsule(s) ruptured, or with ascites containing malignant cells or with positive peritoneal washings
III	Tumour involving one or both ovaries with peritoneal implants outside the pelvis or positive retroperitoneal or inguinal nodes; superficial liver metastases equals stage III; tumour is limited to the true pelvis but with histologically verified malignant extension to small bowel or omentum
IIIA	Tumour grossly limited to the true pelvis with negative nodes but with histologically confirmed microscopic seeding of abdominal peritoneal surfaces
IIIB	Tumour of one or both ovaries; histologically confirmed implants of abdominal peritoneal surfaces, none exceeding 2 cm in diameter; nodes negative
IIIC	Abdominal implants greater than 2 cm in diameter or positive retroperitoneal or inguinal nodes
IV	Growth involving one or both ovaries with distant metastases; if pleural effusion is present, there must be positive cytological test results to allot a case to stage IV; parenchymal liver metastases equals stage IV

can be managed by unilateral procedures plus complete surgical staging in younger patients wishing to retain their fertility, and total abdominal hysterectomy and bilateral salpingo-oophorectomy in women who have completed their families. While case studies of ovarian cystectomy alone have been reported with good results, this should only be considered in patients without a contralateral ovary or in instances of bilateral tumour involvement in the younger patient. In cases of mucinous tumours, whether benign, borderline or malignant, appendectomy should be performed. When cases of metastatic disease to the ovary from a non-gynaecological primary site (breast, gastrointestinal tract) are encountered, typical ovarian cancer surgical staging is not necessary and oophorectomy with removal of gross pelvic disease is usually sufficient.

Surgical mismanagement

Surgical mismanagement of ovarian carcinoma unfortunately occurs with glaring frequency, and misstaging of ovarian cancer is possible whether the initial approach is laparoscopy or laparotomy. The consequences of surgical mismanagement are profound, and directly affect patient care. If effective cytoreduction is not accomplished, undiscovered residual disease will leave the patient in a suboptimal state after adjuvant cytotoxic chemotherapy. Understaging may also lead to undertreatment, and prevent advance-stage patients from receiving appropriate standard therapy or benefiting from experimental protocols. In addition, reoperation for complete staging may be considered, exposing the patient to a second major operative procedure. Finally, accurate prognosis counselling will be hampered, which may lead to unrealistic expectations and poor compliance.

Many studies have documented the misstaging of ovarian cancer and the impact of specialty training. McGowen *et al.* [1] examined the thoroughness of intraoperative evaluation of 191 women with ovarian cancer, and found that while gynaecological oncologists performed appropriate surgical staging in 97% of cases, gynaecologists and general surgeons adequately surgically evaluated only 56% and 35% of patients respectively. Community hospital surgeons were more likely to incorrectly stage patients than those in teaching hospitals. In a significant number of cases handled by general surgeons or general gynaecologists, no stage was noted in the medical records. This data has important implications concerning the laparascopic approach to the adnexal mass, as most endoscopists performing such procedures are not gynaecological oncologists. The most common procedure omitted in determining extent of disease was the evaluation of diaphragmatic undersurfaces, but other commonly omitted procedures included peritoneal biopsies, cytology, omental, bowel and pelvic biopsies, and lymph-node evaluation. Young *et al.* [2], in a study of ovarian cancer patients believed to have stage I or II disease after initial surgery, found that rigorous staging laparotomies upstage the disease for many patients initially thought to have a localized problem. Almost one-third of patients were upstaged after re-exploration, three-quarters of whom actually had stage III disease. In addition, only 25% had the vertical supraumbilical incision felt adequate for proper staging. Results from other studies confirm these concepts. Bagley *et al.* [3] found an approximately 30% discrepancy between reported surgical findings by non-oncological surgeons and the definitive stage demonstrated after reoperation by a gynaecological oncologist. Piver *et al.* [4] reported that unsuspected diaphragmatic and para-aortic nodal metastases resulted in upstaging in 11% of stage I and 23% of stage II patients.

A study by Mayer *et al.* [5] examined not only the issue of physician's specialty in ovarian cancer staging but also its impact on survival. Twenty-six patients with ovarian cancer operated on by gynaecological oncologists were compared with 21 patients operated on by gynaecologists or general surgeons, with all patients receiving adjunctive combination chemotherapy with cisplatin, doxorubicin and cyclophosphamide postoperatively. Five-year actuarial survival and disease-free survival, respectively, for stage I and II patients surgically staged by a gynaecological oncologist were 83% and 76%, compared with 59% ($P < 0.05$) and 39% ($P < 0.03$) for the group operated on by non-oncologists. All patients operated on by gynaecological oncologists were left with no residual disease, compared with about half the patients operated on by non-oncologists. The only significant poor prognostic factor identified in the study was the specialty of the operating surgeon. This study highlights the potential negative impact of initial suboptimal surgical management of ovarian carcinoma.

Laparoscopic approach to the adnexal mass

While some issues concerning the surgical mismanagement of ovarian cancer are common to both laparotomy and laparoscopy, there are unique problems and considerations specific to the laparoscopic approach. Despite the initial absence of data comparing operative laparoscopy with laparotomy for this indication, enthusiasm for the significant technological advances led to dramatic increases in such therapeutic procedures. The benefits of the laparoscopic approach for benign ovarian lesions are numerous. Patient morbidity may be dramatically reduced by avoidance of an abdominal incision, prolonged hospitalization may be avoided, and postoperative pain significantly lessened. In addition, overall medical costs may be substantially decreased. Because most cystic adnexal masses are benign, proper application of this method has a definitive positive impact on the gynaecological health care of women. However, many physicians have been concerned that perhaps, in this setting, technology has progressed faster than education and proper indications for utilization. In a survey of members of the Society of Gynecologic Oncologists (SGO), 29 surgeons reported 42 cases of laparoscopic excision of ovarian neoplasms subsequently found to be malignant [6]. Potential problems with the laparoscopic management of pelvic masses include inappropriate surgical procedures, incomplete surgical staging, inadequate patient preparation and delays in definitive therapy. What has evolved from these concerns is a consensus need for strict preoperative criteria and intraoperative protocols that can guide the laparoscopist and promote optimal patient care.

Adverse outcomes from laparoscopic excision of ovarian neoplasms, which are subsequently found to be malignant, can come from three potential sources: improper patient selection, incorrect application of the principles of surgical oncology and complications associated with the laparoscopic procedure, such as abdominal wall metastases via laparoscopic puncture sites or poorer prognosis from capsular rupture. Careful patient selection is the critical issue. Numerous authors have demonstrated that the inadvertent finding of ovarian malignancy can be minimized by applying cautious preoperative criteria. Nezhat *et al.* [7] diagnosed only four ovarian cancers during laparoscopic management of 1011 women with adnexal masses. In studies of postmenopausal women, Mann and Reich [8] found only one of 44 patients to have ovarian cancer at the time of proposed laparoscopic adnexectomy, while Parker and Berek [9] reported 25 consecutive cases of benign ovarian lesions. Thus, strict preoperative selection criteria may substantially reduce the chance of encountering a malignancy.

A strong family history of ovarian cancer, or a personal or family history of breast, endometrial or colon cancer, should be taken very seriously, and should be considered a relative contraindication to the laparoscopic approach. Three distinct types of hereditary ovarian cancer have been identified. Site-specific ovarian cancer, in which two first-degree relatives have had the disease, may be associated with an autosomal dominant trait that places an individual at a 50% chance of developing ovarian cancer. Women who develop such familial ovarian cancer are usually diagnosed 10–15 years younger than the typical patient who develops the disease. Another familial pattern occurs in women who develop ovarian cancer with a strong familial predisposition for breast cancer. Such women may be at three to five times the risk for the development of ovarian cancer. The third syndrome, the Lynch type II cancer family syndrome, is characterized by the inheritance of non-polyposis colorectal cancer, endometrial cancer and ovarian cancer [10]. Affected women may be at two to four times the risk for ovarian cancer. Even women with non-autosomal dominant genotypes with only one first-degree relative with ovarian cancer are at increased risk, probably at least two to three times normal. Although familial ovarian cancer probably only occurs in 5% of cases overall, laparotomy may be the safer approach in such individuals with morphologically abnormal ovarian masses.

The incidence of epithelial ovarian cancer increases with age, with a median age of diagnosis of 61 years. Therefore, a far more cautious approach to the operative laparoscopic route must be taken in the postmenopausal or perimenopausal patient than in women in their reproductive years. However, it must be recognized that ovarian cancer is not rare in women under the age of 50, especially in those who are nulliparous. In addition, nonepithelial ovarian malignancies occur at younger ages, with the average age of women with malignant germ cell tumors being only 19. In the Society of Gynecologic Oncologist's survey study [6], the average age of patients who subsequently had malignancy was 44 for epithelial tumours and 31 for germ cell tumours, significantly younger and older than the national averages, respectively. Laparoscopic surgeons must fully realize, therefore, that while age is an important part of the patient selection equation, there is no age group in which ovarian cancer does not occur.

In this age of increasing reliance on technology, the value of pelvic examination in the evaluation of an adnexal mass is too often overlooked. Palpation of an asymptomatic adnexal mass during routine pelvic examination is still the most common method of detection for early-stage ovarian cancer. The information obtained during pelvic examination may be complementary and additive to the morphological assessment provided by ultrasonography. Location, mobility, degree of tenderness and consistency are important clinical parameters that aid in the diagnosis. In addition, pelvic examination is invaluable in differentiating a uterine from an ovarian mass. Metastatic ovarian cancer may be diagnosed by finding vaginal or cervical lesions, enlarged inguinal or supraclavicular lymph nodes, evidence of an umbilical hernia or new onset pelvic relaxation. These findings may occur in the absence of ascites or intraperitoneal spread. It is critical to understand that extraovarian disease can occur even with slightly enlarged or normal size ovaries, and therefore the isolated use of sonography as the sole method of evaluating the patient may often be misleading.

Pelvic ultrasonography is probably the most important diagnostic tool in determining whether the laparoscopic approach to an adnexal mass is appropriate. Transvaginal sonography, by virtue of higher frequency transducers, has produced a significant improvement in image resolution and morphological detail compared with transabdominal ultrasound. In general, the sonographic patterns listed below are necessary prerequisites to insure a high probability of benign pathology.

1 *Size.* Although there is no absolute 'cut-off point', ovarian cysts should be less than 8–10 cm. There is a positive correlation between increasing size and increasing risk of malignancy.

2 *Septations.* If present, these should be thin and simple. Complex thick septa (>2 mm) suggest malignancy.

3 *Cystic vs solid.* The mass should be purely cystic with no solid areas. Solid areas imply malignancy. The exception to this is the mature cystic teratoma (dermoid cyst) which has a characteristic sonographic appearance based on the interface of highly echogenic areas such as bone or teeth with sebaceous material and fat.

4 *Borders.* The borders should be regular and even. Irregular borders or unclear margins suggest cancer.

5 *Laterality.* Bilaterality implies malignancy. The mass should be unilateral with a well-visualized normal contralateral ovary. While many benign lesions are bilateral, the frequency of bilaterality increases as we go from benign to borderline to frankly invasive tumours.

6 *Free fluid.* There should be little or no free pelvic fluid. Ascites is an absolute contraindication to the laparoscopic approach.

7 *Papillations.* There should be no evidence of papillary excrescences, either internal or external. Internal excrescences alone suggest tumours of low malignant potential, while surface excrescences or nodularity suggest frankly invasive tumours.

8 *Supporting structures.* Matted loops of intestine or complex and extensive adhesions suggest malignancy.

Ultrasonography is more accurate in predicting which masses are benign than which masses are malignant. Using such strict criteria, some authors have accurately predicted benign masses in 92–96% of cases. However, Benacerraf *et al.* [11] reported that sonography was frankly misleading in 15% of cases, while Herrmann *et al.* [12] reported only a 73% positive predictive value in diagnosing malignancy. Luxman *et al.* [13] found two of 33 patients with a simple cyst smaller than 5 cm in diameter had malignant ovarian tumours. DePriest *et al.* [14] utilized a morphology index to characterize the sonographic appearance of ovarian tumours and included a quantitative scoring system examining volume, cyst wall and

septa structure. Tumours with a score of less than five were uniformly benign, while an index score greater than 5 had a positive predictive value for malignancy of 45%. In the Society of Gynecologic Oncologists survey study [6], 31% of cases found to be malignant were reported to have so-called 'benign' characteristics. Therefore, it must be recognized that finding ovarian malignancy is possible even when stringent ultrasonographic criteria are applied, and the ability to diagnose and surgically manage patients immediately and effectively is mandatory.

Appropriate serum tumour markers should be sent on all patients for whom the laparoscopic approach is considered, for two reasons: (i) as a complimentary test to sonography to aid in diagnosis; and (ii) as a baseline value to assist in follow-up should malignancy be found. The choice of tumour marker depends on the age of the patient and the suspected ovarian neoplasm based on other clinical parameters. Young patients in whom germ cell tumours are suspected should be tested for beta-human chorionic gonadotrophin (β-HCG), alpha-fetoprotein and lactate dehydrogenase. If stromal tumours are considered, then androgen and oestrogen levels are appropriate. CA-125 levels, which are elevated in the serous subtype of epithelial ovarian cancer in 85% of cases, should be evaluated in every patient, and carcinoembryonic antigen (CEA) analysed if a mucinous tumour is in the differential diagnosis. The addition of a normal CA-125 to benign ultrasound evaluation in preoperative screening may significantly increase the predictive value of a negative test; this value increased from 71% to 100% in postmenopausal women in one study [15]. CA-125 is elevated in a variety of conditions other than ovarian cancer, such as peritonitis, liver and renal disease, adenocarcinoma of non-ovarian origin and pregnancy. In premenopausal women, there is a higher prevalence of benign gynaecological conditions, such as leiomyomata uteri, endometriosis and pelvic inflammatory disease, that produce elevated CA-125 levels. Therefore, CA-125 is of limited value as a screening test in women of reproductive age unless an extremely high level is encountered. However, these other benign conditions tend to drop out in the postmenopausal patients. The combination of an adnexal mass and elevated CA-125 (>35) in the postmenopausal patient represents a contraindication to the laparoscopic approach, and prompt surgical evaluation via laparotomy is indicated.

Frozen-section analysis of ovarian tumours adds an extremely important element to the diagnostic evaluation, and should be carried out in virtually all cases of laparoscopic excision of ovarian neoplasms. Multiple studies have shown that the accuracy of this technique is consistently over 90% [16]. It does have limitations, however, particularly in differentiating benign from borderline and borderline from frankly malignant epithelial ovarian tumours. This can be partially overcome by serial sectioning and sampling in difficult or equivocal cases [12]. The additive information conveyed by frozen section may, in properly prepared patients with appropriate informed consent, obviate the need for a second surgery by changing the immediate operative strategy. If malignancy is histologically confirmed intraoperatively, laparotomy and surgical staging are indicated through a midline vertical incision. In all cases of invasive cancer and in most cases of tumours of low malignant potential (except in patients without a contralateral ovary who want to retain their fertility), one must proceed from ovarian cystectomy to oophorectomy. Decisions concerning the preservation of other reproductive structures, removal of the appendix in mucinous tumours and surgical management of endometriosis can also be made. In complicated or equivocal cases, the surgeon should discuss the findings in depth with the pathologist and consult a gynaecological oncologist before committing to definitive surgery.

Perhaps the most controversial issue concerning the laparoscopic approach to ovarian masses is that of capsular rupture. Capsular rupture can and should be avoided in the majority of cases. Attempts at ovarian cystectomy with the inherent risk of capsular rupture should be considered only in selected patients. In all postmenopausal and perimenopausal women, and some younger women, there may be no role for ovarian cystectomy. In addition, if any pelvic or peritoneal signs of malignancy are present, or if external ovarian excrescences are visible, ovarian cystectomy and laparoscopic puncture are contraindicated. It is only in the younger reproductive age patient with a supposedly benign cyst, dermoid cyst or endometriosis, that this issue is appropriate.

There are three theoretical reasons for avoiding laparoscopic violation of the ovarian capsule. First, if a borderline or frankly malignant ovarian tumour is encountered, capsular rupture may adversely alter the prognosis. This concept is controversial and the data are conflicting. Several studies have found no change in prognosis from intraoperative tumour rupture [17], while other studies suggest that rupture may adversely affect prognosis [18]. In the most recent study, Sainz de la Cuesta *et al.* [19] concluded that intraoperative rupture of malignant epithelial ovarian neoplasms worsened the prognosis of patients with stage I disease, with an associated hazard ratio exceeding 6.5 and a comparative reduction in survival. Virtually all authors agree that if spillage of ovarian contents occurs, copious irrigation and suction, followed by immediate surgical management, are necessary. A critical issue, therefore, is immediate, not delayed, surgical treatment and staging, for there is no evidence to support the

safety of delayed definitive management after capsular rupture of ovarian neoplasia. Unfortunately, this lack of preparation and poor operative judgement was evident in the cases in the Society of Gynecologic Oncologists' survey study [6], where the mean interval to subsequent laparotomy after laparoscopic diagnosis was 4.8 weeks.

Second, capsular rupture of ovarian cancer at the time of laparoscopy may alter the pattern of subsequent recurrence. This concept, too, is controversial, but some investigators have reported aggressive tumour implantation after laparoscopic biopsy, and tumour seeding of the laparoscopic tract, umbilicus and suprapubic trocar sites. Recently, Gleeson *et al.* reported three cases of abdominal wall metastases at the site of insertion of laparoscopic trocars, one of which occurred in a tumour of low malignant potential [20]. Such cutaneous implants in laparotomy scars after surgery for ovarian cancer are virtually unheard of. However, Childers *et al.* [21] have reported that tumour implantation at the abdominal wall puncture site is an infrequent occurrence after laparoscopy in patients with ovarian cancer (0.2%), and recommended irrigation of all abdominal puncture sites to decrease its likelihood. The proposed mechanisms for this occurrence after laparoscopy include increased abdominal pressure from pneumoperitoneum or displacement of malignant cells outside the protected intraperitoneal environment and its restraining factors.

Third, intraoperative spillage of even benign tumours can have adverse consequences. This complication is probably rare, it can occur even at the time of laparotomy, and it can theoretically occur in two disease processes.
1 Spillage of gelatinous material in mucinous tumours may initiate pseudomyxoma peritonei, a chronic debilitating and potentially fatal disease that occurs in both benign and malignant tumours.
2 Rupture of ovarian teratomata, which can induce severe chemical peritonitis, granulomata and adhesions.

In both examples, copious irrigation, peritoneal lavage and appropriate surgical treatment carried out immediately after diagnosis may make the risk of such spillage negligible.

Simple aspiration of ovarian cysts, without cyst removal or histological analysis, has recently been attempted and is to be condemned. A benign ovarian cystadenoma may recur if the cyst wall is not removed, and such high recurrence rates (54%) have been demonstrated by some authors [22]. In addition, lack of histology cannot ultimately reassure the physician of a non-malignant diagnosis. Finally, the accuracy of cytological analysis of cyst fluid is unreliable and inaccurate. The absence of malignant cells in aspirated fluid does not guarantee benignity, and false-positive results may lead to an unnecessary radical approach. If the ovarian cyst is functional, then one must question the need for any surgical intervention, as most will spontaneously resolve over time. Because it is unknown whether benign ovarian neoplasms of epithelial origin undergo malignant transformation, simple cyst fluid aspiration, with retention of the cyst wall, in general, cannot be justified.

Proper counselling and informed consent is critical to the concept of surgeon and patient preparation. While strict preoperative selection criteria will lead to properly executed operative laparoscopy in the majority of cases, the possibility of both exploratory laparotomy and ovarian cancer must be discussed with the patient and be included in the consent form. Laparotomy may be necessary, not only if ovarian cancer is detected, but also if laparoscopic complications such as haemorrhage or intestinal injury are unexpectedly encountered. Patients should be prepared for the possibility of hysterectomy and staging, even if the chances seem remote. In addition, they should understand that the type of operation may be dictated, in part, by the frozen-section analysis and that immediate definitive surgery is preferable to delayed treatment if cancer is found. The type of incision that may be necessary should also be discussed. As an increasing number of laparoscopic procedures are performed as outpatient procedures, full facilities for performing ovarian cancer surgery remain an important prerequisite. Frozen-section analysis, blood product administration and the necessary surgical instruments for the completion of oncological procedures must be at hand. If the laparoscopist has no special expertise in the management of gynaecological malignancy, intraoperative consultation with a gynaecological oncologist should be available.

When approaching the adnexal mass by laparoscopy, the steps listed below are recommended.

1 Peritoneal washings should be obtained.

2 The upper abdomen should be explored, including diaphragmatic undersurfaces, the liver, intestinal and peritoneal surfaces and the omentum. Any abnormal areas should be biopsied, and the diagnosis of malignancy will necessitate laparotomy through a vertical incision.

3 The pelvis, including cul-de-sac, bladder undersurface and serosa of sigmoid colon, should be explored.

4 The ovarian mass can then be investigated with frozen-section analysis.

The laparoscopic approach to the pelvic mass offers the potential for safe and effective minimally invasive surgery. The rational application of such techniques is one of the true recent surgical advances in gynaecology. The use of strict preoperative criteria and intraoperative protocols can minimize the chance of inadvertent management of ovarian cancer. Regardless of the level of caution exercised, the possibility that an apparently benign ovarian mass will prove to be malignant exists, and sound surgical and oncological principles must always be applied.

References

1 McGowan L, Parent-Lesher L, Norris HJ, Barnett M (1985). Misstaging of ovarian cancer. *Obstet Gynecol* **65**:568–572.

2 Young RC, Decker DG, Wharton JT *et al* (1983). Staging laparotomy in early ovarian cancer. *JAMA* **250**:3072–3076.

3 Bagley CM, Young RC, Schern PS, Chabner PS, Devita VT (1973). Ovarian carcinoma metastatic to the diaphragm frequently underdiagnosed at laparotomy: a preliminary report. *Am J Obstet Gynecol* **116**:397–400.

4 Piver MS, Barlow JJ, Lele SB (1978). Incidence of subclinical metastases in stage I and II ovarian carcinoma. *Obstet Gynecol* **52**:100–104.

5 Mayer A, Chambers S, Graves E *et al* (1992). Ovarian cancer staging: does it require a gynecologic oncologist? *Gynecol Oncol* **47**:223–227.

6 Maiman M, Seltzer V, Boyce J (1991). Laparoscopic excision of ovarian neoplasms subsequently found to be malignant. *Obstet Gynecol* **77**:563–565.

7 Nezhat F, Nezhat C, Welander CE, Benigno B (1992). Four ovarian cancers diagnosed during laparoscopic management of 1011 women with adnexal masses. *Am J Obstet Gynecol* **167**:790–796.

8 Mann WJ, Reich H (1992). Laparoscopic adnexectomy in postmenopausal women. *J Reprod Med* **137**:254–256.

9 Parker WH, Berek JS (1990). Management of selected cystic adnexal masses in postmenopausal women by operative laparoscopy: a pilot study. *Am J Obstet Gynecol* **163**:1574–1577.

10 Lynch HS, Beurta C, Lynch JF (1986). Familial ovarian carcinoma. *Am J Med* **81**:1073.

11 Benacerraf B, Finkler N, Wojciechowski C, Knapp R (1990). Sonographic accuracy in the diagnosis of ovarian masses. *J Reprod Med* **35**:491–495.

12 Herrmann V, Locher G, Goldhirsch A (1987) Sonographic patterns of ovarian tumours: prediction of malignancy. *Obstet Gynecol* **69**:777–781.

13 Luxman D, Bergman A, Sagi J, David M (1991). The postmenopausal adnexal mass: correlation between ultrasonic and pathologic findings. *Obstet Gynecol* **77**:726–728.

14 DePriest PD, Shenson D, Fried A *et al* (1993). A morphology index based on sonographic findings in ovarian cancer. *Gynecol Oncol* **51**:7–11.

15 Finkler N, Benacerraf B, Lavin F, Wojciechowski S, Knapp RC (1988). Comparison of serum CA125, clinical impression and ultrasound in the preoperative evaluation of ovarian masses. *Obstet Gynecol* **72**:659–663.

16 Obiakor I, Maiman M, Mittal K, Awobuluyi M, DiMaio T, Demopoulos R (1991). The accuracy of frozen section in the diagnosis of ovarian neoplasms. *Gynecol Oncol* **43**:61–63.

17 Dembo AJ, Davy M, Stenwig AE, Berle EJ, Bush RS, Kjorstad K (1990). Prognostic factors in patients with stage I epithelial ovarian cancer. *Obstet Gynecol* **75**:263–273.

18 Hsiu J, Given F, Kemp G (1986). Tumor implantation after diagnostic laparoscopic biopsy of serous ovarian tumors of low malignant potential. *Obstet Gynecol* **68**:905–935.

19 Sainz de la Cuesta R, Goff B, Fuller A, Nikrui N, Eichhorn J, Rice L (1994). Prognostic importance of intraoperative rupture of malignant ovarian epithelial neoplasms. *Obstet Gynecol* **84**:1–7.

20 Gleeson N, Nicosia SV, Mark JE, Hoffman MS, Cavanagh D (1993). Abdominal wall metastases from ovarian cancer after laparoscopy. *Am J Obstet Gynecol* **169**:522–523.

21 Childers J, Aqua K, Surwit E, Hallum A, Hatch K (1994). Abdominal-wall tumor implantation after laparoscopy for malignant conditions. *Obstet Gynecol* **84**:765–769.

22 Lipitz S, Seidman DS, Menczer J *et al* (1992). Recurrence rate after fluid aspiration from sonographically benign-appearing ovarian cysts. *Reprod Med* **37**:845–848.

15   Complications of laparoscopic surgery in gynaecology and gynaecological oncology

Matthew O. Burrell, Joel M. Childers, Mark D. Adelson, Camran Nezhat, Farr Nezhat and Ceana H. Nezhat

Introduction

Laparoscopy, once the sole purview of gynaecologists for almost 20 years, has now become commonplace in the practice of urologists and general surgeons. By the same token, the number of reports of complications have correlated well with the expansion of applications. It would seem that some perverse Murphy's law is in force, for example, 'if something can go wrong, it will'. Without question, the chief problem is the operating surgeon. Several reports corroborate that there is a learning curve, not only for each new gynaecological surgeon, but also for each new procedure [1,2]. The next problem is the patient who, by virtue of past abdominal surgery, obesity or compromised pulmonocardiovascular function, seems destined for disaster [3]. Lastly, there is the opportunity for blaming either the instruments, the anaesthetic staff or the nursing staff, for a variety of problems ranging from minor frustration to major injury.

It seems artificial to separate the complications of general gynaecology arising during laparoscopy for endometriosis, adnexal cysts, tubal sterilization and myomectomies from those of gynaecological oncology occurring during extensive dissection and lymphadenectomies. Indeed, the majority of complications are encountered as often by general gynaecologists as by gynaecological oncologists. They both will experience the same high-risk patients, adhesions, adnexal masses, port-entry problems, potential bowel and vascular injuries. Some problems, however, will be uniquely experienced by the gynaecological oncologist. Therefore, the remainder of this chapter has been partitioned into section A, reporting on complications of laparoscopy encountered both by the general gynaecologist and the gynaecological oncologist, and section B, focusing on the problems unique to the gynaecological oncologist using laparoscopy.

A: Complications of laparoscopy in both general gynaecology and gynaecological oncology

Smith et al. [4] have recently reported on the complications encountered by 42 board-eligible or board-certified gynaecologists performing 127 advanced gynaecological laparoscopies at a general hospital in Seattle. He defined 'interruptive' complications as including haemorrhage, perforation, anaesthesia problems, fluid overload and technical problems. 'Technical' problems referred to difficulty with instrumentation or other procedures, resulting in a prolongation of operative time or failure to complete the proposed surgery. 'Postoperative' complications included unplanned prolonged patient stay in hospital, the need for transfusion, and febrile or infectious episodes. These complications occurred in 13% of 46 patients treated for ectopic pregnancy, no patients out of 11 treated for non-ovarian adnexal masses, 17% of 38 patients treated for ovarian pathology, 31% of 16 patients treated with myomectomy, 60% of 15 laparoscopally assisted vaginal hysterectomies and 55% of nine patients treated for lysis of dense adhesions. The author reflects the opinions of many, in stating that the benefits often do not outweigh the risks. Before dismissing all such procedures as too risky, it must be recognized that only one-third of the gynaecologists performed more than five procedures. With experience, the incidence of time delays, entry problems and postoperative morbidity can be expected to decrease. This chapter reflects the need to better 'grade' complications. Table 15.1 outlines the grading of complications.

National statistics

The serious complication rate, involving grades IV, V and VI in Table 15.1, have remained low in many national surveys despite the increased use of laparoscopy. The American Association of Gynecologic Laparoscopists carried out a membership survey on complications in 1988 [5]. A total of 880 respondents (24%) performed 36928

Table 15.1 Severity of complications associated with laparoscopy.

Grade	Complications
I	Not involving direct injury to patients: prolonged operating time, injury to personnel from cuts, burns, viral transmission, frustration/stress associated with malfunctioning equipment or poor visualization
II	To the patient but corrected immediately without laparotomy: excessive bleeding, most subcutaneous emphysema, corrected vascular injuries, transient anaesthesia problems
III	Resulting in prolonged morbidity but not prolonged hospitalization: postoperative pain, neural injuries, persistent trophoblastic tissue, neoplastic implantation, some hernias
IV	Resulting in hospital stays greater than 72 hours not involving a laparotomy: prolonged ileus, serious cardiovascular problems, bowel, bladder or ureteral injuries repaired laparoscopically, postoperative febrile episodes
V	Switch to a laparotomy not resulting from injury: massive adhesions, poor visualization, equipment failure, recognition that a laparotomy is more appropriate for the pathology
VI	Death or immediate or delayed injuries resulting in a laparotomy: many ureteral, bowel or bladder injuries, trocar or needle injuries to bowel or major vessels, postoperative obstruction due to adhesions or herniae; fatal events such as pulmonary embolism, overwhelming sepsis

operative laparoscopies, including the therapy of endometriosis (36.1%), lysis of adhesions (22.3%), management of ovarian cysts (13.7%), uterosacral nerve ablation for pelvic pain (12.1%), ectopic pregnancy (5.2%), management of hydrosalpinx (3.7%), myomectomy (3.0%), pelvic abscess (0.7%) and others (3.2%). Their grade VI complications (in number per 1000 procedures) included laparotomy for haemorrhage or bowel or urinary tract injuries (4.2%) and death (0.054%). Grade IV complications include prolonged hospitalizations greater than 72 h (4.2%) and hospital readmission (3.1%). Grade III complications included nerve injuries (0.5%), spill of unsuspected ovarian cancer cells (0.5%) and persistent human chorionic gonadotrophin (HCG) titre after ectopic pregnancy (63.2%). The two deaths were a result of bowel injury. There was no information on laparotomy for failure to complete the procedure (grade V). At that time, 60% of the respondents were using laser, 52% used unipolar coagulation, 87% used bipolar coagulation and 25% used sutures.

The American Association of Gynecologic Laparo-

scopists in 1988 also conducted a membership survey on complications of tubal sterilization and diagnostic laparoscopy [6]. Eight hundred and sixteen respondees reported on 30 480 sterilizations and 41 160 diagnostic laparoscopies. The number of laparoscopic sterilizations represented a steady decline over a 10-year period among the sterilization techniques. Fifty-four per cent of laparoscopic sterilizations were performed with bipolar cautery, 25% with the ring, 11% with the Hulka clip and 10% by unipolar coagulation. There was no information given on grade IV or V complications, but complications requiring laparotomy (grade VI) were 2.1 per 1000. No deaths were reported. Surprisingly, diagnostic laparoscopy was associated with a higher grade VI complication rate of 3.1.

Slightly earlier in the USA, the Collaborative Review of Sterilization reported on 5027 women between 1978 and 1982 in 11 institutions in five cities undergoing laparoscopic tubal sterilization [7]. The grade VI complication rate was 2.4 and the grade V failure to complete 7.8. Contributing to the grade V complications were adhesions, hydrosalpinx and difficulty in entering the peritoneal cavity. Four women in this group underwent a laparotomy at a delayed interval. Within the grade VI complication cohort, two were treated with subsequent total abdominal hysterectomy and three required bowel resections. A second hospitalization and a second anaesthetic, presumably for bowel problems, occurred in the remaining six. Previous surgery, intrauterine device (IUD) or pelvic inflammatory disease (PID) all increased the relative risk for grades V and VI complications.

A French multicentre study from 1987 to 1991 reported on 17 521 procedures completed at seven referral centres in France [8]. Only the grade VI complication rates were reported. Diagnostic laparoscopies (23.6%) had a complication rate of 1.7 per 1000. Laparoscopies for minimal adhesiolysis, obstruction of minimal foci of endometriosis, ovarian biopsy, ovarian puncture, tubal sterilization and assisted fertility procedures (24%) had a complication rate of 0.5 per 1000. More major procedures, including extensive adhesiolysis, tuboplasty, uterine suspension, management of ectopic pregnancy and salpingitis, ovarian cystectomies and moderate or severe endometriosis ablation (47.1% of the total), had a combined complication rate of 4.8 per 1000. Advanced laparoscopic procedures, including haemostasis of large vessels, hysterectomy, adnexectomy, myomectomy, bladder neck suspension and lymphadenectomies (5.1% of total), had a disproportionate grade VI complication rate of 8.9. These rates are quite comparable to the American experience, although the American Association of Gynecologic Laparoscopists did not report on advanced procedures. There was no information about the techniques used or on the failure to complete.

A German survey has reported data on 219 314 laparoscopies from 354 clinics and 40 892 laparoscopies from 161 private practices between 1949 and 1988 [9]. Laparoscopy was performed in 98.9% of the clinics and 90.9% of the private practices. The clinic laparoscopies were for diagnosis only (45.4%), sterilization (29.7%) and other operative procedures (24.9%). The private practices had relatively fewer diagnostic procedures (36.5%) and more sterilization procedures (43.5%). Grade VI complications requiring a laparotomy were 2.2 for the clinics and 3 per 1000 for the private practices. Most of these laparotomies were for injuries to the abdominal wall, mesosalpinx, or mechanical damage to the bowel or ureter. Coagulation injuries were approximately 0.5 per 1000 in both groups. The ectopic pregnancy rate after tubal sterilization was 2.1 and 2.5 per 1000 for the clinics and private practices respectively. The grade V complication, failure to complete the intended procedure, could not be gleaned from this survey.

The data from all three national surveys are quite similar in demonstrating a laparotomy rate of less than 5 per 1000. This rate increases with the inexperience of the surgeon and the difficulty of the procedure.

Specific complications: aetiology and management

A logical approach to any discussion of complications would categorize them into those originating in the preoperative, intraoperative or postoperative periods.

Preoperative complications

OPERATOR

Training the operator has already been mentioned and alluded to in this chapter. A thorough understanding of the principles of laparoscopy, learned at a formal teaching course, followed by preceptor-type practical training, is an obvious requisite. Even then the published data indicates that practice makes perfect [1–3].

PATIENT

A second controllable factor originating long before the procedure is patient selection. Patients who are obese and have cardiac or respiratory problems, or who have had previous operations, represent a high-risk situation. As reviewed in Chapter 14, Mitchell Maiman re-emphasizes that we should not repeat history. Operating on obvious malignant adnexal masses, or those that potentially could be so, is acceptable only in investigational settings.

INSTRUMENTATION

The complications of cost, as it applies to instruments, is worth mentioning. It should be emphasized that the prevention of wasted time, caused by malfunctioning instruments and various other frustrations, should be available by having easily available instruments in proper working order. Laser couplers, power supplies, electrical cords, insufflators and trocars should all be checked well before the operation begins.

OPERATING TEAM

Lastly, the operating team needs to be experienced. Failure to dedicate a group experienced in coping with monitors, recorders, cameras, electrical or laser instruments, and the appropriate operative assistance, will invariably lead to delays and costs.

NEUROLOGICAL INJURIES

Femoral neuropathy has been described by Hershlag *et al.* during laparoscopy with a patient in extreme hip flexion, abduction and lateral rotation [10]. It was postulated that nerve stretching or compression contributed to the problem. Nerve palsies have been reported to occur as well, as a result of pressure on the medial or lateral aspects of the knee and ankle in less than one in 1000 [11]. These problems can be prevented by placing the patient with her legs lowered and slightly flexed in well-padded Allen stirrups and with the weight of her leg supported by the bottom of her foot. During surgery, personnel should avoid applying pressure to any part of the lower limbs.

Intraoperative complications

TROCAR AND NEEDLE INJURIES

A survey of 407 Canadian obstetricians and gynecologists revealed that 68.17% of respondents do not use an open laparoscopy technique [12]. At least one incident had occurred in the careers of 26.8% in the survey, during which a Veress needle injury had led to the need for a laparotomy, and an almost equal number (24.4%) could recall an incident related to insertion of the primary trocar. Understandably, insertion of a second trocar under direct vision led to a laparotomy in the experience of far fewer.

In the Canadian survey, the Veress needle and the primary trocar were equally responsible for neurovascular injuries. Injuries were twice as common when excessive force was necessary for insertion of the primary trocar. Corson *et al.* [13] have shown the force necessary to perform primary trocar insertion of a re-sharpened reusable 10-mm primary trocar is twice as great as that necessary for the insertion of the surgi-port, a disposable trocar.

It is likely that the incidence of traumatic injury to bowel has been underreported according to information noted in a survey by Levy *et al.* [14]. Any injuries that were assumed to be of electrosurgical origin may have been related to the traumatic puncture of either the Veress needle or trocar and gone unrecognized from 1 to 9 days.

Needle/trocar abdominal wall vessel injury

Lacerations of the inferior and superior epigastric arteries are the most common vascular injury (2.5–25 per 100 000) [11]. Difficulties of poor visualization from dripping blood or the formation of abdominal wall haematomata occur commonly, even to the most experienced of laparoscopists. Common methods of avoiding this problem involve transillumination of the abdominal wall where possible and, more reliably, according to Hurd *et al.* [15], placing the lateral trocars 8 cm from the midline and at least 5 cm superior to the symphysis. A variety of manoeuvres have been used to treat this complication, including the use of a Foley balloon compressed internally on the bleeding site, mattress sutures through the abdominal wall and the use of a bipolar cautery directed transabdominally or transperitoneally.

Needle/trocar bowel injury

The reported instance of 0.6–3 per 1000 laparoscopies is probably low, because for medical/legal reasons in the USA this complication is underreported. Needle and trocar placements, intraoperative dissection, and thermal trauma from the use of the laser and monopolar or bipolar electricity are all causes of intraoperative bowel injury [11]. A majority are unrecognized at the time of occurrence, as Soderstrom *et al.* have chillingly reported in their review of 66 cases of bowel injury related to laparoscopy [16]. Only six of the 66 were related to electrical dissection and 60 were in fact related to traumatic puncture from the Veress needle or trocar tip. Disposable trocars are not foolproof, and 12 of the 60 cases involved disposable trocars. It has been previously underappreciated that the onset of symptoms in this survey was delayed from 1 to 9 days (average 3 days). Thirty-nine of the 66 patients had a normal white cell count and 22 had temperatures less than 37.8°C (100°F) at the time of presentation of peritoneal signs. All of the patients with large bowel trauma had both an elevation of white cell count and temperature. Free air was shown in 13 of 50 patients who had abdominal X-rays. In 43 patients with abdominal ultrasound for abscesses, only 18 were confirmed. Deaths related to a laparoscopic bowel injury occurred only when the large bowel was injured and were caused by sepsis, disseminated intravascular coagulation, shock and adult respiratory distress syndrome. The three deaths reported in Soderstrom's series were all explored more than 72 hours after the onset of symptoms. This chapter re-emphasizes the difficulty in recognizing early that bowel perforation has occurred.

Strategies to prevent bowel injuries include the avoidance of placing primary trocars or needles at the site of previous scars [17], using the left upper quadrant for initial trocar placement [18] and using sharp trocars and/or safety shield trocars [19]. Direct placement of trocars without a pneumoperitoneum reduce the likelihood of needle injury and has also been advocated [20]. A common approach is to use the open laparoscopy technique.

Management of traumatic bowel injuries is best made at the time of surgery if possible. Both Nezhat *et al.* [21] and Reich [22] have advocated laparoscopic repair, either with suturing or stapling techniques, followed by copious irrigation. Several authors have reported a significantly lower morbidity and hospital stay in patients treated with primary closure than with colostomy [23].

Needle/trocar bladder injuries

The sudden appearance of distending carbon dioxide in the Foley bag is a sure sign of a bladder perforation [11]. This can typically result from the improper angulation of a suprapubic trocar into an undrained bladder. The bladder frequently has been distorted and angulated by prior C-sections. This complication, occurring in 0.2–2 per 1000 laparoscopies, obviously can be avoided by always draining the bladder and by always inserting the suprapubic trocar under direct visualization. A more subtle appearance may be haematuria. A minilaparotomy with the offending trocar in place for open repair or, when skilled laparoscopists are at hand, a laparoscopic repair in one or two layers can be performed. In all cases, Foley catheter drainage should be in place for at least 7 days [24].

Delayed recognition may lead to bloody urine, suprapubic bruising and abdominal swelling. Peritoneal signs may not occur in the absence of infection. Intraperitoneal leaks are repaired and drained well. Extraperitoneal leaks are merely drained [24].

Needle/trocar major vascular injuries

Virtually every large vessel within reach of the anterior abdominal wall has been injured at laparoscopy, but a combined literature review is less than nine per 1000 [25]. In a thin patient, the distance from the aortic arch to the umbilicus may only be 1.5 cm. An improper Veress needle and trocar placement is the most common cause of aortic injury or vena caval injury. The injuries associated with nodal dissection will be covered below in section B. The prevention of the traumatic injury starts with inserting the Veress needle, parallel to the elevated skin in the midline for a distance of 2–4 cm, and then aiming posteriorly at a 45° angle. Diagnosis may involve the rush of blood up the open Veress needle, or a sudden depression of vital signs. Repair should always be via laparotomy in the presence of someone skilled in vascular repair [25].

ELECTROCOAGULATION INJURIES

An evolution in safe electrocoagulation has paralleled the evolution of laparoscopy in general. The first high-voltage spark gap devices have given way to solid-state generators with lower voltages, with a peak voltage no greater than 600 volts and a maximum output of 100 watts [26]. At these voltages, spark gaps are rare and then only occur on instruments in the presence of smoke [27]. Following their introduction by Rioux in 1972, bipolar forceps are now used for the most popular method of tubal sterilization in the USA. With bipolar forceps, bowel injury should be rare and, as previously mentioned, a majority of so-called bowel injuries when examined microscopically have been related to needle and trocar injury [14]. Nevertheless, electrical injuries do occur, primarily with the use of monopolar scissors. Whenever a narrow tag of tissue becomes the chief conduit for current, injury several centimetres away does indeed occur [28]. Breaks in insulation and poor visualization can cause burns at points not under direct visualization. An older concern regarding capacitance (the storage of energy in the isolated metallic trocar sleeve) which might then discharge, has been disproven as a source of significant injury [29].

Monopolar bowel injury is often discovered after a delayed time period of 5–15 days. The extent of damage is frequently far greater than first imagined [16]. Two patients in Soderstrom's series had only a wedge resection at the time of bowel repair, but required re-exploration because of a breakdown of the primary repair. A more generous bowel resection at the outset might have been more appropriate. Delayed recognition may lead to widespread peritonitis and may require a colostomy. Always consider placing a nasogastric tube to decompress the stomach. However, bipolar contact to bowel may only require a purse-string suture.

Bowel, pelvic veins and ureters have all been damaged inadvertently through poor visualization. To prevent these problems, ensure adequate visualization, avoid breaks in insulation and do not reuse disposable instruments. Avoid using operative laparoscopes [11]. To replace all electrical functions with scissors, clips, laser or harmonic scalpel is a little extreme in our opinion.

SUTURE AND STAPLE INJURY

Complications of sutures, clips, staples and lasers, major frustrations with intra-abdominal tying, perforation of the bowel by the unprotected needle and loss of needles have all been described [30]. Endoclips need to be applied under direct vision, to ensure other tissues are not incorporated. One major concern with the EndoGIA has been excessive bleeding along the cut edges. A most useful technique is to apply pressure for 5 minutes or to apply auxiliary clips. Bipolar cautery needs to be used judiciously, because desiccation can cause retraction of the vessel and/or conduction of heat laterally. Laser burns to bowel or bladder and major vessels have all been described and are becoming less of a concern, particularly to the gynaecological oncologist.

URETERAL INJURY

In 1990, 13 cases of ureteral injury occurring during laparoscopy not following laparoscopically assisted vaginal hysterectomy were reported [31]. Over 50% of the cases occurred during division of the uterosacral ligaments and 30% during the treatment of endometriosis. When recognized, stenting the ureter, resuturing the ureter over a stent, and laparoscopic ureteral reanastomosis using fibrin glue have all been described [32]. When delayed, the patient may develop fever, abdominal pain and peritonitis. Confirmation with an intravenous pyelogram followed by stenting is the management of choice. Prevention, of course, depends on adequate visualization [31].

ANAESTHETIC AND CARDIOVASCULAR THORACIC COMPLICATIONS

Between 25% and 30% of grade IV–VI complications are related to cardiovascular thoracic problems [33].

Intra-abdominal pressures can affect pre- and post-load pressures on the cardiovascular system. At intraperitoneal pressures limited to 15–20 mmHg, the overall effect on the cardiovascular system is somewhat hyperdynamic. However, at intra-abdominal pressures of 40 mmHg, a tension pneumoperitoneum exists. Venous return and cardiac blood pressure decrease precipitously and deaths have been reported [3]. Therefore, patients with cardiomyopathy, moderate to severe ischaemic heart disease or massive obesity represent relative contraindications.

Pressure gauge breakdown, or vagal stimulation secondary to peritoneal irritation, may lead to cardiac arrhythmias. Relative venostasis has occurred during even normal laparoscopy and this can be avoided with the use of pressure boots. The head-down position may lead to an increase in cerebral volume, pressure and subsequent strokes [3].

Hypothermia has been extensively investigated by Ott, who estimated that the core temperature decreases by 0.3°C for every 15 litres of carbon dioxide used [33]. He recommended that the gas is warmed before insufflation. Heated blankets and pads should be standard equipment.

Hypercapnia in excess of 16 mmHg pressure has a direct cardiodepressive effect [3]. Severe acidosis and secondary fatal dysrrhythmias are the two conditions which most commonly follow carbon dioxide absorption in the presence of excessive intra-abdominal pressure. Patients with pulmonary disease may not be able to exchange the increased level of carbon dioxide, despite intermittent desufflation.

Pneumothorax and pneumomediastinum are potentially the most dangerous extraperitoneal gas collections. These situations have led to cardiac or respiratory insufficiency in 0.8 and 0.3 per 1000 cases [3]. These gas collections can occur through persistent congenital connections through the diaphragm and also via barotrauma.

Subcutaneous emphysema which follows incorrect needle placement or leakage around the laparoscopic port is generally innocuous occurring in 6.3–20 per 1000 procedures [11]. When massive, emphysema can contribute to inadequate ventilation and subsequent hypercapnia [3].

Venous carbon dioxide embolism reported in 0.02–0.2 per 1000 cases is usually due to the direct injection of gas into the venous system via the Veress needle. Embolism can be fatal as a result of blockage of the right heart outflow, leading to subsequent hypoxia, hypercapnia and circulatory collapse [3]. The sudden onset of hypotension, cyanosis, dysrrhythmias, pulmonary oedema, and a 'mill-wheel' murmur, accompanied by a sudden change in end-tidal carbon dioxide tracing, aid in the diagnosis. Treatment must be swift, including release of the pneumoperitoneum, application of 100% oxygen and placement of the patient in the head-down position. Prevention, of course, can be expedited by minimizing intra-abdominal pressure to less than 20 mmHg, immediately closing open-ended vessels, and shortening the length of surgery.

Intra-abdominal explosion has occurred in older reports where oxygen or nitrous oxide have been used [3]. Helium has recently been suggested as an alternative to carbon dioxide, in an effort to obviate hypercapnia [34]. Unfortunately, helium carries a higher risk of gas embolism [35]. The generation of smoke due to tissue combustion and low oxygen concentration causes the production of carbon monoxide. Ott has recently reported that all 25 patients exposed to laparoscopic smoke for 15 minutes showed carbon monoxide concentrations three times the accepted minimum and that only 44% had returned to normal by 6 hours postoperatively [36]. Some of the effects of this intra-abdominal smoke exposure were associated with postoperative nausea, headache and dizziness. Prevention involves the immediate evacuation of smoke.

Standard anaesthetic concerns are exacerbated in laparoscopy not only by hypercapnia, intra-abdominal pressure and the lithotomy position, but also by excessive absorption of fluid [3]. Postoperative oedema and postoperative expiratory difficulties have been reported. Furthermore, anasarca has been reported by one author in 7% of his laparoscopic hysterectomies [37]. In all cases, over 3000 ml of irrigating fluid had been used in 3 hours. It is possible that there is a subcutaneous extension of fluid from the port sites in such cases. Anasarca will always resolve spontaneously.

Postoperative complications

PAIN

Postoperative pain occurs 100% of the time in laparoscopic procedures. The pain is increased by the production of carbonic acid, which is quite irritating [38]. This in turn is related to the residual carbon dioxide and peritoneal fluid within the abdominal cavity at the end of the procedure. Trauma to the peritoneum and residual blood is also irritating. The problem can be avoided by limiting the length of the procedure, and by taking the patient out of the Trendelenburg position to evacuate all residual fluid and gas [38]. Pain has been prevented by the intraperitoneal infusion of local anaesthetics, local anaesthetics at the trocar sites and a thorough lavage before exiting the procedure [39].

POSTOPERATIVE INFECTIONS

Trocar-site infections occurring in 8–13 per 1000 procedures [11] are obviously exacerbated by excessive trauma and predisposing factors such as obesity and diabetes. Prophylactic antibiotics have been successful, and management with antibiotics and drainage is usually successful as well.

Bacterial contamination of the abdominal cavity obviously can occur with bowel injury but it has also been reported with a contaminated dye injection [40]. Huezo *et al.* have reported pelvic infections in three to four cases per 1000 procedures. Very rarely necrotizing fasciitis has been reported [41]. A case of non-menstrual toxic shock syndrome followed aspiration of an ovarian cyst [42].

POSTOPERATIVE ADHESION FORMATION

A controlled study has demonstrated a significant reduction in adhesions with the use of laparoscopy over laparotomy [43]. Nevertheless, adhesions occur with subsequent concerns of pain, possible tubal occlusion and, to a much less extent, bowel obstruction. The most efficacious method, according to Danniell and Kurtz, is to limit the trauma at the time of the initial operative procedure. Handling should be meticulous, irrigation copious, and residual clot and fibrinous exudate should be minimized. Products such as Interceed® and Goretex® fail in the presence of blood or in areas where they can be removed easily. Stapling devices and the use of second-look laparoscopy can help reduce adhesions [44].

INCISIONAL HERNIAS

The American Association of Gynecologic Laparoscopists reported instances of postoperative hernias in 0.21 per 1000 procedures [45]. Three per cent of these occurred at sites where ports 10mm or larger had been placed. However, 10.9% occurred at ports 8mm in diameter and 2.7% occurred at sites where ports were less than 8mm. Seventy-five per cent of the hernias occurred at the umbilicus. The most common symptom was a palpable mass or fascial defect. However, 16.8% reported bowel obstruction related to incarceration with strangulation, pain and nausea subsequently occurring.

Prevention obviously involves closure of fascial defects, principally those 10mm or larger. Unfortunately, 18% of the fascial defect closures do not prevent herniation. It can only be surmised that inadequate closure had in fact occurred. In three of the 133 hernias reported in this survey, either intestine or the ileoinguinal nerve were incorporated into the suture. There are a number of devices now available that attempt to prevent this complication [45].

POSTLAPAROSCOPIC BLADDER RETENTION

This complication, which is of unknown incidence, is most commonly caused by postoperative pain or trauma of the pelvic structures, but it can also be influenced by diabetes, multiple sclerosis, mental retardation, recurrent urinary infections, ingestion of multiple pharmacological agents and past spinal cord injury. The management obviously involves the prolonged use of Foley drainage [46].

Complications of laparoscopically assisted vaginal hysterectomy

Although no nationwide surveys of complications have been published, there are several individual series. Schwartz reported no grade V or VI complications in a group of 45 laparoscopically assisted vaginal hysterectomies, performed in the year ending in November 1992 [37]. Grade III complications involving bladder perforation by laser tip (repaired intraoperatively), abdominal wall bleeding and subcutaneous emphysema occurred in 11%. The 7% of anaesthetic complications involved excessive intraperitoneal fluid with anasarca. The 16% of postoperative complications primarily involved cellulitis or continued bleeding following a hysterectomy. There were 4% minor neural apraxias, and in 56% an instrument-related delay. No ureteral injuries occurred in his series.

Shearer reported that three of his first 35 patients could not be completed laparoscopically. Twenty-nine of the remaining 32 were discharged in under 3 days and three required laparotomy [47]. Other case reports warn of the damage resulting from cautery or stapling injury to the ureter [48,49].

B: Feasibility and complications of laparoscopic surgery in gynaecological oncology

The relative risk of all of the complications mentioned in section A above increase as a surgeon undertakes the more extensive and prolonged surgery involved with gynaecological oncology. In addition, there are a unique set of complications associated with lymphadenectomy. The complications will be coded in percentage terms rather than as an incidence per 1000, because thousands of cases have not yet been performed.

Complications of lymphadenectomy using the transperitoneal approach

Bleeding problems, feared because of dissection close to vessels, have not materialized. Diffuse oozing has generally stopped, in part because of the pressure of the pneumoperitoneum [50]. Injury to the external iliac vein is the most serious potential risk of pelvic lymphadenectomy. At intraperitoneal pressures greater than 16mmHg, the vein may quiver but not bleed. Frequently such an injury can be controlled with clips [51].

Pelvic plexus bleeding occurs with the inappropriate retraction of the obturator vein or branches of the pelvic plexus. When encountered, tamponade with a closed forceps may sometimes be successful. It is often necessary to resort to the use of clips or bipolar cautery [50]. Some injuries are less likely to occur because of the anatomical knowledge of the operating gynaecological oncologist, namely obturator nerve and ureteral injuries. Both structures obviously have to be dissected free prior to any intended pelvic lymphadenectomy [50].

In the small reported case studies, pelvic haematomata are not common during gynaecological pelvic lymphadenectomies, nor are lymphocysts common because the pelvic peritoneum is left open. Should a lymphocyst develop, aspiration under ultrasound monitoring is safe [50].

A survey has been reported of urological departments, in six major universities, which had attempted dissection of the para-aortic nodes bilaterally for 20 patients with non-seminomatous testicular cancer [52]. The procedure was completed in 18 and abandoned in two (10%), because of an inability to control bleeding from a gonadal vessel injury. A total of six (30%) experienced bleeding greater than 500 ml. Fifteen per cent required blood transfusions. The median operating time was 6 hours and the median estimated blood loss was 250 ml. The stay in hospital was a median of 3 days.

Another series of 372 patients undergoing laparoscopic pelvic lymphadenectomy has been reported from the urological departments of eight medical centres in the USA [53]. An inability to complete surgery, largely due to obesity or technical difficulties, occurred in 16 (4.3%). Fourteen of the 16 failures occurred within the first eight dissections at each institution. Seven laparotomies were undertaken for problems largely related to bleeding at the time of node dissection and six patients underwent a delayed exploration, largely for bowel injury, for an overall grade VI complication rate of 3.5%. Grade III and IV complications were all less than 3%, including deep venous thrombosis, lymphoedema, anaesthetic complications and obturator nerve palsy.

The technique of transabdominal pelvic lymphadenectomy is discussed elsewhere in Chapter 3. In a series of 47 patients with stages IA to IIB carcinoma of the cervix, Querleu found one grade V complication (2.1%), which resulted from intolerance to prolonged pneumoperitoneum requiring the procedure to be abandoned, and one grade II bleeding. The postoperative phase was uneventful, with the exception of one patient who had a pelvic hematoma 5 days postoperatively. Patients were highly selected,

however. Patients with major cardiovascular risk or with CT evidence of positive nodes were excluded [50].

Childers *et al.* have published their experience in 61 women undergoing para-aortic lymphadenectomies for a variety of gynaecological malignancies [54]. In four of the 61 (6.5%) women a grade V complication, namely inability to complete the surgery, occurred. One patient (1.63%) experienced significant bleeding of the vena cava requiring a grade VI laparotomy. The average blood loss for the series was 50 ml per patient and the average hospital stay was 1.3 days.

The use of the laparoscopic clip applicator may be extremely beneficial with vascular injuries. Childers reports (personal communication) that he has experienced two vena cava bleeds; one required a laparotomy and one was repaired with staples. One patient had an external iliac haemorrhage of the mesenteric arteries controlled by clipping.

In a very informative video from the American College of Obstetricians and Gynecologists, numerous complications and their management are demonstrated. These complications come from a single group practice and demonstrate the following injuries and repair: left lumbar ureter injury, large and small bowel enterotomies, liver laceration, bladder perforation, right hemidiaphragm perforation, external iliac vein laceration, vena cava laceration, internal iliac vein laceration, inferior mesenteric artery laceration, inferior epigastric artery laceration and small bowel herniation. With the exception of the last complication, all were managed laparoscopically [55].

Adelson, in a private communication, has reported 44 pelvic lymphadenectomies, 11 para-aortic lymphadenectomies, 10 omentectomies and two colostomies, all performed laparoscopically (M.D. Adelson, personal communication). Blood loss greater than 500 ml occurred in four patients undergoing pelvic lymphadenectomies (9%), and in one patient undergoing a para-aortic lymphadenectomy, One patient had a cystotomy secondary to suprapubic trocar and one patient had an enterotomy repaired after externalizing the bowel through a small infraumbilical incision. No patient required a laparotomy and there were no cases of thrombosis, vessel perforation or infection. Johnson in Western Australia, in a preliminary series, has reported 10 pelvic laparoscopies complicated by one laparotomy for bleeding from the internal iliac vein [56].

A communication from Covens in Canada reports 125 laparoscopies performed for gynaecological oncology indications (A. Covens, personal communication). He experienced four grade VI complications (3.2%). These included two enterotomies occurring during dissection of adhesions, one external iliac vein laceration requiring laparotomy repair and one pneumoperitoneum occurring 6 hours postoperatively. He has noted that all of these occurred within the first year of his experience and none have occurred in the last 6 months.

Burrell reported a personal series of 17 patients undergoing laparoscopically assisted vaginal hysterectomy and bilateral salpingo-oophorectomy with pelvic lymphadenectomies (two para-aortic) for endometrial carcinoma and 21 patients admitted for the re-staging of ovarian cancer [51]. There was one trocar perforation of an unsuspected adherent bowel loop late in his series, and one monopolar injury of large bowel requiring a secondary laparotomy 6 days later. The type V complication rate was therefore 5.2% with three grade IV complications, including one anasarca of the lower abdomen following a second-look laparoscopy, one re-admission for a pelvic cellulitis and one re-admission for deep venous thrombosis occurring in the calf but not the pelvic veins.

In summarizing the limited available data, the failure to complete a transperitoneal pelvic lymphadenectomy in the well-selected patient is very low, probably not more than 4%. On the other hand, the feasibility of completing para-aortic lymphadenectomies ranges from 6.5% in the gynaecological oncology literature to 10% in the urological literature.

Complications of lymphadenectomy using the extraperitoneal laparoscopic approach

This technique, popularized by Dargent and Salvat, has been reported in 46 cases [57]. Four patients had to undergo a laparotomy secondary to the presence of a large tumour preventing the peritoneal dissection (8.7%). There were no major vascular or bowel problems. A laparotomy for a pelvic abscess was carried out in one patient on the eighth postoperative day. Three asymptomatic lymphocysts were discovered postoperatively. There was one inferior epigastric artery haemorrhage, one obturator paresis, one bladder entry and one ureteral entry for an overall grade IV complication rate of 4.2%. Other difficulties have included inadequate carbon dioxide gas tension retroperitoneally, loosening of the peritoneal sac, difficulty in initially locating the anatomical reference points, and difficulties with extractions.

Abdominal wall tumour implantation

The problem of tumour spill from unrecognized ovarian malignancies is discussed in Chapter 14. Childers reviewed laparoscopic procedures on 105 patients with proven malignancies, 88 patients with cytologically and

histologically proven intraperitoneal disease and 17 with retroperitoneal disease [58]. Only one trocar site (0.3%) in one patient (1%) developed an implantation occurring after a second-look laparoscopy for ovarian cancer. Gleeson *et al.* reported two cases of abdominal metastases in the presence of preoperatively proven ascites and one patient with implantation from a borderline tumour having obvious evidence of papillary excrescences of both ovaries [59]. This experience of obvious demonstrable disease and subsequent implantations contrasts to Childers' experience of more occult disease. Laparoscopic inoculation from adenocarcinomata of the gallbladder occurring postextraction have been reported in the surgical literature [60].

Instances of implantation from involved lymph nodes have been reported.

Deep venous thrombosis

As experience increases with the manipulation of veins in high-risk patients, more reports of deep venous thrombosis are to be anticipated. At present, the authors are aware of three cases reported personally, which all responded to standard therapy and were unassociated with any sequelae [51].

Complications of laparoscopically assisted radical hysterectomy

The literature on radical hysterectomies is in its infancy. Nezhat has reported seven patients undergoing laparoscopic radical hysterectomies in whom the ureters were dissected laparoscopically and 11 patients undergoing laparoscopically assisted Schauta hysterectomies, all for stages IA to IIA squamous cell carcinoma of the cervix [61]. A long operating time of 4–8 hours was the chief problem with the first approach, whereas the second approach was completed in 2–3.5 hours. Intraoperative blood loss ranged from 30–250 ml. All patients attempted were completed laparoscopically and there were no subsequent laparotomies. Grades II–III complications included postoperative blood loss from the umbilical vein and a urinary tract infection. The anticipated bladder dysfunction resolved in all patients. Dargent, in an unpublished presentation, reported that his laparoscopically assisted modified Schauta procedures lasted 2–3 hours and were accompanied by minimal morbidity [62]. Unpublished reports from those surgeons beginning to perform laparoscopically assisted radical hysterectomies indicate a higher than usual ureteral complication rate. It can be anticipated that this particular learning curve will improve.

Conclusion

In conclusion, the feasibility of proceeding with completion of a pelvic or para-aortic lymphadenectomy and extended dissection for gynaecological malignancies in patients with good cardiovascular status and weighing less than 81 kg (180 pounds) is 4.0–6.5%. The complication rates requiring progression to laparotomy for repair of bleeding or bowel injury are equally low (0–5.2%). In experienced hands, laparoscopic surgery has staked a legitimate claim to be within the armamentarium of the gynaecological oncologist.

References

1 Capelouto CC, Kavoussi LR (1993). Complications of laparoscopic surgery. *Urology* **42**:2–12.
2 See WA, Cooper CS, Fisher RJ (1993). Predictors of laparoscopic complications after formal training in laparoscopic surgery. *JAMA* **270**:2689–2692.
3 Wolf JS Jr, Stoller ML (1994). The physiology of laparoscopy: basic principles, complications and other considerations. *J Urol* **152**:294–302.
4 Smith DC, Donohue LR, Waszak SJ (1994). A hospital review of advanced gynecologic endoscopic procedures. *Am J Obstet Gynecol* **170**:1635–1642.
5 Peterson HB, Hulka JF, Phillips JM (1990). American Association of Gynecologic Laparoscopist's 1988 Membership Survey on Operative Laparoscopy. *J Reprod Med* **35**:587–589.
6 Hulka JF, Peterson HB, Phillips JM (1990). American Association of Gynecologic Laparoscopists' 1988 Membership Survey on Laparoscopic Sterilization. *J Reprod Med* **35**:584–586.
7 Franks AL, Kendrick JS, Peterson HB (1987). Unintended laparotomy associated with laparoscopic tubal sterilization. *Am J Obstet Gynecol* **157**:1102–1105.
8 Querleu D, Chapron C, Chevallier L, Bruhat M (1992). Complications of gynecologic laparoscopic surgery—a French Multicenter Collaborative Study. *J Gynecol Obstet Biol Reprod* **21**:711.
9 Lehmann-Willenbrock E, Riedel H-H, Mecke H, Semm K (1992). Pelviscopy/laparoscopy and its complications in Germany, 1949–1988. *J Reprod Med* **37**:671–677.
10 Hershlag A, Loy RA, Lavy G, DeCherney AH (1990). Femoral neuropathy after laparoscopy, a case report. *J Reprod Med* **35**:575–576.
11 Montz FJ (1993). Complications in laparoscopic surgery. Presented at the Society of Gynecological Oncologists February 1993, Palm Desert, California.
12 Yuzpe AA (1990). Pneumoperitoneum needle and trocar injuries in laparoscopy. A survey on possible contributing factors and prevention. *J Reprod Med* **35**:485–490.
13 Corson SL, Batzer FR, Gocial B, Maislin G (1989). Measurement of the force necessary for laparoscopic trocar entry. *J Reprod Med* **34**:282–284.
14 Levy BS, Soderstrom RM, Dail DH (1985). Bowel injuries during laparoscopy. Gross anatomy and histology. *J Reprod Med* **30**:168–172.
15 Hurd WW, Bude RO, DeLancey JOL, Newman JS (1994). The location of abdominal wall blood vessels in relationship to abdominal landmarks apparent at laparoscopy. *Am J Obstet Gynecol* **171**:462–466.
16 Soderstrom RM (1993). Bowel injury litigation after laparoscopic laparoscopy. *J Am Assoc Gynecol Laparoscopists* **1**:74–77.
17 Kaali SG, Barad DH (1992). Incidence of bowel injury due to dense adhesions at the sight of direct trocar insertion. *J Reprod Med* **37**:617–618.
18 Childers JM, Brzechffa PR, Surwit EA (1993). Laparoscopy using the left upper quadrant as the primary trocar site. *Gynecol Oncol* **50**:221–225.
19 Oshinsky GS, Smith AD (1992). Laparoscopic needles and trocars: an overview of designs and complications. *J Laparoendoscop Surg* **2**:117–125.
20 Nezhat FR, Silfen SL, Evans D, Nezhat C (1991). Comparison of direct insertion of disposable and standard reusable laparoscopic trocars and previous pneumoperitoneum with Veress needle. *Obstet Gynecol* **78**:148–149.
21 Nezhat C, Nezhat F, Pennington E (1992). Laparoscopic treatment of infiltrative rectosigmoid colon and rectovaginal septum endometriosis by the technique of videolaparoscopy and the CO_2 laser. *Br J Obstet Gynaecol* **99**:664–667.
22 Reich H (1992). Laparoscopic bowel injury. *Surg Laparosc Endosc* **2**:74–78.
23 Childers JM (1997). Laparoscopic bowel injuries. (Personal communication.)
24 Martin DC (1993). Trocar injuries to the bladder. In: Corfman RS, Diamond M, DeCherney A, eds. *Complications of Laparoscopy and Hysteroscopy*. Boston: Blackwell Science, 56.
25 Wheeler JM (1993). Major vascular injury at laparoscopy. In: Corfman RS, Diamond M, DeCherney A, eds. *Complications of Laparoscopy and Hysteroscopy*. Boston: Blackwell Science, 64.
26 Soderstrom RM (1993). Electro-coagulation injuries during laparoscopic sterilization procedures. In: Corfman RS, Diamond M, DeCherney A, eds. *Complications of Laparoscopy and Hysteroscopy*. Boston: Blackwell Science, 84.
27 Saye WB, Miller W, Hertzmann P (1991). Electrosurgery thermal injury—myth or misconception? *Surg Laparos Endosc* **1**:223–228.
28 Ata AH, Bellemore TJ, Meisel JA, Arambulo SM (1993). Distal thermal injury from monopolar electrosurgery. *Surg Laparos Endosc* **3**:323–327.
29 Grosskinsky CM, Ryder RM, Pendergrass HM, Hulka JF (1993). Laparoscopic capacitance: a mystery measured. *Am J Obstet Gynecol* **169**:1632–1635.
30 Milad MP, Corfman RS (1993). Complications of laparoscopic suturing and clip applications. In: Corfman RS, Diamond M, DeCherney A, eds. *Complications of Laparoscopy and Hysteroscopy*. Boston: Blackwell Science, 113.
31 Grainger DA, Soderstrom RM, Schiff SF, Glickman MG, DeCherney AH, Diamond MP (1990). Ureteral injuries at laparoscopy: insights into diagnosis, management, and prevention. *Obstet Gynecol* **75**:839–843.
32 McKay TC, Albala DM, Gehrin BE, Castelli M (1994). Laparoscopic ureteral reanastomosis using fibrin glue. *J Urol* **152**:1637–1640.
33 Ott DE (1991). Laparoscopic hypothermia. *J Laparoendoscop Surg* **1**:127–131.
34 Leighton TA, Liu SY, Bongard FS (1993). Comparative cardiopulmonary effects of carbon dioxide versus helium pneumoperitoneum. *Surgery* **113**:527–531.

35 Wolf JS, Carrier S, Stoller ML (1994). Gas embolism: helium is more lethal than carbon dioxide. *J Laparoendoscop Surg* **4**:173–177.

36 Ott DE (1994). Smoke poisoning at laparoscopy. Presentation at the American Fertility Society 50th Annual Meeting, 5–10 November.

37 Schwartz RO (1993). Complications of laparoscopic hysterectomy. *Obstet Gynecol* **81**:1022–1024.

38 Alexander JI, Hull MGR (1987). Abdominal pain after laparoscopy: the value of a gas drain. *Br J Obstet Gynaecol* **94**:267–269.

39 Benhamou D, Narchi P, Mazoit JX, Fernandez H (1994). Postoperative pain after local anesthetics for laparoscopy sterilization. *Obstet Gynecol* **84**:877–880.

40 Pyper RJD, Ahmet Z, Houang ET (1988). Bacteriological contamination during laparoscopy with dye injection. *Br J Obstet Gynaecol* **95**:367–371.

41 Huezo CM, De Stetano F, Rubin GL, Ory HW (1983). Rate of wound and pelvic infection after laparoscopic tubal sterilization: instrument disinfection vs. sterilization. *Obstet Gynecol* **61**:598–602.

42 London SN (1991). Nonmenstrual toxic shock syndrome after aspiration of an ovarian cyst—a case report. *J Reprod Med* **36**:885–886.

43 Luciano AA, Maier DB, Koch EI, Nulsen JC, Whitman GF (1989). A comparative study of postoperative adhesions following laser surgery by laparoscopy versus laparotomy in the rabbit model. *Obstet Gynecol* **74**:220.

44 Daniell JF, Kurtz BR (1993). Techniques in laparoscopy that reduce postsurgical adhesions. In: *Gynecologic Surgery and Adhesion Prevention*. New York: Wiley–Liss, 59–63.

45 Montz FJ, Holschneider CH, Munro MG (1994). Incisional hernia following laparoscopy: a survey of the American Association of Gynecologic Laparoscopists. *Obstet Gynecol* **84**:881–884.

46 Thatcher SS, Joshi PN (1993). Acute urinary retention after laparoscopy. In: Corfman RS, Diamond M, DeCherney A, eds. *Complications of Laparoscopy and Hysteroscopy*. Boston: Blackwell Science, 30.

47 Shearer RA (1993). Laparoscopic-assisted vaginal hysterectomy: report on 32 initial cases. *Surg Laparosc Endosc* **3**:191–193.

48 Woodland MB (1992). Ureter injury during laparoscopy-assisted vaginal hysterectomy with the endoscopic linear stapler. *Am J Obstet Gynecol* **167**:756–757.

49 Kadar N, Lemmerling L (1994). Urinary tract injuries during laparoscopically assisted hysterectomy: causes and prevention. *Am J Obstet Gynecol* **170**:47–48.

50 Querleu D, LeBlanc E (1993). Complications of laparoscopic pelvic lymphadenectomy. In: Corfman RS, Diamond M, DeCherney A, eds. *Complications of Laparoscopy and Hysteroscopy*. Boston: Blackwell Science, 48.

51 Childers JM, Lang J, Surwit EA (1995). Laparoscopic staging of ovarian cancer *Gynecol Oncol* **59**:25–33.

52 Gerber GS, Bissada NK, Hulbert JC et al (1994). Laparoscopic retroperitoneal lymphadenectomy: multi-institutional analysis. *J Urol* **152**:1188–1192.

53 Kavoussi LR, Sosa E, Chandhoke P et al (1993). Complications of laparoscopic pelvic lymph node dissection. *J Urol* **149**:322–325.

54 Childers JM, Hatch KD, Tran AN, Surwit EA (1993). Laparoscopic para-aortic lymphadenectomy in gynecologic malignancies. *Obstet Gynecol* **82**:741–747.

55 Childers JM (1995). Complications—management of advanced operative laparoscopy. Film library of the American College of Obstetrics and Gynecology.

56 Johnson N (1994). Laparoscopic versus conventional pelvic lymphadenectomy for gynecological malignancy in humans. *Br J Obstet Gynaecol* **101**:902–904.

57 Salvat J, Vincent-Genod A, Guilbert M (1993). Intra-abdominal complications associated with extra-peritoneal dissection of the lymphatic nodes. In: Corfman RS, Diamond M, DeCherney A, eds. *Complications of Laparoscopy and Hysteroscopy*. Boston: Blackwell Science, 250.

58 Childers JM, Aqua KA, Surwit EA, Hallum AV, Hatch KD (1994). Abdominal-wall tumor implantation after laparoscopy for malignant conditions. *Obstet Gynecol* **84**:765–769.

59 Gleeson NC, Nicosia SV, Mark JE, Hoffman MS, Cavanagh D (1993). Abdominal wall metastases from ovarian cancer after laparoscopy. *Am J Obstet Gynecol* **169**:522–523.

60 Lucciarini P, Konigsrainer A, Ebert T, Margreiter R (1993). Tumour inoculation during laparoscopic cholecystectomy. *Lancet* **342**:8759.

61 Nezhat C, Nezhat F, Teng NNH et al (1994). The role of laparoscopy in the management of gynecologic malignancy. *Semin Surg Oncol* **10**:431–439.

62 Dargent D (1993). The laparoscopically assisted modified Schauta hysterectomy. Scientific Presentation at International Society of Gynecologic Oncologists. Stockholm, Sweden, September 1993.

Section 4
Laparoscopic Surgery in
the Management of
Gynaecological Cancers

16   Microinvasive carcinoma of the cervix

John Monaghan

Introduction

In the last decade laparoscopic surgery in gynaecology has moved from being a simple diagnostic device, with occasional uses in the management of endometriosis and infertility, towards becoming probably the most vital surgical tool that is currently available in this field. It was also inevitable that the role of the laparoscope should be extended towards gynaecological oncology which, while remaining to a large extent the area requiring maximal access, it has become clear that minimal access techniques have an important and developing role to play.

Definition of microinvasive carcinoma of the cervix

The International Federation of Gynecology and Obstetrics (FIGO) recommended in 1995 that the terminology for early invasive cancer of the cervix should be modified, and that the 'catch-all phrase'—microinvasive carcinoma of the cervix—should be replaced with the following definition.

Stage IA1 should now consist of those cases where early invasive cancer of the cervix reaches from the basement membrane or deepest part of an affected gland to a depth of no more than 3 mm, with a lateral extension of no more than 7 mm.

Stage IA2 is present when the depth of invasion lies between 3 and 5 mm of invasion, the lateral boundaries of these invasive processes should be no more than 7 mm.

There is a considerable degree of logic in these new definitions, as it is generally felt that where there is invasion of less than 3 mm, the risk of lymph-node metastases is minimal or close to zero, but beyond 3 mm there is a progressive and increasing concern about the risk of lymph-node metastases. The risk of metastases is also increased where the tumour is poorly differentiated or lymphatic channel involvement is seen, or there is a low level of lymphocytic response from the host.

Diagnosis

It is important to stress that the diagnosis of early invasive carcinoma of the cervix can only be made by using an adequate biopsy technique, i.e. it is not possible to confidently and comprehensively identify this condition utilizing a small punch biopsy. The diagnosis must be made on a wedge or cone biopsy, using either a knife, a laser or the much more popular loop diathermy cone biopsy. If an adequately large biopsy is produced, the pathologist is able to determine accurately the depth of invasion from the basement membrane. Care must be taken not to misdiagnose glandular involvement by cervical intraepithelial neoplasia (CIN3), or to mistakenly exaggerate the depth of invasion because of tangential sectioning.

Treatment options

Very often the simple performance of a cone biopsy, either with knife, laser or loop diathermy, will be all that is required for the treatment of stage IA1 carcinoma of the cervix [1]. As long as the margin of the lesion is completely removed and the patient is comfortable with conservative therapy, then no further action is necessary as the risk of metastases is extraordinarily small. However, for the patient in whom the margins are not confidently clear or the stage is IA2, further and better therapy is necessary. Traditionally this has involved a total abdominal or vaginal hysterectomy, with or without assessment of the pelvic lymph nodes.

From time to time a management dilemma will occur where the 'microinvasive' lesion, or CIN3, extends to the endocervical resection margin of the cone biopsy specimen. The concern is whether the resection margin represents the upper limit of the lesion identified, or whether the margin represents the lower margin of a much more significant lesion lying further into the cervix.

It is prudent, before moving to definitive therapy, to take further and better biopsies in the form of deeper cone biopsies.

In the younger patient with stage IA2 cancer or even early stage IB cancer, who is very anxious to preserve their fertility, conservative therapy in the form of trachelectomy, as advocated by Dargent, may be the most appropriate therapy (see Chapter 10). For the older patient definitive therapy, involving removal of the cervix and uterus, is essential. The advantages of using a vaginal approach, whether by standard vaginal hysterectomy or a laparoscopically assisted vaginal hysterectomy, are considerable, as the lesion can be very accurately defined on the cervix and in that tiny percentage (2.5%) of patients where the transformation zone extends onto the fornices of the vagina [2]. The entire abnormality on the cervix and vagina can be mapped prior to treatment and a confident removal performed. It is an unfortunate fact that the patient who has a total abdominal hysterectomy for the management of early invasive disease is at significant risk of residual cytological and histological abnormality because of incomplete or inadequate removal of the entire cervix up to the vaginal fornices. These technical difficulties can be effectively avoided when a vaginal or laparoscopically assisted vaginal hysterectomy is performed.

Risk of nodal metastases

There is a general acceptance that the risk of nodal metastases with invasive depths of less than 3 mm is infinitesimally small. There is no real consensus about the importance of lymphatic channel involvement and the risk of node metastases. Armed with this knowledge, it is thus recommended, and indeed practised [3], that lesser degrees of invasion can be treated conservatively. There is less agreement when the lesion extends down to 5 mm.

Laparoscopic possibilities

The great advantage of using laparoscopic minimal access techniques in the management of early invasive cancer of the cervix is the ease with which lymph-node assessment can be made and the markedly reduced affect upon the patients.

The techniques of lymphadenectomy are well documented (see Chapters 3 and 4).

Stage IA1

For patients who desire to have a hysterectomy for the coincidental management of menorrhagia, fibroids, etc., the standard laparoscopically assisted vaginal hysterectomy technique will be ideal. Also, depending on their personal circumstances and desires, the ovaries may be preserved or removed. Visual assessment of the lymph nodes can be performed and, where appropriate, sampling can be carried out. As already mentioned, this procedure allows considerable accuracy in dealing with any vaginal extensions of the lesion or the precancer condition.

Stage IA2

As noted above, these patients have a small but significant risk of lymph-node metastases. In the early stages of the development of any cancer which spreads primarily by the lymphatic route, the initial mode of spread is embolic and therefore the necessity to carry out a true en bloc dissection is removed. It is now generally accepted that in cancers of the cervix, vulva and vagina a separate dissection of the lymph nodes will be extremely effective in early disease because of this embolic phenomenon. Thus a laparoscopically assisted vaginal hysterectomy, utilizing stapling or diathermy techniques, will effectively remove the entire organ at risk and thereafter laparoscopic node sampling or even comprehensive lymphadenectomy can be carried out without undue difficulty.

Technique: laparoscopically assisted vaginal hysterectomy

Laparoscopic node removal (pelvic)

The pelvic side wall structures are usually easily visible laparoscopically in most patients. The external iliac artery and the ureter is seen through the peritoneum.

The lymph nodes of the external iliac system are approached first.

Opening the pelvic side wall

The uterus is moved over to the opposite side to be dissected by the uterine manipulator. (The author prefers not to use an intrauterine device.) The round ligament may be divided, this may be done using uni- or bipolar diathermy or by surgical clips or any combination. The uterine end of the round ligament is then grasped and drawn medially. This opens up the soft fascia of the pelvic side wall, allowing the infundibulopelvic ligament to be defined and divided at an appropriate place, depending on the desire to preserve or remove the ovaries. This procedure can be carried out with the ureter in full view on the inner side of the peritoneum.

Separating the nodes from the vessels

Once the peritoneum has been separated and drawn away the nodes can be removed from the artery, beginning laterally using the genitofemoral nerve as the lateral limit of dissection (see Chapter 3). If the fascia is divided along the line of the artery on the medial side of the genitofemoral nerve, then by putting medial tension on the fascia the entire block of nodes and lymphatic channels can be completely removed, leaving the artery clean.

Keeping tension on the fascial tissue the external iliac vein is cleaned in a similar manner, exposing the obturator node and nerve in the fossa. This scissor dissection, aided by unipolar diathermy or surgical clips, is then carried forward to the inguinal ligament and backwards to the common iliac artery and the internal iliac system.

Ideally, the nodes should be removed as one block. However, if fragmented they can be placed in the opposite iliac fossa for retrieval at the end of the procedure. Techniques of placing the nodes in 'bags' for later removal may also be used.

There is no need to attempt to close the peritoneum following the procedure, and the laparoscopic vaginal hysterectomy is then performed in the usual way.

Number of nodes

Most surgeons find that very rapidly a similar node number can be removed laparoscopically as at the open procedure.

Follow-up of patients

Subsequent management will depend to a large extent on the histological report of the lymph nodes. As long as the lymph nodes are negative, and the vast majority will be, then no further therapeutic action will be necessary. If the lymph nodes are found to be positive, there remains the dilemma of adjuvant therapy. It is generally accepted worldwide that adjuvant radiation to the pelvic side wall is of questionable value, and may in fact jeopardize the patient's future. In some centres, if only one or two nodes are positive then irradiation is dispensed with. The role of chemotherapy/radiation remains controversial. For the assessment of the vault in follow-up, cytology is all that is required and should be carried out, first at 3 months after the procedure, and then at 1 year. If complete removal with good margins has been reported, a less rigorous review may be used. If there is any abnormality or the margins are not clear, a comprehensive colposcopic assessment of the vault must be performed and further therapies instituted as appropriate.

Conclusion

Laparoscopic surgery should become the standard therapy in the management of stages IA1 and IA2 carcinoma of the cervix for those patients requiring a hysterectomy. The ease of performance and the reduction in morbidity by far outweigh any cost disadvantage. At the present time, one of the major difficulties in applying this generally is the limited skills available among gynaecologists for the performance of such complex surgery.

References

1 Burghardt E, Monaghan JM (1993). Treatment of microinvasive cancer of the cervix. In: Burghardt E, Webb MJ, Monaghan JM, Kindermann G, eds. *Surgical Gynaecological Oncology*. Stuttgart: Thieme, 260.
2 Nwabineli NJ, Monaghan JM (1991). Vaginal epithelial abnormalities in patients with CIN: clinical and pathological features and management. *Br J Obstet Gynaecol* **98**:25–29.
3 Morgan PR, Anderson MC, Buckley CH *et al* (1993). The Royal College of Obstetricians and Gynaecologists micro-invasive carcinoma of the cervix study: preliminary results. *Br J Obstet Gynaecol* **100**:664–668.

17   Invasive carcinoma of the cervix

Daniel Dargent

Introduction

Defining the place of laparoscopic surgery in the management of cancer of the cervix presuppose having answered three questions: (i) what is the place of surgery in the management of cervical cancer?; (ii) what kind of surgery has to be carried out in cases where surgery has a place?; (iii) does laparoscopic surgery fulfil the requirements of such a surgery? A clear answer does not exist to any of these questions. Or, rather, many answers exist which are conflicting.

Surgery in the management of cervical cancer

For decades a debate has existed between surgeons and radiotherapists about the treatment of cervical cancer. Both groups agree that the results are similar in 'early cases', and a consensus has emerged in favour of surgery for such cases, especially in young patients whose ovarian function can be spared. For 'advanced cases' radiotherapy is considered to be the treatment of choice, even if convincing comparative studies are still lacking, i.e. studies where the assessment of tumour volume is made by MRI (from the radiobiological point of view it is assumed that the greater the volume of the tumour, the more radiotherapy loses its efficiency).

Despite a lack of scientific evidence, it is now established that surgery has to be withdrawn in favour of radiotherapy or integrated therapies as soon as the case can no longer be classified as early. Today, consideration of medicolegal problems is the main component when medical judgements are made. And, as said by Burghardt [1], 'for reasons that remain unclear surgical complications are judged more severely than complications after radiotherapy'. Under these conditions, the only thing the surgical oncologist can do is to search for a better definition of the boundary between early cases (surgical cases) and late cases (non-surgical cases).

One definition of an early case which can be proposed, and which should be accepted by even the more rigid radiation oncologists, is a patient in whom surgery alone can offer chances of survival reaching or exceeding, 85–90%. At this level of efficiency, improving the results, supposing that this is possible, could only be obtained at the expense of adding more hazards and costs. As a result of some large studies published in recent years, the cases where surgery alone offers such chances of cure are rather easy to define.

Definition of early cases

The three crucial elements in the prognosis of cancer of the cervix are tumour volume, parametrium involvement and lymph-node involvement. These criteria of prognosis are best evaluated at assessment of specimens of radical hysterectomies. However, they can be investigated by various imaging and endoscopic techniques, and this will be discussed later. The most important pathological data will be reviewed here.

The classic publications of Piver et al. [2] and Van Nagell et al. [3] should be considered, because they directly address the problem mentioned above of the definition of surgical and non-surgical cases. Piver and Van Nagell considered tumour diameters of 3 cm and 2 cm, respectively, were the upper limits above which the rate of recurrences could be considered to be too high after surgery only. However, those assertions were based on highly biased data, and the assessment of tumour diameter was purely clinical.

The Gynecologic Oncology Group survey published in 1990 [4] does not escape reproach, as the assessment of tumour volume was based on clinical evaluation. Nevertheless, the depth of tumour invasion and the fractional thickness of cervical involvement were assessed pathologically in the operative specimen in the 732 evaluable patients with a squamous cell carcinoma (who were treated by an abdominal radical hysterectomy combined with a pelvic and aortic lymphadenectomy). The 3-year disease free survivals were 94.6% for the patients with occult tumour (157), 84.5% for the patients with a tumour 3 cm or less in diameter (276) and 68.4% for the patients with a tumour more than 3 cm in diameter (101). In the same way, the rates move from 94.6% for an invasion of 5 mm or less to 86.0% between 6 and 10 mm, 75.2% between 11 and 15 mm, 71.5% between 16 and 20 mm and 59.5% for 21 mm or more. Also 3-year disease-free survivals were 94.1% for superficial third tumour, 84.5% for the middle and 73.6% for the deep third tumours. The effect of parametrial involvement is: 84.9% 3-year disease-free survival for cases with no parametrial involvement vs 69.6% for cases with parametrial involvement. The influence of lymph-node involvement is less (85.6% 3-year disease-free survivals for pelvic pN_0 patients vs 74.4% for pelvic pN_1 patients). This has no influence on the crude survival rates. By contrast, capillary lymphatic space invasion is a significant prognostic factor: 88.9% 3-year disease-free survival for patients without invasion vs 77.0% for patients with invasion. Taking into account the morphometric criteria, five risk groups can be defined, with the 3-year disease-free survival rates being more than 90% for the first two groups (233 cases), more than 80% for the third and fourth groups (258 cases) and falling to under 60% for the fifth group (141 cases).

The survey carried out by the Clinics of Cologne, Heidelberg, Erlangen, Munich and Graz, published in 1992 [5], is based on 1028 cases. All cases were submitted to an abdominal radical hysterectomy combined with a pelvic (±aortic) lymphadenectomy. All specimens were processed in the same way: one sagittal slice which facilitated calculation of the height and thickness of the tumour and serial horizontal slices allowing measurement of the width of the tumour. The effect of tumour volume has been established as a result of the tridimensional evaluation carried out on the operative specimen. The 5-year survival rate ranges from 97% for tumours of less than 2.5 cm³ to 79.2% for tumours of 2.5–10 cm³, 70.4% for tumours of 10–15 cm³ and 63% for tumours of 40–50 cm³, but the difference is not statistically significant. The 5-year survival rate with involvement of the parametrium was 86.7% for pIB cancers, 85.4% for pIIA cancers and 62.7% for pIIB cancers. The influence of lymph-node involvement depends, among other factors, on the number of positive lymph nodes (5-year survival rates of 89.3% for pN_0 patients vs 69.8% for pN_1 patients with one positive lymph node, 62.1% for pN_1 patients with two or three positive lymph nodes and 36.9% for pN_1 patients with four or more positive lymph nodes). The rate of lymph-node involvement is related to the tumour volume and, more precisely, to the tumour–cervix quotient (volume of the tumour related to the volume of the cervix). By combining tumour–cervix quotient and lymph-node involvement, a category of patients can be defined whose chances of survival exceed the 84% threshold: tumour–cervix quotient less than 81% and negative lymph nodes. This sub-

population accounts for half of the stage I and II cancers (215 cases among 419 in the Burghardt series).

Our series [6] is based on 253 observations, in which the patients were treated using either abdominal radical hysterectomy combined with pelvic (±aortic) lymphadenectomy or a combination of vaginal radical hysterectomy followed by a pelvic (±aortic) lymphadenectomy carried out 6–8 weeks later using an extraperitoneal laparotomy. In all cases the operative specimen was analysed with the same methods as those used in the German survey. The role of tumour volume has been assessed taking into account maximal tumour diameter; a preliminary study established that the linear correlation index between the cube root of the volume and the maximal tumour diameter was 0.93. In the relationship between maximal tumour diameter and 5-year disease-free survival, a cut off is seen at the level of 4 cm. The rate of disease-free 5-year survival moves from $84 \pm 3.8\%$ for the early cases to $52 \pm 5\%$ for the late cases. The influence of parametrial involvement depends on the tumour volume. For the early cases the chances of disease-free 5-year survival move from $87 \pm 4\%$ to $71 \pm 8\%$, depending on the state of the parametrium; for more advanced cases (tumour diameter > 4 cm) the rates are $72 \pm 8\%$ and $44 \pm 6\%$ respectively. Five-year disease-free survival rates are $77 \pm 4\%$ for pN_0 patients vs $43 \pm 7\%$ for pN_1 patients. By combining tumour volume (diameter < or >4 cm), parametrial involvement (present or not) and lymph-node involvement (present or not), eight subpopulations can be defined. From the practical point of view, tumour diameter and lymph-node involvement are the two most relevant criteria because they can be evaluated before the therapeutic regimen is fixed (see below). Considering these two criteria, two subpopulations can be defined: (i) pN_0 tumours of less than 4 cm and (ii) pN_1 tumours of any diameter or tumours of more than 4 cm whatever the lymph-node status. In the first subpopulation the chances of disease-free 5-year survival are 89%, in the second 51%. The early cases account for a little less than a third of stages I and II cancers (68 among the 227 cases where all the morphometric data are available).

The three reports analysed, if slight methodological differences are discounted, lead to very similar conclusions, and it can be stated that the pN_0 cancers of less than 4 cm are the genuine early cases, which can be treated by surgery only without any adjunctive radiotherapy.

Place of surgery in advanced cases

If we admit that there is no longer a place for surgery alone in the treatment of advanced cases, does this mean that surgery has no place at all in the treatment of these cases? The answer is no.

STAGING SURGERY

Surgery has been used for assessing aortic lymph nodes before undertaking radiotherapy in advanced invasive cancers. The concept was later extended to early cases for which aortic and pelvic lymph-node assessment was used, in order to select the indications for radical hysterectomy. Unfortunately the results obtained were far below those expected. The overall results showed no improvement. Sixty-four and a half per cent and 57.1% of patients surgically explored for stage IIB and stage III survived, vs 92.8% and 60% of patients not surgically explored [7]. The rate of complications in patients submitted to periaortic radiation therapy was prohibitive in surgically assessed patients [8]. The use of a retroperitoneal approach significantly reduced the complication rate: 3.9% vs 11.5% major complications in the prospective randomized trial involving 284 patients undertaken by the Gynecologic Oncology Group [9]. However, even knowing that the use of an extraperitoneal approach reduces complications, iatrogenic morbidity is excessive considering that the chances of survival are enhanced for only a limited subpopulation and not for the whole population. As a consequence, pretreatment staging surgery disappeared. Laparoscopic techniques have completely reversed the situation and staging surgery is now fashionable again. Moreover, its indications are broader: laparoscopic staging surgery is indicated not only for high-risk patients but also for the low-risk patients, in order to identify the node-positive subset — a subset of patients who can no longer be considered to be at low risk.

ADJUVANT SURGERY

Adjuvant surgery may be considered in the management of advanced cases, whereas, in our opinion, laparoscopy has no place in the treatment of these cases. Adjuvant surgery, or intervention surgery, is performed after radiotherapy, either for all patients or only for the non-responders or poor responders. Technically, it is a sort of debulking surgery which is carried out in risky conditions. A large amount of data exists about this surgery and its efficacy remains controversial. Einhorn *et al.* [10] found that adjuvant surgery increases the cure rate and increases it exponentially as the tumour volume becomes larger. Perez *et al.* [11] found no significant differences in survival or recurrence rates in patients treated either with irradiation alone or with irradiation followed by surgery. However, both these papers are based only on comparative retrospective surveys [10] and/or short series [11]. As stated by Himmelmann [12], a prospective trial including about 1100–1200 patients is needed to answer the question of the efficacy of adjuvant surgery. Obviously, the hazards

of this surgery have been underlined in all the publications devoted to the issue. These are related to the dose of irradiation the patient has received and to the extent of the surgical procedure to which the patient is submitted (radical hysterectomy is obviously more hazardous than simple extrafascial hysterectomy). Overall, the rate of complications after adjuvant surgery is about twice that after primary surgery.

Types and techniques of surgery in the management of cervical cancer

Using halstedian radical surgery endorses, in the treatment of cervical cancer, the distal-type radical hysterectomy combined with systematic pelvic and aortic lymphadenectomy as a treatment of choice. In 'Piver 4' radical hysterectomy the sacrouterine ligaments are cut at the level of their pelvic origin and half of the vagina is removed. However, most importantly, the cardinal ligament is divided at the level of its insertion on the pelvic wall. This means that the visceral branches of the hypogastric artery are cut at the level of their origin and the tributaries of the internal iliac vein are divided at the point they flow into it. In Burghardt's technique the vessels are carefully dissected, then clipped and cut one after the other, rather than clamped and cut *en bloc* as they are in the classic technique. Benedetti-Panici *et al.*, in a randomized controlled study, removed a 33-mm wide piece of paracervix by clamping and a 52-mm wide piece of paracervix by clipping ($P < 0.05$). Positivity rates were 64% and 44%, respectively [13].

Systematic pelvic and aortic lymphadenectomy is supposed to remove all the lymph nodes potentially involved in cancer of the cervix. The interiliac lymph nodes are removed (see Chapters 3 and 4). In addition, other pelvic lymph nodes are removed: hypogastric nodes (including the nodes, satellites of the superior and inferior gluteal vessels); the presacral nodes (including the nodes located in the concavity of the sacrum, at the level of emergence of the roots of the sciatic plexus); and the lumbosacral nodes (located behind the common iliac vein in the space limited by the psoas muscle laterally, the last lumbar vertebra medially and the cranial aspect of the wing of the sacrum dorsally). Aortic lymphadenectomy completes pelvic lymphadenectomy. Some surgeons limit the aortic dissection to the area located below the level of the origin of the inferior mesenteric artery, others extend it to the level of the left renal vein [14–17].

Modification of radical hysterectomy

As demonstrated by Piver and Rutledge, morbidity for distal (type 4) radical hysterectomy is much higher than that for less radical variants of the same operation (types 1–3). The question is whether increased morbidity is justified by better oncological outcomes. Only prospective and randomized studies can answer this question; the results of two such studies [18,19], published in the literature, are discussed below.

Stark [18], in Nüremberg, published data that included 210 patients affected by cervical cancer stage IB. The Te Linde operation was performed for 102 patients and the Meigs operation for the remaining 108. There were two postoperative fistulae in the Te Linde group and 11 in the Meigs group. The number of patients suffering postoperative problems (dysuria, incontinence, dyspareunia) was four in the Te Linde group and 12 in the Meigs. On the other hand, the rate of local recurrences, either isolated or combined with distant metastases, was exactly the same in the two populations—15.6%.

Mangioni [19] in Monza used the Piver 2 operation in 48 patients and the Piver 3 operation in 49 patients selected randomly from a population of women presenting with stage IB and IIA cervical cancers. No postoperative fistula was observed in the first group versus one in the second one. Urinary incontinence developed in six of the patients in the first group versus 16 in the second one; urinary retention developed in one and nine, respectively. After a 36 months follow-up the number of failures was 12 in the first group versus 13 in the second one (10 and eight, respectively, if only the pelvic recurrences were considered).

Two conclusions can be drawn from these prospective trials.

1 The more radical operations, while increasing morbidity, do not increase the chances of cure or reduce the risk of recurrence—an important argument in favour of modification.

2 When considering the definition of the different types of radical hysterectomies, differing terminology only confuses which type of operation is to be performed. Stark names the most radical operation as 'Meig's operation' and the less radical as 'Te Linde's operation'. Mangioni uses Piver terminology, and calls the most radical operation 'type 3' and the less radical 'type 2'. The conclusion is that between type 1 (extrafascial hysterectomy + colpectomy) and type 5 (radical hysterectomy + partial cystectomy), it is better to distinguish only two types of radical hysterectomy: proximal (modified radical) and distal (radical).

Modification of lymphadenectomy

Morbidity after systematic pelvic and aortic lymphadenectomy is obviously greater than after interiliac lymphadenectomy only. However, the difference is not as great as it is between the two types of radical hysterectomy. The arguments in favour of the most radical approach are very weak: whether one should remove only the interiliac nodes, or perform a systematic pelvic lymphadenectomy, or even include the para-aortic lymph nodes, is debatable and will only be answered by future studies.

In cases where interiliac lymph nodes are negative, systematic lymphadenectomy is not worth the effort and the hazards of the procedure. From reported research on systematic lymphadenectomy in cases where the pelvic lymph nodes are not involved, the rate of positive aortic lymph nodes lies between 1 and 2%. The first study on this topic, published by the team of the Fondation Curie in Paris [20] in 1977, found that the rate of positive common iliac lymph nodes is less than 2% in cases where the interiliac lymph nodes are not involved. Pilleron and Durand found positive common iliac lymph nodes in conjunction with negative interiliac lymph nodes only in stage IIB and/or bulky cases of cervical cancer. This suggests that only advanced tumours can bypass the sentinel nodes and metastasise directly to the common iliac and/or aortic nodes. This can be related to the fact that bulky and/or extended tumours may be neglected tumours, but most are fast growing aggressive diseases. This may also occur in other morphotypes of cancer (e.g. adenocarcinoma, massive lymphovascular spaces involvement), but cervical cancer extension generally follows the orthodox pathway, and systematic lymphadenectomy does not appear mandatory when interiliac assessment is negative.

When considering whether to perform systematic lymphadenectomy or selective lymphadenectomy, the value of lymphadenectomy itself should be discussed. Lymphadenectomy is obviously of no therapeutic value in pNo patients. For pN1 patients, data provided by Burghardt (see above) showed that removing positive lymph nodes has a definite value in cases where lymph-node involvement is limited: about two out of three patients are cured if one to three lymph nodes are involved. However, surgery is not effective in cases where four or more lymph nodes are positive. In the Gynecologic Oncology Group (GOG) study published by Fuller *et al.* [21], the cut-off limit is different (three positive lymph nodes), but the difference is of a similar magnitude (60% of cure in low-risk cases, 0–20% in high-risk cases). This report shows that lymphadenectomy has a therapeutic role. In fact, this study was a randomized trial which opposed postoperative radiotherapy vs no postoperative radiotherapy. No difference was found between the two arms, either in the favourable cases (one or two positive lymph nodes) or in the poor cases (three or more positive lymph nodes). This suggests that the high survival rate we observe after lymphadenectomy performed in patients with limited lymph-node involvement is related to lymphadenectomy itself rather than to radiotherapy which traditionally is given postoperatively.

Assuming that lymphadenectomy has a therapeutic value in selected cases, a question still remains open: which type of lymphadenectomy should be performed to obtain the best therapeutic effect? Some reports have established that the more complete the lymphadenectomy, the higher the chances of cure. Crouet *et al.* [22] reported that the chances of 5-year disease-free survival in stage IB or early stage II are 80% if 20 lymph nodes or more are removed vs 63% if 12 lymph nodes or less are removed. Knapstein *et al.* [23] made the same statement with another cut-off: in a series of 122 stage IB–IIIB cases, the rate of 5-year disease-free survival moved from 79% to 54%, depending on the number of lymph nodes removed: >35 or ≤35. However, in the institutions where the latter surveys were made the number of retrieved nodes depends on the individual characteristics of each patient rather than on the surgeon's skill. Kjorstad [24] counted the number of lymph nodes left behind (by preoperative lymphangiography and postoperative X-ray). He did not find any significant difference in recurrence between the cases where no lymph nodes remained (81 cases, 17% recurrence rare) and the cases where one to three lymph nodes were left (143 cases, 11%). Only in cases where four or more lymph nodes were left (69 cases) did the rate of recurrence increase dramatically—to 28%.

Finally, the number of retrieved nodes is not the relevant issue. The template of node dissection is much more important.

1 If no metastasis is found after a correctly performed interiliac lymphadenectomy (seven lymph nodes on each side on average), it is not necessary to perform the 'upper' lymphadenectomy neither for diagnosis nor for therapeutic purposes: the risk of common iliac and/or aortic lymph-node involvement is negligible.

2 If one or two interiliac lymph nodes are metastatic it is necessary to perform a systematic lymphadenectomy. If no diseased extrapelvic lymph nodes are found the chances of cure are two out of three. The extent of lymph-node removal is certainly not the cause of this result, but there is no other method of being sure that lymph-node involvement is limited. The prognosis of the patients who are affected by extrapelvic lymph-node metastases is poor. However, the only patients who can be cured are the those submitted to systematic lymphadenectomy and especially the patients whose lymph-node metastases are purely microscopic, hence detectable only by systematic lymphadenectomy.

3 If three or more interiliac lymph nodes are positive the prognosis is very poor and the place of the upper lymphadenectomy should be questioned. Potish [25] has shown

that the patients affected by aortic lymph-node metastases do better if debulking is performed. Even if this assertion is largely biased (the only patients who were debulked were those who were debulkable), performing systematic lymphadenectomy may make sense.

Routes used for radical hysterectomy

Historically, radical surgery for cancer of the cervix has been carried out either through the abdominal route or through the vaginal route. Almost one century after the mythic fight opposing Schauta and his former pupil Wertheim, the controversy is still not dead.

In the very early days, surgery for uterine cancer was performed transvaginally. Surgical morbidity and mortality were high and the outcomes were very poor. In 1895 some pioneers, Clark, Latzko, Ries and Rumpf, started performing abdominal hysterectomies for uterine cancer. On 16 November 1898, Ernst Wertheim performed his first abdominal radical hysterectomy. The patient died 8 hours later. However, Wertheim reported to the Society of Practitioners in Vienna on 14 October 1904 a series of more than 200 cases [26]. The mortality was 30 for the first 100 cases and 22 for the following 100 cases. At this time Friedrich Schauta had less experience; he had performed his first vaginal radical hysterectomy on 1 June 1901. The patient did well and his postoperative mortality was 14 for the 113 cases operated in the years 1901–3 (12.4%). During the discussion which followed the presentation made by his pupil, Schauta used as an argument the differences in the postoperative mortality. However, most of the controversy was over the lymphadenectomy. Schauta stated that selective lymphadenectomy (removing the enlarged lymph nodes), which was put forward by Wertheim as a decisive advantage in favour of the abdominal approach, was useless, as almost all the patients affected by lymph-node metastases in Wertheim's series recurred.

During the following decades only a few reports on the use of vaginal surgery were published. In 1956 Van Bouwdijk Bastianse [27] reported 76 patients who were operated on during the years 1947 and 1948, with a 75% and 65% disease-free survival rate in stage I and stage II, respectively. Navratil reported in 1963 [28] on 808 cases operated in the years 1947–56, with 83.3% 5-year disease-free survival for stage I, 79.9% for stage IB and 51.7% for stage II cases. In the same year, McCall [29] reported on 50 patients with stage IA, IB and IIA cervical cancer operated on 5 or more years before; 45 survived. Ingiulla in 1966 [30] reported results on 327 patients: the 5-year disease-free survival was 81% in stage I and 56% in stage II cases. Massi *et al.* published in 1993 [31] the results of their experience concerning 458 patients operated during the years 1968–83. They found similar 5-year disease-free survival rates after Schauta (*n* = 356) or Wertheim (*n* = 288) radical hysterectomies (79.5% and 76.7% respectively).

Combining the data of published reports, it appears that Schauta's statement is still timely: evidence is lacking for the need to combine lymphadenectomy with radical hysterectomy, at least for early cases in which the rates of cure are the same after radical vaginal hysterectomy and after radical abdominal hysterectomy. If, in such cases, the rate of positive lymph nodes is about 15%, including 10% of cases in which a systematic lymphadenectomy can cure two out of three patients (no more than one or two positive lymph nodes), the rate of cure should be 5–10% more after the abdominal operation, which is not the case. This could be interpreted as evidence that the vaginal operation is more radical, which could balance the absence of lymphadenectomy. The assumption that vaginal radical hysterectomy has at least the same value as the abdominal procedure is still valid. We chose to adopt it in conjunction with laparoscopic lymphadenectomy to fulfil two apparently contradictory goals: minimizing surgical trauma and increasing radicality.

Place of laparoscopy in the surgical management of cancer of the cervix

In accordance with the data analysed in the first part of this chapter, early cases (stage IA2 and IB1) and advanced cases (stages IB2 and others) are dealt with separately.

Early cervical carcinoma

In early cases, laparoscopy selects patients who require radical hysterectomy, while at the same time technically preparing the way for radical surgery. Before undertaking laparoscopy, it is important to ensure that the case is an early one. This is not a problem for patients previously submitted to conization; the assessment of their specimen gives the diagnosis (stage IA2 or stage IB) and assesses the tumour volume. In other cases, an MRI is routinely performed as it gives a relatively precise evaluation of the status of the paracervix and enables us to measure the tumour diameter with great accuracy. In a few cases, hypertrophy of the pelvic lymph nodes is seen and a stereotaxic puncture is recommended. If this is positive the case is moved to the advanced category (see later).

LAPAROSCOPY AS A SELECTION TOOL FOR RADICAL SURGERY

In early cases laparoscopy can assess both the peritoneal cavity and the retroperitoneal space. The former is not as important as the latter, but it should not be neglected. Three questions have to be answered when assessing the retroperitoneal space.

How significant is the lymph-node assessment?

The extent of the lymph-node assessment has been widely discussed in the first part of this chapter. With a few exceptions (adenocarcinoma, lymph vascular space involvement) the assessment should be limited to the interiliac area and extended higher only in cases where the interiliac lymph nodes are positive.

Are frozen sections adequate?

Frozen sections do not provide the same diagnostic safety as assessment performed on embedded specimens. They have the advantage that a decision can be made immediately and a radical operation can be performed under the same anaesthesia. This approach could be thought of as more patient friendly. However, the rate of false negatives is relatively high, leading to re-operation and/or radiotherapy, which is problematical for the patient and the surgeon. For this reason we prefer the two-step procedure. After the first short hospital stay, the patient is recalled and the therapeutic policy is discussed with her after full documentation: lymph nodes involved or not? number of involved nodes? macro- or micro-metastasis? capsular rupture? Laparoscopic preparation for radical surgery (see later) can be carried out during the initial surgery—at the end of laparoscopic lymph-node dissection—and still helps the secondary surgery provided it is undertaken within 10 days.

What should be done post laparoscopy?

The first aim of laparoscopic staging is to select the candidates for radical surgery. It is generally accepted that node-negative patients are good candidates for surgery but that the indications for the need for surgery in node-positive patients is open to discussion. Two patient groups may be defined in the pN1 population: less than three positive lymph nodes (pN1A) and three or more positive lymph nodes (pN1B).

For the pN1A patients radical surgery offers good chances of cure, and should be considered. The hysterectomy is straightforward, but the type of lymphadenectomy and the approach has to be discussed. In this situation, a systematic lymphadenectomy has to be carried out. It can be performed by using the laparoscope. However, the operation takes a long time, because all the lymph nodes need to be removed between the left renal vein and the femoral ring, and there are obviously hazards. Therefore, in my opinion, the surgery is better performed using laparotomy, and this is particularly true when the positive interiliac lymph node(s) is(are) enlarged and fixed to the big vessels. In this circumstance open lymphadenectomy offers some chance of cure.

LAPAROSCOPY AS PREPARATION FOR RADICAL SURGERY

Which route should be chosen for performing radical hysterectomy after laparoscopic staging?

Three options are available.

1 Laparotomy, for many gynaecological oncologists, is the only way a radical hysterectomy can be performed. Should this be the case, presurgical laparoscopic staging would not be cost effective. The only patients who can take advantage of surgical staging are the node-positive patients for whom radiotherapy can be directly undertaken, while avoiding laparotomy and its associated radiation complications. However, these patients represent only about 15% of all the node-positive patients or only 5% if only the patients with massive metastases (pN1B) are managed by radiation therapy. For all the other patients (85%), laparoscopic staging leads to a laparotomy by means of which the lymphadenectomy could have been faster and cheaper.

2 Full laparoscopic radical hysterectomy is an option for some surgeons, and it has the advantage of great consistency: it starts and finishes with laparoscopy. However, the radicality of the radical laparoscopic hysterectomy is more than questionable. It is very easy to divide laparoscopically the cranial part of the paracervix at the level of its origin, but doing the same to the caudal part is very difficult because of the huge amount of plexoid veins which are present at this level. As a result the specimens produced at radical laparoscopic hysterectomy, in the rare instances where the laparoscopic surgeons present them, are far from equivalent to those obtained after a century of classical radical surgery. We believe this procedure needs to be refined more before it can be endorsed.

3 The vaginal approach does not incur the same reproaches as its radicality cannot be questioned. In fact it is almost too radical, as it often leads to well-documented urinary bladder dysfunction. However, the radicality of the radical vaginal hysterectomy can be modified (see below).

How radical should surgery be?

The chances of survival in stages IB and IIA cervical cancer are similar whatever the extent of radical hysterectomy:

these are the conclusions of the two prospective and randomized reports discussed above [18,19]. Can these conclusions be extrapolated to radical vaginal hysterectomy? We believe the answer is yes. The modified Stoeckel vaginal radical hysterectomy [32] probably provides the same outcome as the classic Schauta–Amreich procedure. However, data establishing this concept are lacking. In this context, a separation between tumours less than 2 cm in diameter and those 2–4 cm in diameter seems to be sensible.

1 For tumours less than 2 cm in diameter, proximal radical hysterectomy is adequate, whatever the route used for performing the surgery. If the amount of removed paracervical tissues is added to that of the uninvolved cervical tissues, the space between the tumour and the margins of the specimen is large enough. The Schauta–Stoeckel operation is appropriate.

2 For tumours 2–4 cm in diameter, proximal radical hysterectomy is adequate if we operate through the abdominal route. The transverse diameter of the pelvic cavity is, at the level of the pelvic brim, more than 12 cm. Putting the clamps at a distance of more than 2 cm from the tumour, while keeping some space between the clamp and the pelvic wall, is possible. Vaginal access to the paracervical ligament is obtained at the level of the narrowest diameter of the pelvic cavity: the bi-ischiatic diameter is no more than 10 cm. The particular anatomy of the vaginal approach thus leads to the performance of distal radical hysterectomy.

How much use should be made of the laparoscope?

The role of laparoscopic assistance in the two variants of laparoscopically assisted vaginal radical hysterectomy has been described in Chapters 7 and 8. This role is summarized below.

1 In proximal laparoscopically assisted vaginal radical hysterectomy, the laparoscopic development of the paravesical and pararectal spaces, and the laparoscopic division of the uterine arteries at the level of their origins, improve downwards mobility of the genitalia and facilitates clamping of the paracervix, which is done from below at the appropriate 'intermediate' level.

2 In distal laparoscopically assisted vaginal radical hysterectomy, the role of laparoscopy is not only to prepare the paravesical spaces and divide the uterine arteries, but also to divide the paracervix at the appropriate distal level, which can be done much more easily from above. A paravaginal incision (Schuchardt), which is mandatory in the Schauta–Amreich procedure, can be avoided.

Comparison of our personal data from two periods — 1986–92 (laparoscopic lymphadenectomy + classic vaginal radical hysterectomy) and 1992–6 (laparoscopically assisted vaginal radical hysterectomy)—does not demonstrate any advantage of the most recent policy over the previous one. The vaginal step of the laparoscopically assisted vaginal radical hysterectomy is easier to perform and can be performed in a shorter time than the classic vaginal radical hysterectomy. However, the laparoscopic step of the combined procedure is not without difficulties, and can lead to complications which do not exist in a simple laparoscopic lymphadenectomy. Moreover, it was a great disappointment to discover that the distal laparoscopically assisted vaginal radical hysterectomy led to the same rate of bladder retentions and secondary dysurias as did the classic Schauta–Amreich procedure.

The bladder problem is the most embarrassing drawback of distal vaginal radical hysterectomy, but laparoscopy may provide the optimal answer. The bladder dysfunction we observe after distal radical hysterectomy results from distal division of the caudal (nervous) part of the paracervix; they are not observed (or only very transiently) after proximal radical hysterectomy. However, cutting the paracervix at the level of its origin is carried out with the aim of removing all the adipose tissue and lymphatic structures which are lying in it. Laparoscopic magnification is an invaluable help in completing a precise dissection of the distal part of the paracervix, while preserving the vascular and, more importantly, the nervous part. After completion of a laparoscopic paracervical lymphadenectomy (see Chapter 3) there is no need to perform a distal laparoscopically assisted vaginal radical hysterectomy: the proximal type vaginal procedure is enough. That is the rationale for the laparoscopic-vaginal radical hysterectomy we developed jointly with Denis Querleu: this new procedure is currently undergoing prospective trials in our institutions.

Advanced cervical carcinoma

Performing a laparoscopically assisted vaginal radical hysterectomy on a tumour of more than 4 cm seems to be technically possible, but we do not consider it to be a reasonable option. When balancing costs and benefits, radiation therapy with or without chemotherapy is the method of choice in such cases. In some protocols this is followed by a modified radical hysterectomy done as 'closure surgery' or intervention surgery: using a laparoscopic and/or laparoscopic-vaginal approach for this kind of surgery is potentially dangerous and we do not recommend its use. As a consequence, in advanced cases laparoscopic surgery plays no more than the role of a staging procedure.

WHICH ROUTE SHOULD BE CHOSEN FOR LAPAROSCOPIC STAGING?

The retroperitoneal route can be advocated to reduce de novo postoperative adhesions. This advantage is of crucial importance to patients who will be, with no exception, submitted to radiation therapy.

The transumbilical examination of the peritoneal cavity is advised as advanced malignancies can involve the intraperitoneal structures (pelvic peritoneum, rectosigmoid, ileum and/or right colon, ovaries and tubes).

A combination of transperitoneal and retroperitoneal approaches fulfils the double goal of laparoscopic staging in the face of advanced cervical cancer. We advise that a transumbilical transperitoneal laparoscopic assessment is first performed, then move to the retroperitoneal approach (see Chapter 5).

PELVIC ± AORTIC STAGING?

The rationale for aortic staging in advanced cervical cancer is that (i) aortic nodes may be involved even in the absence of pelvic node metastasis, (ii) extended-field radiation therapy is not necessary in the case of negative aortic nodes, and (iii) pelvic exenteration, when required locally, is considered to be contraindicated when the aortic nodes are positive. In addition, the clinical significance of common iliac involvement is generally considered as similar to aortic involvement. For these reasons, we recommend aortic and common iliac dissection in all cases of advanced cervical carcinoma, provided that the age or medical condition of the patient does not contraindicate extended-field radiation therapy or exenteration.

The question is whether or not to add a pelvic (external and internal iliac) dissection and, if the answer is yes, whether to start with pelvic or aortic dissection. Two categories of patients may be defined after preoperative imaging. If radiologically enlarged nodes are visible, surgical debulking of the nodes is considered, and laparoscopic surgery may not be the best tool. If the imaging does not detect any enlarged node, the dose and template of pelvic radiation therapy which will be used for the control of the central disease is supposed to control microscopic involvement of nodes at the same time. In neither category is laparoscopic pelvic dissection of use in planning management protocol. In addition, some of the patients with tumours larger than 4 cm, especially IB2 patients, will have radical surgery after external radiation therapy. In such cases, a previous retroperitoneal dissection, by whatever approach, leaves a dense and extensive fibrosis that makes radical surgery more difficult. As a consequence, we do not perform staging external and internal iliac dissection in advanced carcinoma of the cervix.

Conclusion

There are many areas in this field which are subject to personal or institutional preferences or policies. The philosophy of oncology from different countries and centres accounts for the multiple options when it comes to individualized management. Laparoscopy increases the number of available management options. Whatever the agenda and extent of pretherapeutic laparoscopic staging, and how how the treatment ends (secondary surgery or not), staging lymphadenectomy has to be as complete as possible. In patients who will be submitted to radiation therapy only, its diagnostic value is suboptimal if only a few nodes are retrieved. In patients who will be submitted to surgery as part of their management, the fibrosis induced by a simple sampling procedure makes the completion of a systematic lymphadenectomy extremely difficult. As a consequence, laparoscopic staging may well be a 'targetted' dissection in a limited area, but a complete lymphadenectomy should always be performed in the corresponding area.

References

1 Burghardt E (1993). *Surgical Gynecologic Oncology*. Stuttgart: Thieme.

2 Piver MS, Rutledge FN, Smith JP (1974). Five classes of extended hysterectomy for women with cervical cancer. *Obstet Gynecol* **44**:265–270.

3 Van Nagell JR, Raddik JW, Lowin DM (1971). The staging of cervical cancer—inevitable discrepancies between clinical staging and pathologic findings. *Am J Obstet Gynecol* **110**:973–978.

4 Delgado G, Bundy BN, Fowler WC *et al* (1989). A prospective surgical pathological study of Stage I squamous carcinoma of the cervix: a gynecologic oncology group study. *Gynecol Oncol* **35**:314–320.

5 Baltzer J, Lohe KJ, Kaufmann C *et al* (1982). Histological criteria for the prognosis in patients with operated squamous cell carcinoma of the cervix. *Gynecol Oncol* **13**:184–194.

6 Dargent D, Keita N, Mathevet P *et al* (1993). Histoire naturelle du cancer du col: confrontation entre les données morphologiques et les chances de survie. *Ref Gynecol Obstet* **1**:548–554.

7 Nelson JH, Macaset MA, Lu T *et al* (1974). The incidence and significance of laparoscopic lymph nodes metastases in late invasive carcinoma in the cervix. *Am J Obstet Gynecol* **118**:749–756.

8 Nelson JH, Boyce J, Macaset M *et al* (1977). Incidence, significance and follow up of paraaortic lymph nodes metastases in late invasive carcinoma of the cervix. *Am J Obstet Gynecol* **128**:336–340.

9 Weiser FB, Bundy BN, Hoskins WJ *et al* (1989). Extraperitoneal versus transperitoneal selective para-aortic lymphadenectomy in the treatment surgical staging of advanced cervical cancer (a GOG study). *Gynecol Oncol* **33**:283–289.

10 Einhorn N, Patek E, Sjoberg B (1985). Outcome of different treatment modifications in cervix carcinoma, Stage IB and IIA: observation in a well defined Swedish population. *Cancer* **55**:949–955.

11 Perez CA, Camel HM, Kao MS, Askin F (1987). Randomized study of preoperative radiation and surgery or in radiation alone in the treatment of Stage IB and IIA carcinoma of the uterine cervix: final report. *Gynecol Oncol* **27**:129–140.

12 Himmelmann A, Holmberg E, Janson I *et al* (1985). The effect of post operative external radiotherapy in cervical carcinoma Stage IB and IIA. *Gynecol Oncol* **22**:73–84.

13 Benedetti-Panici P, Scambia G, Baiocchi G *et al* (1993). Radical hysterectomy: a randomized study comparing two techniques for resection of the cardinal ligament. *Gynecol Oncol* **50**:226–231.

14 Winter R (1993). Cervical cancer. Lymphadenectomy. In: Burghardt E, ed. *Surgical Gynecologic Oncology*. Stuttgart: Thieme.

15 Di Re F, Lupi G, Fontanelli R *et al* (1989). I tumori dell utero e della vulva. In: Veronesi V, ed. *Trattato di Chirurgia Oncologica*. Torino: UTET, 493–508.

16 Benedetti-Panici P, Scambia G, Bariocchi G *et al* (1991). Technique and feasibility of systematic para-aortic and pelvic lymphadenectomy in gynecologic malignancies—a prospective study. *Int J Gynecol Cancer* **1**:133.

17 Michel G, Morice Ph, Castaigne D *et al* (1998). Lymphatic spread in stage IB and II cervical carcinoma: anatomy and surgical implications. *Am J Obstet Gynecol* **91**:360–363.

18 Stark G (1987). Zum operativen Therapie des Collum Karzinoms Stadium IB. *Geburtshilfe Frauenheilkd* **47**:45–48.

19 Maneo A, Landoni F, Milani R *et al* (1996). Radical hysterectomy in cervical cancer stage IB–IIA. A randomized study. In: Benedetti-Panici P, Scambia G, Maneschi F, Sevin BU, Mancuso S, eds. *Wertheim's Radical Hysterectomy*. Rome: Societa Editrice Universo, 93–100.

20 Pilleron JP, Durand JC, Hamelin JP (1974). Prognostic value of node metastasis in cancer of the uterine cervix. *Am J Obstet Gynecol* **119**:458–462.

21 Fuller A, Elliot N, Kosloff C *et al* (1982). Lymph nodes metastases from carcinoma of the cervix stages IB and IIA: implications for prognosis and treatment. *Gynecol Oncol* **13**:164–174.

22 Crouet H, Mace-Lesc'h J, Heron JF (1994). Cancer du col utérin au Stades opérables—Influence de la qualité du prélèvement ganglionnaire. Presented to Congrès de la Société Française d'Oncologie Gynécologique, Lille, 16 Septembre 1994.

23 Knapstein PG, Balhlmann F, Beck T *et al* (1996). Mikroinvasive Chirurgie—ein Ausblick. *Zentralbl Gynakol* **118**:110–112.

24 Kjorstad KE (1988). The rationale of pelvic lymphadenectomy in patients with Stage IB cancer of the cervix: a diagnostic or therapeutic procedure? *Baillieres Clin Obstet Gynaecol* **2**:905–918.

25 Potish R, Downey G, Adcoch L *et al* (1989). The role of surgical debulking in cancer of the uterine cervix. *Int J Radiat Oncol Biol Phys* **17**:979–984.

26 Wertheim E (1904). Bericht über die mit der erweiterten Uteruskreboperation zu erwartenden Dauerhellungen. *Wien Klin Wochenschr* **42**:1128 and **43**:1153.

27 Van Bouwdijk Bastianse MA (1956). Treatment of cancer of the cervix uteri. *Am J Obstet Gynecol* **72**:100–118.

28 Navratil E (1963). Indications and results of the Schauta Amreich operation with and without postoperative roentgen treatment in epidermoid carcinoma of the cervix of the uterus. *Am J Obstet Gynecol* **86**:141–150.

29 McCall ML (1963). A modern evaluation of the radical vaginal

operation for carcinoma of the cervix. *Am J Obstet Gynecol* **85**:295–301.

30 Ingiulla W (1966). Five year results of 327 Schauta Amreich operations for cervical carcinoma. *Am J Obstet Gynecol* **96**:188–191.

31 Massi G, Savino L, Susini T (1993). Schauta Amreich vaginal hysterectomy and Wertheim Meigs abdominal hysterectomy in the treatment of cervical cancer: a retrospective analysis. *Am J Obstet Gynecol* **3**:928–934.

32 Stoeckel W (1928). Die vaginale Radikaloperation des Collumkarzinoms. *Zentralbl Gynakol* **1**:39–63.

18 Endometrial carcinoma

Magdy W. Nour and Joel M. Childers

Introduction

Since the turn of the century, physicians have known that most women with early endometrial carcinoma can be cured by hysterectomy and removal of the adnexa. Abdominal hysterectomy has been the technique most frequently employed. In 1900 Thomas Cullen recommended in his book *Cancer of the Uterus* that abdominal hysterectomy was the treatment of choice for patients with endometrial carcinoma [1]. This chapter will summarize the current literature on the use of laparoscopy in patients with endometrial cancer and present a brief historical overview of traditional surgical management to aid in understanding why laparoscopy logically has a place in the surgical management of these patients. We believe that operative laparoscopy will probably play a significant role in the management of these patients in the future.

From clinical to surgical-pathological staging

It has been recognized for a number of years that patients with early endometrial cancer and/or well-differentiated malignancies have done better than patients with more advanced disease and/or less differentiated carcinoma. Unfortunately, early literature on survival rates did not differentiate for factors such as grade of the tumour or depth of myometrial invasion. As survival data became available, investigators noted a clear relationship between survival and differentiation of tumour [2].

Individual investigators and literature reviews have also indicated that the survival of patients with endometrial carcinoma decreased as myometrial invasion increased [2]. Cheon reported an increased percentage of deep myometrial invasion with decreased differentiation of tumour [3]. Creasman *et al.* studied the relationship between nodal metastases and histological grade of myometrial involvement. They discovered as tumours decreased in differentiation and increased in myometrial invasion, the incidence of nodal metastases increased. This was true for both pelvic and para-aortic lymph nodes [4]. Following this, the Gynecologic Oncology Group

(GOG) initiated prospective surgical-pathological studies in clinical stage 1 subjects. This group's original limited institutional study, as well as a group-wide study involving 621 patients with clinical stage 1 carcinoma of the endometrium, substantiated the previously reported relationships between grade of tumour and depth of myometrial invasion [5,6]. It was also noted that as the depth of invasion increased within each grade category, so did the chances of lymph-node metastases.

Surgical-pathological staging studies have clearly demonstrated the inaccuracies of clinical staging [4–11]. Because clinical evaluation is unable to identify most adnexal metastases, intraperitoneal implants and nodal metastases, between 15% and 28% of patients with clinical stage 1 endometrial carcinoma are understaged. Realizing clinical staging was potentially quite inaccurate when treatment results were analysed, the cancer committee of the International Federation of Gynecology and Obstetrics (FIGO) changed their classification for endometrial carcinoma from a clinical to a surgical-pathological staged disease [12]. Because, grade for grade, survival rates did not seem to be affected by whether the patient had received preoperative radium and surgery or surgery alone [13–15], and because potential important prognostic factors such as depth of invasion, vascular space invasion, true tumour grade, peritoneal cytology, oestrogen-progesterone receptor status and DNA ploidy are potentially unevaluable in patients who have received preoperative radiotherapy, surgical-pathological staging made sound scientific sense. For all these reasons, the once common practice of administering preoperative radiation therapy to patients with endometrial carcinoma has now largely been abandoned for primary surgical-pathological staging. Currently, adjuvant treatment recommendations are clearly influenced by the information obtained from surgical staging [16].

Vaginal hysterectomy in endometrial cancer

The use of vaginal hysterectomy by physicians treating patients with adenocarcinoma of the endometrium has

148

been limited, because it was thought survival could be compromised. However, there are several reports on the use of vaginal hysterectomy in patients with endometrial cancer. European reports date back several decades. Van Bouwdijk Bastianse, in a retrospective study of 217 patients, reported on the use of total vaginal hysterectomy to treat patients with all stages and grades of endometrial carcinoma [17]. This study, which was published in 1952, reported a survival rate of 72%. This uncorrected survival rate is similar to the 73% survival rate reported by Ingiulla *et al.* in their retrospective study of 112 patients treated with total vaginal hysterectomy and bilateral salpingo-oophorectomy [18]. They, too, treated patients of all stages and grades.

The largest American experience using vaginal hysterectomy to treat patients with endometrial cancer has been at the Mayo Clinic [19–22]. In four separate reports that cover the years from 1930 to 1972, with very little overlap, they reported the use of total vaginal hysterectomy in 263 patients. The first of these publications reports a 5-year survival of 82.7% (67/81) of patients [19]. The second report, and the only publication from this institution devoted solely to the use of vaginal hysterectomy in endometrial cancer, is also the largest American series on this surgical approach to endometrial cancer [20]. This retrospective study of 100 patients comprised 15% (100/659) of the patients with endometrial cancer treated at the Mayo Clinic during the decade 1945–54. In 44 patients a vaginal hysterectomy was utilized for medical reasons. Forty-three of these patients had ovaries which, for technical reasons, were not removed. In this publication, Pratt *et al.* reported an 89% corrected 5-year survival (95% for grade 1 tumours and 72.7% for grade 3 tumours). Three patients required morcellization of the uterus and none of these three died of the disease. In four of the 10 patients who died of the disease within 5 years, the ovaries were not removed.

The third publication on the Mayo Clinic's experience with vaginal hysterectomy and endometrial cancer reports similar 5-year survival rates [22]. Malkasian *et al.* reported a study on patients with endometrial cancer who were managed between 1962 and 1972; 67 patients were treated by total vaginal hysterectomy. The 5-year survival for the patients with grade 2 and 3 tumours did not differ from that of patients treated with abdominal hysterectomy during the same period, and the outcome for patients with well-differentiated tumours was higher than predicted by the actuarial tables.

This similarity in 5-year survival rate between patients with stage 1 endometrial carcinoma treated with total vaginal hysterectomy, and those treated with total abdominal hysterectomy, is confirmed in a report by Candiani *et al.* [23]. These authors published results on 425 patients treated in the decade between 1970 and 1980. Three different surgical approaches were utilized: total abdominal hysterectomy with bilateral salpingo-oophorectomy and selective pelvic lymphadenectomy (245 patients), total abdominal hysterectomy and bilateral salpingo-oophorectomy (100 patients) and total vaginal hysterectomy with bilateral salpingo-oophorectomy (80 patients). A similar corrected 5-year survival rate was observed in each of these groups (81%, 90% and 88%, respectively). Unfortunately, the number of grade 2 and 3 lesions was not evenly distributed (69%, 35% and 43%, respectively), and therefore sound conclusions concerning survival and surgical approach cannot be reached.

Cliby *et al.* [24] reported a retrospective study of 54 patients treated at the Mayo Clinic for uterine prolapse and coexistent endometrial cancer. All patients underwent vaginal hysterectomy between the period 1950 and 1993. In 19 patients bilateral oophorectomy was not performed. The 5-year survival rate was 83%, 4/53 patients had a recurrence (two with grade 2, one with grade 1 and one with grade 3). The disease-free survival for all patients was 92% at 5 and 10 years. This report compares favourably with other reports for stage 1 endometrial cancer.

The recent literature on the use of vaginal hysterectomy in the treatment of patients with endometrial carcinoma is scant. There are only three reports in the literature on this topic in the last 10 years. The report by Candiani *et al.* is the only one of these publications that did not limit this surgical approach to medically compromised patients [23]. It is also the only European report. The remaining two publications are both retrospective American studies addressing the use of vaginal hysterectomy for the management of medically compromised patients with clinical stage 1 endometrial cancer.

Peters *et al.* combined experiences from the University of Virginia and the University of Michigan over the 27 years from 1955 to 1981 [25]. Vaginal hysterectomy was performed in 56 patients because of obesity or major medical problems. The 5-year survival for all patients was 94%. The 5-year survival was 98% with grade 1 tumours, 78% with grade 2 tumours and 84% with grade 3 tumours. The adnexa were removed in only 10 of the patients (18%) in this report. Thirty-two patients received adjuvant radiotherapy. Several of the surgical techniques discussed in this report are worthy of mention. These authors were the first to describe procurement of pelvic washings upon entering the cul-de-sac. While the clinical significance of malignant peritoneal cytology in patients with early endometrial carcinoma has not been completely defined, and is certainly beyond the scope of this chapter, most investigators believe that this information is worth retrieving [26]. To assist in removal of the uterus, they used Schuchardt incisions in five patients and uterine morcellization in seven.

Bloss *et al.* reported the only other recently published experience on vaginal hysterectomy in endometrial carcinoma [27]. They combined the experience of three southern Californian institutions from 1970 to 1990. All 31 of their patients had clinical stage 1 endometrial carcinomata and were treated with total vaginal hysterectomy, because they were considered to be at high risk for morbidity and mortality from an abdominal approach. The risk factors included morbid obesity, hypertension, diabetes mellitus and cardiovascular disease. Thirty-five per cent of their patients received adjuvant radiotherapy because of deep myometrial invasion or an unfavourable histology. They reported a 5-year survival rate of 93%. The only cancer-related death occurred 4.5 years following surgery in a patient with a poorly differentiated carcinoma. Three patients experienced serious postoperative complications which extended their time spent in hos-pital (haemorrhage requiring abdominal exploration, pulmonary embolism and myocardial infarction). There were no postoperative deaths.

The authors listed several recommendations for safely accomplishing vaginal hysterectomies in these high-risk patients. Episiotomy (either unilateral or bilateral) and suturing the labia to the inner thighs was recommended to improve exposure. Preoperative ultrasound assessment was recommended to identify large uteri. They believed morcellization of the uterus, which was not used in any of the patients in their series, should be avoided. While removal of the adnexa was recommended and was performed in 11 (35%) of their patients, they did not believe that failure to do so warranted abdominal exploration.

There are several drawbacks to vaginal surgery for the treatment of endometrial cancer. Obviously, the surgeon is unable to assess the intraperitoneal cavity for extra-uterine disease. The lymph-nodes status will also remain unknown. For a number of reasons, the adnexa may not be able to be removed. It is even possible that a large uterus, or a uterus fixed high in the pelvis by inflammation, endometriosis or other factors, may not be able to be removed. These, and other factors, mean vaginal hysterectomy can be legitimately limited to those patients who are morbidly obese, medically compromised or have well-differentiated carcinomata. In the latter case, frozen section should be performed intraoperatively and lymph-node sampling should be performed depending on the grade of the tumour and the depth of invasion.

Rationale for laparoscopy in endometrial cancer

The components required for surgical staging of endometrial cancer, hysterectomy, adnexectomy and pelvic and para-aortic lymphadenectomy were all individually discussed in early reports on operative laparoscopy [28–40]. Numerous authors have reported their initial experience with laparoscopic hysterectomy and laparoscopically assisted vaginal hysterectomy for benign disease.

Fewer investigators reported on laparoscopic lymphadenectomy, and initial reports on laparoscopic lymphadenectomy were limited to pelvic lymph nodes; however, laparoscopic removal of para-aortic lymph nodes soon became feasible [37]. Shortly after these three procedures, hysterectomy and pelvic and para-aortic lymphadenectomy, were combined for the management of patients with stage 1 endometrial carcinoma (Figs 18.1 & 18.2) [38]. These investigators believed that operative laparoscopy could overcome the surgical limitations of the pure vaginal approach in patients with stage 1 endometrial cancer. Laparoscopy was used to: (i) assess the intraperitoneal cavity; (ii) obtain washings; (iii) guarantee removal of the adnexa; (iv) perform pelvic and para-aortic lymph-node sampling; and (v) guarantee vaginal removal of the uterus.

There are currently only a handful of reports addressing the role of operative laparoscopy in endometrial cancer [38,40–44]. Laparoscopy has been used to surgically stage patients with their uterus *in situ* and patients whose uterus has been removed. First reports involved patients with clinical stage 1 disease in whom hysterectomy had not yet been performed. These patients underwent laparoscopic surgical staging, including laparoscopically assisted vaginal hysterectomy, salpingo-oophorectomy and lymphadenectomy. The second group of patients, in which investigators have found a role for operative

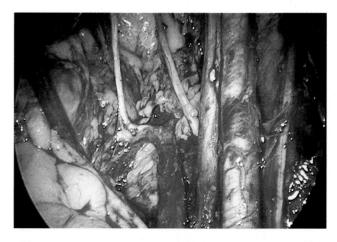

Fig. 18.1 Photograph following completion of a right laparoscopic pelvic lymphadenectomy. The right external iliac artery can be seen adjacent to the psoas muscle. The obturator nerve can be seen in the top portion of the centre of the photograph between the external iliac artery and the obliterated umbilical artery.

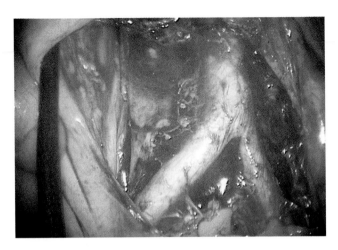

Fig. 18.2 Photograph following completion of a bilateral laparoscopic para-aortic lymphadenectomy. Note the nodal tissue below the inferior mesenteric artery has been completely removed.

laparoscopy, are those in whom surgical staging was not performed at the time of their hysterectomy [40]. In these patients, laparoscopic surgery was used to obtain peritoneal cytology, remove regional lymph nodes and remove remaining adnexa in some patients.

Experience with operative laparoscopy in endometrial cancer

Our experience at the University of Arizona with our first 100 patients with clinical stage 1 adenocarcinoma of the endometrium has been published in two separate reports [42,44]. The first report described the management algorithm and experience with 59 patients. The second report analysed the learning-curve parameters of the first 100 patients. This is a consecutive series of patients managed by two oncological surgeons. The overall arrangements for diagnosis and treatment were identical to those utilized prior to laparoscopic management. Patients with well-differentiated malignancies and invasion to less than one-half of the myometrium are at low risk for metastatic disease, and traditionally lymphadenectomy has been omitted during these staging procedures. Typically, intraoperative frozen section has been used to minimize understaging of those patients whose preoperative diagnosis indicated a well-differentiated tumour. We strongly believe that laparoscopy should not change individual surgeons' oncological beliefs. Philosophies on cancer management vary from country to country and from individual to individual. Laparoscopy is only an 'access' window to the abdomen. Oncological philosophies should not be changed because the size of the abdominal incision changes. This cannot be stressed enough.

Using the schema described above, over a 4-year period 100 consecutive patients, referred to us with clinical stage 1 adenocarcinoma of the endometrium, were managed. The mean age of these patients was 69.4 years, with a range from 29 to 88 years. There was no statistical difference in the ages of the patients over the 4 years when analysed using linear regression analysis. Their mean weight was 161 pounds (73 kg), with a range from 97 to 328 pounds (44–150 kg). Their Quetelet index ranged from 19.1 to 56.4, with a mean of 28.5. There was no statistical significance in the weight or Quetelet index of these patients over the 4-year period. Fifty-three patients had well-differentiated tumours while 30 had moderately differentiated tumours and 17 patients, on final pathological diagnosis, had poorly differentiated tumours.

Para-aortic lymphadenectomy could not be performed in three patients who should have had lymphadenectomy according to our schema. In all cases this was due to obesity. Furthermore, intraoperative frozen section was misleading in four patients. This was because of an error either in the depth of invasion or the grade of the tumour.

Overall, 50 patients had laparoscopically assisted surgical staging that included lymphadenectomy, and 50 had laparoscopically assisted surgical staging without lymphadenectomy. Metastatic disease was discovered in 27.6% (13/47) of the patients with grade 2 or 3 lesions; 16.7% (5/30) of the patients with grade 2 tumours had metastatic disease; and 47.1% (8/17) of the patients with poorly differentiated tumours had metastatic disease. The ability to discover metastatic disease did not vary significantly throughout the duration of the study. Intraperitoneal disease was discovered in the pelvic peritoneum, the ovary, the omentum and the right hemidiaphragm. Retroperitoneal disease was both macroscopic and microscopic, and included both pelvic and para-aortic lymph nodes. The estimated blood loss did not vary statistically between those patients undergoing staging with lymphadenectomy and those whose staging was without lymphadenectomy, and was 257 ± 155 ml. The blood loss difference from the first patient to the 100th patient was not statistically significant. The operating times for the patients undergoing staging without lymphadenectomy decreased significantly as the series progressed, from a mean of 163 minutes to 103 minutes ($P < 0.001$). Operating times for staging of patients with lymphadenectomy also decreased significantly, from a mean of 192 minutes to 160 minutes ($P < 0.02$).

The most impressive improvement in our experience was the length of time spent in hospital. Overall, this ranged from 0 to 6 days. The mean hospital stay for the initial 25 patients was 3.2 days; this decreased to a mean of 1.7 days in the last 25 patients. The linear regression analysis of hospital stay relative to our operator experience was statistically significant ($P < 0.0001$). These times for hospital stay compared favourably to those of recent studies utilizing an abdominal approach to surgical staging of patients with endometrial cancer. Orr *et al.* reported a mean time in hospital of 6 days in 149 patients who were surgically staged [11]. Homesley *et al.*, in a retrospective study evaluating the morbidity of selective lymphadenectomy in the surgical staging of endometrial cancer, reported a mean postoperative stay of 10 days for their 281 patients [45]. These reports were published in 1991 and 1992, respectively.

There were no complications related to the lymphadenectomy. There were five major operative complications: two cystotomies, one colotomy, one enterotomy and one ureteral injury. The ninth patient in the series had her left ureter transected with a stapling device during transection of the left uterine artery. This technique was discontinued immediately after this incident. Two injuries occurred in the first 25 patients, and two in the final quarter of our study. The first two injuries required laparotomy for repair. The last three injuries (an enterotomy during adhesiolysis, a transverse colotomy from the primary trocar insertion and a cystotomy from the suprapubic trocar) were all repaired laparoscopically. There was no appreciable difference in the rate of major complications throughout the study. However, the laparotomy rate dropped impressively from 8% (2/25) in the first quarter to 0% (0/75) in the final three-quarters of the study.

Spirtos *et al.* [43] recently reported the use of laparoscopy in 35 patients with gynaecological malignancies. Twenty-three patients with untreated endometrial cancer underwent laparoscopically assisted vaginal hysterectomy and bilateral salpingo-oophorectomy, together with pelvic and para-aortic lymph-node sampling. Seven patients with endometrial cancer and previous hysterectomy and bilateral salpingo-oophorectomy underwent laparoscopic pelvic and para-aortic lymph-node sampling. Four patients with ovarian cancer and one patient with fallopian tube cancer underwent laparoscopic node dissection. All the patients had a Quetelet index equal or less than 30. In two patients, para-aortic lymph-node sampling was inadequate. Five patients converted to laparotomy. Two patients had uncontrollable bleeding, one from a perforator arising from the vena cava and the second from a perforator arising from the right iliac vessel; two other patients had unsuspected intra-abdominal metastasis; and equipment failure necessitated laparotomy in the fifth patient. The average lymph-node count was 27.7 (pelvic 20.8 and para-aortic 7.9); two patients with endometrial cancer had positive nodes, one had a single positive pelvic node and the other had positive aortic and pelvic nodes. The mean operative time was 3 hours and 13 minutes with an estimated blood loss less than 100 ml. The

hospital stay ranged from 1 to 6 days with an average of 2.69 days. Four patients had postoperative complications: two had deep venous thrombosis including one with vena caval injury, and the other two had small bowel obstruction secondary to herniation of the small bowel through the 12-mm trocar sites.

These experiences mirror our initial experience with laparoscopic staging of the unstaged patient with clinical stage 1 endometrial cancer [40]. In this study, laparoscopic staging for 13 patients with incompletely staged adenocarcinoma of the endometrium was performed. The patient's mean age was 64 years (range 36–74) and mean weight 147.5 pounds (67 kg) (range 132–201 pounds, 60–91 kg). The interval between hysterectomy and laparoscopic staging ranged from 14 to 63 days, with an average of 47. Nine patients had disease limited to the inner half of the myometrium, five with grade 1 and four with grade 2. Four patients had disease invading the outer half of the myometrium, one with grade 1 and three with grade 2. All patients underwent inspection of the entire intraperitoneal cavity, pelvic washings and/or pelvic or para-aortic lymphadenectomy. The adnexa were removed in two patients with remaining ovaries. The mean lymph-node count was 17.5.

Three patients had extrauterine disease. One of them, with disease limited to the inner half of the myometrium and vascular space involvement, had intraperitoneal washings that were positive for well-differentiated adenocarcinoma together with negative pelvic nodes. The second patient, with disease limited to the superficial third of the endometrium and vascular space involvement, had a right obturator node positive for adenocarcinoma together with 24 negative nodes removed. The last patient, with extrauterine disease, had moderately well-differentiated tumour invading the outer half of the myometrium; all her para-aortic lymph nodes were negative but a left obturator node was positive for microscopic adenocarcinoma.

There were no intraoperative complications; one patient developed a postoperative deep venous thrombosis. The estimated blood loss was less then 50 ml. The mean hospital stay was 1.5 days (range 0–3 days).

Laparoscopically assisted surgical staging

Our current algorithm for the management of patients with clinical stage 1 adenocarcinoma of the endometrium includes selective laparoscopic lymph-node sampling based on grade of tumour, depth of invasion and the presence of extrauterine disease (Fig. 18.3). Patients with well-differentiated lesions have laparoscopically assisted vaginal hysterectomy first, while patients with grade 2 or 3 lesions undergo lymphadenectomy prior to the

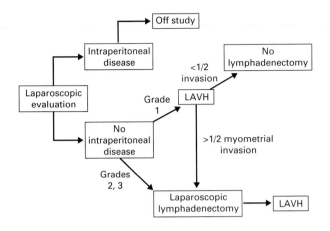

Fig. 18.3 The laparoscopically assisted surgical staging schema.

hysterectomy. Patients with well-differentiated lesions invading greater than one-half of the myometrium, as determined by frozen section, undergo laparoscopic lymphadenectomy. All lymphadenectomies are bilateral, including para-aortic lymph-node sampling, thus adhering to the current Gynecologic Oncology Group surgical procedures manual [46]. Before we had developed the technique of left-sided para-aortic lymphadenectomy, right-sided-only sampling was performed [39].

Conclusion

While reports are limited, it appears that laparoscopy is able to play an important role in the management of patients with endometrial cancer. By avoiding an abdominal incision, patients benefit from a shorter stay in hospital and probably a more rapid recovery time. The literature indicates that vaginal hysterectomy has less morbidity and mortality than abdominal hysterectomy [47–49]. This may hold true for patients with endometrial cancer who have abdominal procedures converted to laparoscopically assisted vaginal procedure. The limited data currently available supports the fact that laparoscopically assisted surgical staging procedures are relatively safe and, with experience, complications may be managed laparoscopically.

More importantly, it appears that metastatic disease can be discovered laparoscopically with an accuracy equal to laparotomy [4–11]. It could be argued that an even better evaluation of the peritoneum, especially in the pelvis and over the diaphragm, can be obtained laparoscopically.

The most important data is still lacking. The survival rates of patients managed laparoscopically must be comparable to those of patients managed via laparotomy. These numbers will not be available for several years and even then will reflect the small numbers of the initial studies. None the less, the 5-year survival data should be

available before large-scale recommendations are made to laparoscopically manage patients with endometrial cancer.

Virtually all operative laparoscopists are aware of the 'learning curve' confronted in acquiring the new haptic skills required for endoscopic surgery. This is certainly true for laparoscopic staging of endometrial cancer. It is comforting to know that the lymphadenectomy skills are acquired fairly quickly and that the ability to detect metastatic disease is not affected by experience if one has prior oncological surgical experience. Also, it is not surprising that patients managed laparoscopically require a shorter stay in hospital, they can be ambulated, fed and discharged home sooner. It is interesting to note that this hospital-stay learning curve, in our experience, was quite long, possibly reflecting the learning curve of other personnel such as residents and hospital nurses.

Overall, the initial reports are encouraging and indicate that further investigation into the laparoscopic management of endometrial cancer is indicated.

References

1 Cullen TH (1900). *Cancer of the Uterus*. Philadelphia: Saunders.
2 Jones HW (1975). Treatment of adenocarcinoma of the endometrium. *Obstet Gynecol Surv* **30**:147–169.
3 Cheon HK (1969). Prognosis of endometrial carcinoma. *Obstet Gynecol* **34**:680–684.
4 Creasman WT, Boronow RC, Morrow CP, Di Saia PJ, Blessing J (1976). Adenocarcinoma of the endometrium: its metastatic lymph node potential. *Gynecol Oncol* **4**:239–243.
5 Boronow RC, Morrow CP, Creasman WT *et al* (1984). Surgical staging in endometrial cancer: clinical pathological findings of a prospective study. *Obstet Gynecol* **63**:825–832.
6 Creasman WT, Morrow CP, Bundy BN, Homesley HD, Graham JE, Heller PB (1987). Surgical–pathological spread patterns of endometrial carcinoma: a Gynecologic Oncology Group study. *Cancer* **60**:2035–2041.
7 Lewis BV, Stallworthy JA, Cowdell R (1970). Adenocarcinoma of the body of the uterus. *J Obstet Gynaecol Br Common* **77**:343–348.
8 Musumeci R, DePalo G, Conti U *et al* (1980). Are retroperitoneal lymph node metastases a major problem in endometrial carcinoma? *Cancer* **46**:1887–1892.
9 Chen SS (1985). Extrauterine spread in endometrial carcinoma clinically confined to the uterus. *Gynecol Oncol* **21**:23–31.
10 Cowles TA, Magrina JF, Masterson BJ, Capen CV (1985). Comparison of clinical and surgical staging in patients with endometrial carcinoma. *Obstet Gynecol* **66**:413–416.
11 Orr JW, Holloway RW, Orr PF, Holimon JL (1991). Surgical staging of uterine cancer: an analysis of perioperative morbidity. *Gynecol Oncol* **12**:209–216.
12 Sheperd JH (1989). Revised FIGO staging for gynecologic cancer. *Br J Obstet Gynaecol* **96**:889–892.
13 Frick HC, Munnell EW, Richart RM, Berger AP, Lawry MF (1973). Carcinoma of the endometrium. *Am J Obstet Gynecol* **115**:663–676.
14 Salazar OM, Bonfiglio TA, Patten SF *et al* (1978). Uterine sarcomas: natural history, prognosis. *Cancer* **42**:1152–1160.

15 Wharam MD, Phillips TL, Bagshaw MA (1976). The role of radiation therapy in clinical stage 1 carcinoma of the endometrium. *Int J Radiat Oncol Biol Phys* **1**:1081–1089.

16 Gretz HF, Economos K, Husain A *et al* (1996). The practice of surgical staging and its impact on adjuvant treatment recommendations in patients with stage 1 endometrial carcinoma. *Gynecol Oncol* **61**:409–415.

17 Van Bouwdijk Bastianse MA (1956).Treatment of cancer of the cervix uteri. *Am J Obstet Gynecol* **72**:100–118.

18 Ingiulla W, Cosmi EV (1968). Vaginal hysterectomy for the treatment of cancer of the corpus uteri. *Am J Obstet Gynecol* **100**:541–543.

19 Pratt JH (1954). The surgical treatment of cancer of the cervix and uterine fundus. *J Fla Med Assoc* **40**:463–470.

20 Pratt JH, Symmonds RE, Welch JS (1964). Vaginal hysterectomy for carcinoma of the fundus. *Am J Obstet Gynecol* **88**:1063–1068.

21 Malkasian GD, McDonald TW, Pratt JH (1977). Carcinoma of the endometrium: Mayo clinical experience. *Mayo Clin Proc* **52**:175–180.

22 Malkasian GD, Annegers JF, Fountain KS (1980). Carcinoma of the endometrium: Stage 1. *Am J Obstet Gynecol* **136**:872–883.

23 Candiani GB, Belloni C, Maggi R, Colombo G, Frigoli A, Carinelli SG (1990). Evaluation of different surgical approaches in the treatment of endometrial carcinoma at FIGO stage 1. *Gynecol Oncol* **37**:6–8.

24 Cliby WA, Dodson MK, Podratz KC (1995). Uterine prolapse complicated by endometrial cancer. *Am J Obstet Gynecol* **172**:1675–1683.

25 Peters WA, Andersen WA, Thornton N, Morley GW (1983). The selective use of vaginal hysterectomy in the management of adenocarcinoma of the endometrium. *Am J Obstet Gynecol* **146**:285–291.

26 Lurain JR (1992). The significance of positive peritoneal cytology in endometrial carcinoma. *Gynecol Oncol* **46**:143–144.

27 Bloss JD, Berman ML, Bloss LP, Buller RE (1991). Use of vaginal hysterectomy for the management of stage 1 endometrial in the medically compromised patient. *Gynecol Oncol* **40**:74–77.

28 Reich H, DeCaprio J, McGlynn F (1989). Laparoscopic hysterectomy. *J Gynecol Surg* **5**:213–215.

29 Mage G, Canis M, Wattiez A, Pouly J-L, Bruhat M-A (1990). Hystérectomie et coelioscopie. *J Gynecol Obstet Biol Reprod* **19**:569–573.

30 Minelli L, Angiolillo M, Caione C, Palmer V (1991). Laparoscopically assisted vaginal hysterectomy. *Endoscopy* **23**:64–66.

31 Liu CY (1992). Laparoscopic hysterectomy: a review of 72 cases. *J Reprod Med* **37**:351–354.

32 Summitt RL Jr, Stovall TG, Lipscomb GH, Ling FW (1992). Randomized comparison of laparoscopic-assisted vaginal hysterectomy with standard vaginal hysterectomy in an outpatient setting. *Obstet Gynecol* **80**:895–901.

33 Padial JG, Sotolongo J, Casey MJ, Johnson C, Osborne NG (1992). Laparoscopy-assisted vaginal hysterectomy: report of seventy-five consecutive cases. *J Gynecol Surg* **8**:81–85.

34 Wurtz A, Mazeman E, Gosselin B, Woelffle D, Sauvage L, Rousseau O (1987). Bilan anatomique des adenopathies retroperitoneales par endoscopie chirurgicale. *Ann Chir* **41**:258–263.

35 Dargent D, Salvat J (1989). *L'Envahissement Ganglionnaire Pelvien*. Paris: McGraw-Hill.

36 Querleu D, Leblanc E, Castelain B (1991). Laparoscopic pelvic lymphadenectomy in the staging of early carcinoma of the cervix. *Am J Obstet Gynecol* **164**:579–581.

37 Childers JM, Hatch KD, Surwit EA (1992). The role of laparoscopic lymphadenectomy in the management of cervical carcinoma. *Gynecol Oncol* **47**:38–43.

38 Childers JM, Surwit EA (1992). Combined laparoscopic and vaginal surgery for the management of two cases of stage 1 endometrial cancer. *Gynecol Oncol* **45**:46–51.

39 Childers JM, Hatch KD, Tran AN, Surwit EA (1993). Laparoscopic paraaortic lymphadenectomy in gynecologic malignancies. *Obstet Gynecol* **82**:741–747.

40 Childers JM, Spirtos NM, Brainard P, Surwit EA (1994). Laparoscopic staging of the patient with incompletely staged early adenocarcinoma of the endometrium. *Obstet Gynecol* **83**:597–600.

41 Photopulos GJ, Stovall TG, Summit RL (1992). Laparoscopic assisted vaginal hysterectomy, bilateral salpingo-oophorectomy and pelvic node sampling for endometrial carcinoma. *J Gynecol Surg* **8**:91–95.

42 Childers JM, Brzechffa PR, Hatch KD, Surwit EA (1993). Laparoscopic assisted surgical staging (LASS) of endometrial cancer. *Gynecol Oncol* **51**:33–38.

43 Spirtos NM, Schlaerth JB, Spirtos WT, Schlaerth BA, Indman PD, Kimball RE (1995). Laparoscopic bilateral pelvic and paraaortic lymph node sampling: an evolving technique. *Am J Obstet Gynecol* **173**:105–111.

44 Melendez T, Harrigill K, Childers JM, Surwit EA (1997). Laparoscopic management of endometrial cancer: the learning experience. *J Laparoscopic Surg* **1**:45–49.

45 Homesley HD, Kadar N, Barret RJ, Lentz SS (1992). Selective pelvic and periaortic lymphadenectomy does not increase morbidity in surgical staging of endometrial carcinoma. *Am J Obstet Gynecol* **167**:1225–1230.

46 Gynecologic Oncology Group (1989). *Surgical Procedures Manual* Washington: American College of Obstetricians and Gynecologists, 48.

47 Pitkin RM (1976). Abdominal hysterectomy in obese women. *Surg Gynecol Obstet* **142**:532–536.

48 Pitkin RM (1977). Vaginal hysterectomy in obese women. *Obstet Gynecol* **49**:567–569.

49 Wingo PA, Huezo CM, Rubin GL, Ory HW, Peterson HB (1985). The mortality risk associated with hysterectomy. *Am J Obstet Gynecol* **152**:803–808.

19   Cancer of the ovary

Earl A. Surwit and Joel M. Childers

Introduction

Modern operative laparoscopy entered the field of oncology with the advent of laparoscopic pelvic lymphadenectomy. This technique, which was originated in France by Daniel Dargent, was performed on patients with early cervical cancer using a retroperitoneal approach [1,2]. The first transperitoneal pelvic lymphadenectomies were reported in 1991 by Querleu, for staging patients with early cervical carcinoma [3].

Laparoscopic para-aortic lymphadenectomy developed simultaneously in France and the USA. Initial case reports included patients with non-Hodgkin's lymphoma, cervical cancer, endometrial cancer and ovarian cancer [4–7]. Reports of small series of patients undergoing laparoscopic para-aortic lymphadenectomy soon followed, suggesting that this procedure was safe and adequate [8–12].

While operative laparoscopy in gynaecological oncology is still in its infancy, there appear to be several clinical situations in which it could be routinely used in the future.

Ovarian cancer is surgically staged according to the International Federation of Gynecology and Obstetrics (FIGO) system. Staging should include a systematic evaluation of the intraperitoneal cavity, including infracolic omentectomy, sampling of the pelvic and para-aortic lymph nodes, multiple biopsies of the pelvic, abdominal, visceral and parietal peritoneum, and peritoneal cytology specimens. Random diaphragmatic biopsies or scrapings for cytology are also recommended [13].

Experience

In 1992, at the University of Arizona, the laparoscopic staging of patients with ovarian carcinoma was undertaken prospectively and was designed to determine the ability to adequately evaluate both the intraperitoneal cavity and retroperitoneal lymph nodes. Two patient populations were evaluated: those with optimally debulked advanced disease undergoing second-look procedures and those with presumed stage I disease requiring surgical staging.

Second-look laparoscopy

The first group, second-look laparoscopies, consisted of 40 women with advanced (stage II–IV) disease who had completed surgical debulking, which was 'optimal' in 39, and had received platinum-based chemotherapy. All patients had negative examinations and serum CA-125s. A total of 44 laparoscopic procedures were performed in this group (four patients had positive second-look laparoscopic procedures followed by third-look laparoscopies after treatment with intraperitoneal monoclonal-tagged yttrium). The mean age of these patients was 60 years, and their weights ranged from 105 to 185 pounds (48–84 kg), with a mean of 137 pounds (62 kg). Twenty-four of the 44 laparoscopic second-look procedures (56%) were positive for persistent disease. Microscopic disease only was discovered in five patients (21%), located in the omentum, para-aortic nodes (two patients), pelvic peritoneum and peritoneal washings. In two of these patients, the only site of persistent disease was microscopic involvement of para-aortic lymph nodes.

Twenty of the 44 patients (44%) had negative restaging procedures. However, five of these procedures were deemed inadequate at the time of surgery because of intraperitoneal adhesions that were too extensive to allow successful evaluation of the abdominal cavity. Disease recurred in all five of these patients, compared with a 20% recurrence rate in the remaining 15 patients.

Significant complications occurred in six (14%) of the 44 procedures. Three of these patients required laparotomy: one for repair of a hole in the vena cava, one to repair a trocar injury to the transverse colon and one to repair a small-bowel enterotomy.

Excluding the six patients with significant complications, hospital stays for the remaining 39 patients ranged from 0 to 3 days with an average of 1.1 days.

Surgical staging laparoscopy

The second set of patients consisted of 14 women with presumed early ovarian carcinoma. Five patients were referred unstaged after their malignant masses had been removed. These patients underwent laparoscopic staging as their second procedure. The remaining nine patients had malignant ovarian tumours discovered during the laparoscopic management of their adnexal masses and underwent laparoscopic staging at the time of their primary procedures. Twelve of the 14 patients had epithelial ovarian tumours (five well differentiated, three grade II and four grade III tumours). The remaining two patients had a Sertoli–Leydig cell tumour and a dysgerminoma. The ages of these patients ranged from 17 to 75 years, with a mean of 64.5. Their weights ranged from 109 to 200 pounds (50–90 kg), with a mean of 160 pounds (73 kg).

Metastatic disease was discovered in eight (57%) of the 14 patients in this group. Two patients were upstaged to stage IC, based on washings that contained adenocarcinoma; three patients were upstaged to stage II for positive pelvic biopsies; three patients were upstaged to stage IIIC, based on metastatic disease to para-aortic lymph nodes. Two of these patients also had microscopic omental metastases. The hospital stay ranged from 0 to 3 days, with an average of 1.6.

Laparoscopy in ovarian cancer patients was able to detect microscopic disease in high-risk areas—washings, pelvic peritoneum, omentum, and pelvic and para-aortic lymph nodes—at a rate similar to that reported in the current literature. Laparoscopy offers an excellent opportunity to inspect peritoneal surfaces, and especially the diaphragms [4]. Visualization is enhanced because of the magnification offered by endoscopic techniques.

The main advantage of laparoscopic staging is related to the avoidance of a large abdominal incision, which means that the time spent in hospital and the recovery time are significantly shorter. The disadvantages are related to the inherent difficulties in acquiring the laparoscopic skills to accomplish this difficult surgical procedure, particularly the left infrarenal lymphadenectomy. Exposure can be difficult to obtain, and lumbar veins can be difficult to visualize, dissect around and control if injured. Surgical assistants need to be skilled in endoscopic procedures and familiar with the retroperitoneal anatomy.

Laparoscopic cytoreduction after neoadjuvant chemotherapy for advanced ovarian cancer

Chemotherapy before surgery in patients with advanced ovarian cancer has two main advantages.
1 An improvement in the patient's performance status prior to surgery. A reduction in tumour volume, bowel pressure and ascites, with a subsequent improvement in oral intake, enhances the patient's nutritional status.

The decrease in pleural effusion can eliminate the oxygen shunt through the atelectatic lung, improving the patient's oxygenation, thus lowering the anaesthetic risk.
2 The reduction in tumour volume from neoadjuvant chemotherapy requires less extensive cytoreductive surgery and virtually eliminates bowel surgery.

The significant reduction in tumour volume after neoadjuvant chemotherapy led us to investigate the feasibility of laparoscopic cytoreductive surgery in selected patients who had optimal responses to chemotherapy.

Over the past 3 years, 11 patients have had a tumour response that is significant enough to allow us to perform optimal laparoscopic cytoreduction. The CA-125 tumour marker is an accurate predictor of the likelihood of successful cytoreductive surgery in this setting [14]. Laparoscopic debulking would not be considered unless the patient had at least a 1-log decrease in her CA-125 marker in response to neoadjuvant chemotherapy. Examination under anaesthesia and diagnostic laparoscopy select the patients in whom the debulking may be completed laparoscopically. Patients with extensive pelvic disease and densely adherent disease in the abdominal cavity are better debulked by laparotomy.

Dissection was begun in the pelvis and consisted of either a laparoscopically assisted vaginal hysterectomy and bilateral salpingo-oophorectomy or a laparoscopic bilateral salpingo-oophorectomy. After resection of pelvic disease was completed, the omentum was mobilized laparoscopically from the splenic and hepatic flexures. The 12-mm umbilical trocar site incision was extended to 4–5 cm in order to deliver the transverse colon. Resection of the supracolic and infracolic omentum was then completed outside the abdomen. Any pelvic masses were also extracted through this incision.

The mean operating time was 1.9 hours (1.1–3.5), with a mean blood loss of 210 ml (50–500 ml). There were no intraoperative complications and no complications related to the use of laparoscopy itself. One of the patients required postoperative transfusion of 2 units of red blood cells. Febrile morbidity (>36 hours) was noted in one patient and was resolved with antibiotic therapy. One patient had an ileus that resolved spontaneously after 4 days. The mean hospital stay was 3 days (1–8 days).

Currently we are investigating the feasibility of laparoscopic debulking of patients with advanced ovarian cancer after the administration of neoadjuvant chemotherapy, consisting of a combination of taxol and carboplatin. This dose-intensive protocol may increase the proportion of patients that may be debulked laparoscopically.

Laparoscopic cytoreductive surgery after the administration of neoadjuvant chemotherapy for patients with advanced ovarian cancer is feasible, and may offer a selected group of patients with optimal response to chemotherapy an overall improved quality of life.

Suspicious adnexal masses

An endorsed consensus committee of the American College of Obstetrics and Gynecology published guidelines in 1992 for avoiding unsuspected malignancy in the laparoscopic management of adnexal masses [15]. The sonographic criteria require a small mass with thin walls, no solid parts, no internal echoes, septations or excrescences, and no ascitic fluid in the pelvis. No family history of ovarian carcinoma should be noted, and the postmenopausal patient should have a normal CA-125 (<35). Adherence to these guidelines will virtually assure the physician that the mass is benign. In this way, capsular rupture and tumour spill can be avoided, as can cancer mismanagement such as incomplete resection of the mass, incomplete surgical staging and cyst aspiration without cyst removal.

Masses that do not meet these ultrasound and CA-125 criteria can be defined as suspicious, and should be managed only by surgeons who have the skill and knowledge to manage ovarian carcinoma. However, it is possible that some of these masses can be managed laparoscopically.

Capsular rupture should not be a concern for these patients if tumour spill is avoided. Laparoscopy clearly increases the risk of capsular rupture compared with laparotomy, but cyst drainage can be accomplished without tumour spillage.

Therefore capsular rupture and tumour spill should, if possible, be avoided in the laparoscopic management of these patients. However, little data are available to support the concept that capsular rupture and tumour spill worsen patient prognosis or survival. Only one study shows a statistically significant difference in 5-year survival of patients with stage I ovarian carcinoma who had rupture of the tumour capsule versus unruptured capsules [16]. This study, like most studies evaluating the impact of tumour spill, is small, its analysis retrospective and not multivariant. Patients were not surgically staged, and it deals with patients in whom varying adjuvant treatments were administered. In this study, 53 patients were evaluated and categorized into rupture versus non-rupture, but grade of tumour, presence of extracystic excrescences and tumour adherence were not taken into the analysis. More than 50% of the patients had tumour adherence, and patients with extracystic excrescences had worse prognoses, but the report does not define in which groups these patients were categorized. Furthermore, there were more well-differentiated tumours in the non-ruptured group compared with those with rupture.

Five recent studies [17–21] have examined rupture of the tumour capsule in stage I ovarian carcinoma, using multivariant analyses. These studies outline several high-risk factors in stage I ovarian carcinoma, including: tumour adherence, rupture before surgery, high-grade tumours, malignant ascites/cytology and extracystic excrescences. However, all five of these studies, which comprise more than 1600 patients in total, show no statistically significant difference in survival of patients with capsular rupture vs no capsular rupture.

One important factor outlined in the study reported by Sjövall *et al.* [21] is that patients with preoperative rupture had worse survival rates than those with intraoperative rupture (10-year survival = 59% vs 87%). This absolutely mandates the complete resection of all malignancies at the primary procedure. There is no role for tumour spill followed by a delay in definitive management. Copious irrigation should be utilized if spillage occurs.

Spill should be avoided if possible, and this can be accomplished via colpotomy or intraperitoneal sacs. However, surgeons with the skills to carry out resection and management of ovarian carcinoma should not allow the fear of capsular rupture to prevent them from managing suspicious adnexal masses laparoscopically.

Our experience in laparoscopic management of suspicious adnexal masses includes 138 patients whose ages ranged from 9 to 91 years (mean 52 years), and weights from 57 to 338 pounds (26–154 kg), with a mean of 152 pounds (69 kg). One hundred and twenty-seven patients had abnormal imaging studies and 39 had CA-125 levels >35. The CA-125 levels ranged from <5 to 8200, with a mean of 155. The masses ranged in size from 3 to 35 cm.

Eight per cent (11/138) of the procedures were converted to laparotomy, six because of an inability to dissect the mass laparoscopically and five for staging or debulking of the carcinoma. Eighty-three patients underwent unilateral or bilateral salpingo-oophorectomy. Hysterectomies were performed in 27% (26/96) of patients with uteri. Masses were removed vaginally in 40 patients because of their size, or in an attempt to avoid capsular rupture.

Malignancies were discovered in 14% (19/138) of patients; 16 of the 19 were primary adnexal carcinoma. Of these, eight were staged laparoscopically, five underwent laparotomy for resection or staging and three were not staged (two for medical reasons, one missed diagnosis). Capsular rupture was avoided in patients with masses of 10 cm in diameter or smaller. However, drainage was required in six malignant masses of 10 cm and larger. One of these patients, who was unstaged, recurred 6 months after a negative second-look procedure, following an initial treatment with carboplatin for apparent stage I disease (unstaged). She had a poorly differentiated tumour within 0.1 mm of the surface.

Three major complications were encountered: an enterotomy and a lacerated vena cava (both repaired laparoscopically), and a small-bowel herniation through a 5-mm lateral port site (requiring reoperation). Hospital stays ranged from 0 to 11 days, with a mean of 1.5 days. Operating times ranged from 25 to 210 minutes, with a mean of 86 minutes. Over the last 2 years of the study, operating times have decreased to a mean of 63 minutes, and hospital stays have decreased to 1 day.

The laparoscopic management of suspicious adnexal masses is technically feasible with a low morbidity. Hysterectomies can be avoided in the majority of patients, and the hospital stay is remarkably brief. Adnexal carcinomata can be identified and managed appropriately. However, complete avoidance of capsular rupture is impossible, particularly with large masses. Therefore a varying management protocol is recommended, depending on the surgeon's skills and philosophy on capsular rupture. Suspicious masses that can be removed intact, should be. Suspicious masses that must be drained can be managed laparoscopically if the surgeon can drain without spill [7]. If the mass is at risk of rupture because of adherence or if the surgeon believes drainage is unsafe, then laparotomy should be utilized. If rupture does occur, the mass should be resected completely, the patient staged and copious irrigation utilized. There is no role for incomplete resection or cyst aspiration in the laparoscopic management of adnexal masses. This delay would potentially increase the risk of recurrence for these patients.

The myth of abdominal-wall implantation prevents many women from benefiting from laparoscopy. However, we are aware of only four case reports of implantation in women with ovarian cancer [22–25], none of which addresses the incidence of this phenomenon. In our experience, abdominal-wall implantation has developed in only one of our patients, with an incidence of 0.5% of procedures for patients with metastatic gynaecological malignancies. This patient had a grade III papillary carcinoma of the ovary and died of carcinomatosis 7 months after the procedure (microscopic second look). The threat of abdominal-wall implantation in patients with gynaecological malignancies is extremely low and should not deter the continued investigation of laparoscopy in these patients.

Conclusion

Laparoscopy can now be used in the management of patients with cervical, endometrial and ovarian carcinoma, as well as patients with suspicious adnexal masses. Patients with cervical cancer who are candidates

for radical hysterectomy can undergo laparoscopic lymphadenectomy and avoid laparotomy if nodes are positive. Large abdominal incisions can be avoided by laparoscopic radical hysterectomy, laparoscopically assisted radical vaginal hysterectomy or radical vaginal hysterectomy.

Patients with clinical stage I endometrial carcinoma can be managed by laparoscopically assisted surgical staging. Obesity will not be a significant limitation for these patients if lymphadenectomy is not performed on patients with well-differentiated lesions with less than one-half myometrial invasion. Patients referred after hysterectomy who have high-risk endometrial cancers can also undergo laparoscopic staging with minimal morbidity.

Patients with presumed stage I carcinoma of the ovary, who are unstaged at the time of their original surgery, can undergo laparoscopically assisted surgical staging rather than empiric chemotherapy. The laparoscopic management of patients with suspicious adnexal masses will also identify some patients with presumed stage I ovarian cancer, who can be staged at the same time that the mass is being managed laparoscopically.

The advantages of laparoscopic management in any of these procedures is strictly for the patient. These patients benefit from a short time spent in hospital and a more rapid recovery.

One of the disadvantages of laparoscopy in gynaecological malignancies is that the oncological surgeon has to learn new surgical skills. The acquisition of laparoscopic skills is not easy and requires a serious time commitment. This can be particularly arduous for some surgeons for whom laparoscopic hand–eye coordination skills may be difficult to acquire. During the learning process, operating times will be much longer than those of laparotomy. Further, the oncological surgeon will discover that the *assistance* of a skilled surgeon is required. This, too, is an inconvenience when most oncological surgeons can perform cancer operations with an unskilled assistant. It has been our experience, however, that the challenge has been stimulating. Our efforts have been well rewarded by our patients, who are grateful for the more rapid recovery.

Laparoscopy is the future for gynaecological oncology, and the future begins now.

References

1 Wurtz A, Mazman E, Gosselin B *et al* (1987). Bilan anatomique des adénopathies rétropéritonéales par endoscopie chirurgicale. *Ann Chir* **41**:258–263.
2 Dargent D, Salvat J (1989). *L'Envahissement Ganglionnaire Pelvien*. Paris: McGraw-Hill.
3 Querleu D, LeBlanc E, Castelain B (1991). Laparoscopic lymphadenectomy in the staging of early carcinoma of the cervix. *Am J Obstet Gynecol* **164**:579–581.

4 Childers JM, Surwit EA (1992). Combined laparoscopic and vaginal surgery for the management of two cases of stage I endometrial carcinoma. *Gynecol Oncol* **45**:46–51.

5 Childers JM, Surwit EA (1992). Laparoscopic para-aortic lymph node biopsy for diagnosis of a non-Hodgkin's lymphoma. *Surg Laparosc Endosc* **2**:139–142.

6 Nezhat C, Burrell M, Nezhat F (1992). Laparoscopic radical hysterectomy with para-aortic and pelvic node dissection. *Am J Obstet Gynecol* **166**:864–865.

7 Querleu D (1993). Laparoscopic para-aortic lymph node sampling in gynecologic oncology: a preliminary experience. *Gynecol Oncol* **49**:24–29.

8 Childers JM, Surwit EA, Hatch KD (1992). The role of laparoscopy in the management of cervical carcinoma. *Gynecol Oncol* **47**:38–43.

9 Childers JM, Brzechffa PR, Hatch KD, Surwit EA (1993). Laparoscopically assisted surgical staging (LASS) of endometrial cancer. *Gynecol Oncol* **51**:33–38.

10 Childers JM, Hatch KD, Tran AN, Surwit EA (1993). Laparoscopic para-aortic lymphadenectomy in gynecologic malignancies. *Obstet Gynecol* **82**:741–747.

11 Nezhat CR, Nezhat FR, Burrell MO *et al* (1993). Laparoscopic radical hysterectomy and laparoscopic-assisted vaginal radical hysterectomy with pelvic and para-aortic lymph node dissection. *J Gynecol Surg* **9**:105–120.

12 Querleu D, LeBlanc E (1994). Laparoscopic infrarenal para-aortic node dissection for restaging of carcinoma of the ovary or fallopian tube. *Cancer* **73**:1467–1471.

13 Berek JS, Hacker NF (1985). Staging and second-look operations in ovarian cancer. In: Alberts DS, Surwit EA, eds. *Ovarian Cancer*. Boston: Martinus Nijhoff, 109–127.

14 Surwit EA, Childers JM, Atlas I, Nour M, Hatch KD, Alberts DS (1996). Neoadjuvant chemotherapy for advanced ovarian carcinoma. *Int J Gynecol Oncol* **6**:356–361.

15 Maiman M, Boyce F, Goldstein SR *et al* (1992). Laparoscopic surgery in the management of ovarian cysts. *Female Patient* 1716–1723.

16 Webb M, Symmonds R (1980). Site of recurrence of cervical cancer after radical hysterectomy. *Am J Obstet Gynecol* **138**:813–817.

17 Sevelda P, Vavra N, Schamper M, Salzer H (1990). Prognostic factors for survival of stage I epithelial ovarian carcinoma. *Cancer* **65**:2349–2352.

18 Dembo HA, Davy M, Stenwig AE *et al* (1990). Prognostic factors in patients with stage I epithelial ovarian carcinoma. *Obstet Gynecol* **75**:263–273.

19 Vergote IB, Kaern J, Abeler VM *et al* (1993). Analysis of prognostic factors in stage I epithelial ovarian carcinoma: importance of deoxyribonucleic acid ploidy in predicting relapse. *Am J Obstet Gynecol* **169**:40–52.

20 Finn C, Luesley DM, Buxton EJ *et al* (1992). Is stage I epithelial ovarian cancer overtreated both surgically and systemically? Results of a five-year cancer review. *Br J Obstet Gynaecol* **99**:54–58.

21 Sjövall K, Nilsson B, Einhorn N (1994). Different types of rupture of the tumor capsule and impact on survival in early ovarian carcinoma. *Int J Gynecol Cancer* **4**:333–336.

22 Dobronte Z, Wittmann T, Karacsony G (1978). Rapid development of malignant metastases in the abdominal wall after laparoscopy. *Endoscopy* **10**:127–130.

23 Stockdale AD, Pocock TJ (1985). Abdominal-wall metastases following laparoscopy: a case report. *Eur J Surg Oncol* **11**:373–375.

24 Hsiu JG, Given FT, Kemp GM (1986). Tumor implantation after diagnostic laparoscopic biopsy of serous ovarian tumors of low malignant potential. *Obstet Gynecol* **68**:90S–93S.

25 Gleeson NC, Nicosia SV, Mark JE, Hoffman MS, Cavanagh D (1993). Abdominal-wall metastases from ovarian carcinoma after laparoscopy. *Am J Obstet Gynecol* **169**:522–523.

20 Second-look laparoscopy in ovarian cancer

Gérard Mage, Michel Canis, Jean-Luc Pouly,
Arnaud Wattiez, Charles Chapron, Hania Moal and
Maurice-Antoine Bruhat

Introduction

The use of a surgical second look in oncology was used by Wangensteen et al. [1] in 1951, to follow-up colon cancer. Rutledge and Burns [2] then proposed the use of this technique in the follow-up of patients treated for ovarian cancer. A vertical midline incision is the standard approach to reassessment of the peritoneal cavity. However, laparoscopy is an attractive alternative, and its use has been reported by many authors since 1975 [3–13]. Surprisingly, the benefits of laparoscopy, which has often been considered to be routine [14] in clinical practice, have never been clearly demonstrated [14,15]. Creasman, in a recent review [16], confirmed that a second laparotomy provides little, if any, benefit for patients, but it is the standard method for assessing the effectiveness of a medical treatment, and its use is still necessary for studying and improving postsurgical treatments.

The laparoscopic approach is much more attractive when the value of a treatment is questionable, and when it is mainly used to evaluate a new therapeutic protocol. Indeed, in patients with ovarian cancer, all the well-known advantages of laparoscopy over laparotomy are worthwhile and important, allowing faster postoperative treatment, more frequent assessment of the abdomen, better inspection of many peritoneal areas because of the magnification provided by the laparoscope and decreased trauma, which is invaluable in patients with a poor prognosis. It may even be hypothesized that, until now, the benefits of the laparoscopic approach have not been used enough. By using a laparoscopic technique surgical evaluation of the abdomen could become an interval procedure, to assess the efficacy of the treatment used, to assess the feasibility of a secondary debulking procedure or to propose a new treatment when the response is poor.

We have performed second-look operations by laparoscopy for many years [4]. Based on this experience, our current technique, which has been improved following complications that have occurred, will be described. Then the morbidity rates for a laparoscopic second look, which are similar to or lower than those observed at laparotomy, will be detailed. Finally, the reliability of a laparoscopic second look, using a study of the long-term survival rate according to the surgical approach used, will be described.

Fifty-two patients who underwent a laparoscopic second look were included in the study. These patients had the following characteristics.

1 A complete initial surgical treatment comprising hysterectomy, bilateral adnexectomy, omentectomy, removal of all suspicious areas and para-aortic lymph-node excision after 1987.
2 Surgery followed by six multiple-agent chemotherapy treatments including cisplatin.
3 Complete clinical, biological and radiological remission after chemotherapy.

Patient preparation and set-up for laparoscopy

Laparoscopic second look should be considered as a high-risk laparoscopic procedure, as it often includes the treatment of extensive and dense bowel adhesions to the anterior abdominal wall and/or to the sites initially invaded by the tumour, which should be evaluated both visually and by biopsies. Therefore, certain points are essential.

Bowel preparation is similar to that used for colon surgery and primarily uses the laparoscopic 'retractor'. This facilitates manipulation of the bowel loops and the enterolysis required to achieve a complete exploration of the abdominopelvic cavity. Furthermore, this type of preparation minimizes the consequences of bowel injuries, which are not uncommon, and can be repaired safely and immediately, by laparoscopy or by laparotomy, without colostomy.

To ensure complete inspection of the peritoneal cavity in every patient, it should be possible to alter the angle of the operating table in the various planes. In the same way, two or three video screens should be available, allowing the surgeon to operate comfortably in the left paracolic gutter and in the right upper quadrant as well as in the pelvic area. Consequently, all the cables connected to the laparoscope should be long enough to allow the surgical team to change position easily. The light source and the electronic insufflator are placed on a cart. Ideally, both arms are fixed alongside the patient's body. When necessary it should be possible to insert the laparoscope in several trocars. To minimize cutaneous scars, a 5-mm 0° lens is often used. Several laparoscopes should be available, including a 30° lens which allows better vision when operating far away from the trocar entry sites on organs which are parallel to the direction of the trocar. This indication for a 30° laparoscope has been re-emphasized recently by general surgeons, who sometimes encounter this problem when dissecting the hepatic pedicle which may be parallel to the umbilical trocar [17]. Finally, a complete set of instruments is required, including curved scissors, bipolar forceps, reliable needle holders and an efficient aspiration lavage instrument.

Technique

These patients often have extensive abdominal wall—bowel adhesions. The location of the adhesions may be related to the previous surgical procedures and/or to unfavourable evolution of the disease during the six courses of postoperative chemotherapy. Therefore their location is not always accurately deduced from the cutaneous scars or from the operative reports. Consequently, extreme care must be taken when setting up for laparoscopy, knowing that the umbilicus has been chosen as the insertion point of the primary trocar mainly for cosmetic reasons. The Veress needle and the primary trocar can be inserted at different sites without any added morbidity, except for the cutaneous scar. As demonstrated below from our experience, most complications are the consequences of these initial steps in laparoscopy. For this reason, we currently begin all second-look procedures with a needlescope [18–21], as recommended by Berek [14]. He used a 1.7-mm laparoscope, and significantly reduced the rate of complications, from 18.9% with a conventional technique to 1.2% (in 82 patients) with a needlescope ($P < 0.05$). Using this endoscope, the abdominal cavity can be explored to locate areas free of any adhesions where the first trocar can be introduced without any risk. Our approach is slightly different from that proposed by Berek. The needlescope is inserted directly through the Veress needle. Before insufflating the carbon dioxide, the surgeon lifts the abdominal wall with one hand below the needle entry site. It is then possible to check the intra-abdominal position of the needle before creating the pneumoperitoneum. After insufflation, the needlescope is used to introduce the first 5- or 10-mm trocar under visual control. The diameter of the needlescope used should be large enough to provide good vision of the abdomen, and small enough to avoid the need for suture when the bowel has been injured by the scope. It is well known that bowel injuries induced by the Veress needle have no postoperative consequences and do not need to be repaired [22]. For this reason, the instrument currently used is inserted through a pneumoperitoneum needle of 1.2-mm diameter.

When this instrument is not available, the following procedure is recommended, as proposed by Ozols [9] and Lele [23]. For patients who have undergone previous midline laparotomy and omentectomy, insert the Veress needle in the left upper quadrant, halfway between the umbilicus and the edge of the ribs. This area is unlikely to have adhesions in patients who have undergone a vertical midline laparotomy. The needle is inserted perpendicular to the abdominal wall. Three planes are palpated. The peritoneum is the last plane and the abdominal wall is lifted after the second plane. As in any laparoscopic procedure, insufflation must be preceded by all the safety tests to ensure that the needle is in the peritoneum. During insufflation, it is essential to check the intra-abdominal pressure, and if the pneumoperitoneum cannot be carried out in total safety (intra-abdominal pressure must remain below 15mmHg) the laparoscopic procedure must be stopped.

The insertion of the primary trocar is performed when the pneumoperitoneum is satisfactory. A safety test, such as the 'needle test' previously described by our group, should be routinely performed before introducing the laparoscope trocar [4]. A 20-ml syringe filled with 10ml of saline and fitted with an 18-gauge needle is used. The needle is slowly inserted perpendicular to the abdominal wall, while aspirating slightly to measure the depth at which the carbon dioxide is found. If the depth at which carbon dioxide is obtained is consistent—is the same in the area tested—the trocar can be safely inserted. It is essential to check an area large enough to ensure that a bowel loop is not transfixed with the needle. Indeed, when 20–30cm of bowel are fixed to the anterior abdominal wall by dense adhesions, the thickness of the abdominal wall may appear very consistent, although the thickness of the bowel is included in the measurement. To avoid this problem, check the thickness of the abdominal wall in another area, particularly when the depth at which the carbon dioxide is obtained appears surprising given the patient's weight.

If there is any suspicion of adhesions in the periumbilical area, do not hesitate to introduce the laparoscope trocar outside the umbilicus, after establishing an area of at least 5 cm in diameter without any suspected adhesions.

Whatever the technique and the safety tests used, bowel lacerations are possible when inserting the primary trocar.

For this reason, this trocar entry site should always be checked visually by introducing a 5-mm diameter laparoscope via one of the ancillary ports. A bowel laceration is not a significant problem, provided it is diagnosed and repaired immediately; by contrast, a postoperative peritonitis secondary to a small bowel fistula is a life-threatening complication in these often old and already depressed patients. Therefore any doubt is unacceptable, and the least suspicion of bowel injury should be checked and repaired, even if a laparotomy is necessary.

Among 52 cases of second-look laparoscopy performed in patients who had no clinical, radiological or biological evidence of disease after a primary surgical procedure and 6 months' chemotherapy with cisplatin, our study produced three complications: two bowel injuries and one 'impossible' laparoscopy. One case of transverse colon injury occurred at the beginning of our experience in 1982. Although all the safety tests appeared satisfactory, the transverse colon was transfixed by the primary trocar inserted in the umbilicus. However, the thickness of the abdominal wall had not been checked in other areas so the tests were inadequate. In the second case, the tests which showed adhesion in the umbilical area appeared satisfactory in the left hypochondrium. A 5-mm primary trocar was inserted very high in the left hypochodrium. An initial inspection of the abdominal cavity showed multiple peritoneal metastases and many unexpected bowel adhesions to the abdominal wall. It was decided to check the primary trocar entry site, using a 5-mm laparoscope inserted through a secondary trocar, and it was found that the small bowel had been transfixed by the first trocar. Although this complication happened recently, a laparotomy was performed to repair the bowel as an extensive adhesiolysis was required to achieve a satisfactory suture of the bowel. Extensive dense adhesions were found on the midline laparotomy, and a large incision was necessary to find the peritoneal cavity. This case demonstrates that a blind insertion of the first trocar may induce a complication, even when performed carefully and cautiously by an experienced surgeon.

These complications are uncommon (two out of 52 cases, 4%). In our experience, the incidence is lower than that reported here. This is because many patients underwent several laparoscopies (third- and fourth-look procedures) after surgical treatment of an ovarian cancer. Among 32 additional laparoscopies, there were no other bowel lacerations. Overall, the incidence of bowel laceration is 2.4% (two cases out of 84 laparoscopies).

In the third complication the laparoscopy was 'impossible': despite several attempts, the creation of the pneumoperitoneum was impossible because the intraabdominal pressure was always above 15 mmHg. It was decided to proceed to laparotomy and extensive bowel adhesion were found, involving all of the anterior abdominal wall; a tedious and very long enterolysis was required to reach the paracolic gutters, the pelvis and to evaluate the peritoneal cavity.

Our experience shows that laparoscopic second look is technically feasible. However, it is a high-risk procedure: the failure rate ranges between 2% and 13% in the literature [3,23]. In our series, laparoscopy proved to be impossible only once, but evaluation of the abdominopelvic cavity was almost impossible at laparotomy. The complication rate is far higher than that for standard laparoscopic surgery. Three conversions to laparotomy were necessary (3/52 = 5.7%) in complications that were diagnosed immediately. The postoperative course was uncomplicated.

Various techniques have been proposed to avoid the problem with abdominal wall adhesions. Instead of the syringe test, it has been suggested that the adhesions could be identified by ultrasound [24,25]. The preliminary results of this approach are interesting, as in 18 of 42 patients suspected of having bowel adhesions at ultrasound, the positive diagnosis of adhesions was confirmed at surgery in sites corresponding to those suspected during the ultrasound procedure.

Unlike other teams [23,26], 'open laparoscopy' is not used. Whereas this technique avoids almost all risk of complications secondary to large vessel injury [27], it does not completely eliminate that of a bowel injury [28,29]. Indeed, in patients with extensive adhesions, identification of an area free of bowel is very difficult through a 1-cm incision.

Childers *et al.* recently proposed to insert the Veress needle and the first trocar in the ninth or tenth intercostal space [5]. They reported very promising results, because the left upper area quadrant of the abdomen is rarely involved in the dissemination process.

The needlescope appears to be the best alternative. Our last 10 cases were begun with a 1.2-mm laparoscope, which can be inserted as described above, and there was satisfactory vision of the abdomen allowing safe insertion of the first trocar. Whatever the technique, the laparoscope trocar entry site should always be carefully checked.

The operation

The ancillary trocars should be inserted under direct visual control. The entry sites are determined according to the location of the abdominopelvic adhesions, together with that of the lesions at initial surgery. This requires perfect knowledge of the previous operative reports, which should be both detailed and very accurate. At least three operating trocars are required to carry out the operation under optimum conditions. The trocar entry sites should be carefully checked during the surgical procedure when changing the instrument or when the trocar needs to be reinserted; blind 'replacements' of the trocar are also dangerous in patients with extensive abdominal wall adhesions. This point is particularly important if the surgeon operates from several positions, as this always makes it more difficult to identify the direction of a trocar. When bringing an instrument back into the operating field, blind manipulations of the instruments are not uncommon; this should be avoided to decrease the risks of bowel lacerations and, particularly, undiagnosed bowel injuries during the adhesiolysis. To avoid this problem, adhesions close to the trocar entry sites should be treated at the beginning of the procedure.

The first step is aspiration of the peritoneal fluid in the posterior cul-de-sac for cytology. If there is no peritoneal fluid, peritoneal washings are obtained.

The whole abdominopelvic cavity must be explored, effectively carrying out a complete adhesiolysis. The bowel is freed to gain total access to the pelvis, and to any other abdominal areas involved at initial laparotomy, including the paracolic gutters, the diaphragm and all the peritoneum. Bowel adhesiolysis is also essential for inspection of the mesentery and all the bowel loops. When the adhesiolysis and/or the inspection of the peritoneal cavity is too difficult, the laparoscope may be moved to other trocars to obtain better exposure of the adhesions and easier access for inspection. Introducing a 5-mm laparoscope through another trocar sometimes provides better conditions for carrying out the adhesiolysis. It is sometimes useful to use two laparoscopes simultaneously.

Any abnormal or suspicious area should be biopsied. Multiple biopsies of normal areas should also be routinely made. These biopsies should be taken at various locations, including all the areas involved by the tumour at initial surgery, and apparently healthy peritoneum in the paracolic gutters and on the diaphragm. These random biopsies should be large and should be performed with a 5-mm grasping forceps and laparoscopic scissors to excise a large peritoneal area. Hydrodissection can be helpful in obtaining these samples, by making the cleavage plane easier. Biopsy forceps are used to excise very small abnormal areas. Indeed, in such cases the magnification provided by the laparoscope is necessary to see the abnormality, implying that it may be difficult to find it at pathological examination if a large area is excised around the vegetation. By carrying out the biopsy with 1- or 2-mm forceps, the surgeon will excise only the abnormal area, facilitating investigation of the pathology and making the results of the second-look operation more reliable.

In our group of 52 patients, bowel adhesiolysis was necessary to achieve a complete evaluation of the peritoneal cavity in 70% of the cases. Once the laparoscopy had been set up without complications, the whole abdominopelvic cavity could be explored in 51 patients. The other patient, at the beginning of our series, had a highly suspicious diaphragmatic nodule on which we had been unable to perform a biopsy. The adhesions were described as severe and extensive by the surgeon in a third of the cases. Lele and Piver [23] reported, in a series of 51 cases, that they were able to carry out laparoscopic second look in all their patients except one (failure rate 2%). Because of extensive bowel adhesions, Berek *et al.* [3] failed to achieved a complete evaluation of the peritoneal cavity in 13.4% of cases (16/119). These results emphasize that a thorough laparoscopic exploration of the peritoneal cavity often requires a bowel adhesiolysis that is extensive and difficult. Adhesiolysis is the key step in laparoscopic second look, because a complete assessment of the abdominal cavity and multiple biopsies can then be easily performed. This enterolysis is often difficult, particularly on the midline, but it has become easier as a result of technological progress over the past few years. This is confirmed by the lower failure rate observed in more recent studies [4,23] compared with the initial report by Berek *et al.*

In our experience three complications occurred during the surgical evaluation of the abdomen. One bladder injury occurred while excising a suspicious, 2-cm-diameter nodule located on the peritoneal surface of the bladder. Pathological examination of this nodule was negative. Two bowel injuries occurred during the adhesiolysis. All these complications were treated by laparoscopy; the postoperative courses were uneventful without any sequelae. The postoperative course was uneventful for all other patients except one, who was reoperated on postoperative day 8 for the treatment of a bowel occlusion. Most patients left the hospital on day 2.

In summary, seven of the 52 patients had an intra- or an immediate postoperative complication (13.6%). Similar complication rates [3,4,23] have been reported by Berek [3] and Lele [23] based, respectively, on 119 and 51 cases. This complication rate is high and, in the future, should be prevented by avoiding the blind steps of the operation. It should be emphasized that the key point for safe management of these patients is immediate diagnosis and treatment of all the complications. If the diagnosis is doubtful, the organ should be carefully checked. A bladder injury should be suspected when the urine sac is inflated with carbon dioxide and confirmed by filling the bladder with saline and methylene blue. Injuries of the rectosigmoid are obvious when injecting air into the rectum after filling the pelvic cavity with 250ml of Ringer's lactate. Small bowel injuries are more difficult to confirm, and a close inspection of the abnormal area is essential; these injuries may be more easily identified using an underwater inspection. With increased experience in operative endoscopy, bladder and bowel lacerations can be sutured by laparoscopy (three cases in our series), thus keeping the consequences of these complications to a minimum.

Morbidity after laparoscopic second look seems to be lower than that reported after second-look laparotomy. Although we observed only a single case of postoperative occlusion after laparoscopic second look justifying re-operation and with no particular medical problems, the rate for all complications taken together after second-look laparotomy varies between 15.9 and 63%, depending on the series [6,11,12,30–32]. These results are higher than the present results and of those reported by Berek *et al.* [3]. A comparison between these reports is difficult, however, as secondary debulking procedures may have been performed during some second-look laparotomy procedures, whereas laparoscopic second look is only a diagnostic tool.

In conclusion, second look is feasible by laparoscopy. The decreased operative trauma and postoperative morbidity are major advantages for those patients who have already undergone multiple surgical procedures and medical treatment and whose prognosis is very often poor.

Is laparoscopic second look a reliable diagnostic tool?

Some authors consider that the laparoscopic second look is not as reliable as that via laparotomy. To study the prognostic value of a second look performed by laparoscopy, several approaches can be used. We compared the long-term results of patients who underwent a second-look laparoscopy with those of patients who had undergone the same procedure by laparotomy. It was decided not to perform a laparotomy at the end of the laparoscopic pro-

cedure, because of the added morbidity and complications. Indeed, a second-look laparoscopy for an ovarian cancer may be a long procedure (more than 2 hours in some cases) and it appeared difficult to add a laparotomy at the end of the procedure.

To study the reliability of the results obtained when performing a second look by laparoscopy, only patients treated for an epithelial tumour were included, and 27 laparoscopic second looks were compared with 20 cases of second look via laparotomy. As shown in Tables 20.1 and 20.2, the survival rate was related to the results of the second look and to the initial stage of the tumour, but not to the technique used for the second-look operation.

After positive second-look laparotomy (14 cases), 71.4% of patients (10 cases) died within 15.4 ± 3 months. These results are not significantly different from those observed after positive laparoscopic second look (nine cases), in which 66.6% of patients (six cases) died within 26 ± 25 months (Table 20.1). After positive second look, 28.6% (four cases) and 33.3% (three cases) of patients were still alive after second-look laparotomy and laparoscopy, respectively. The average follow-up for each of these groups is, respectively, 52 ± 9.6 months and 42 ± 40 months.

When the second look was negative (24 cases), the prognosis for the patients was similar whether the second look was carried out by laparotomy or by laparoscopy (Table 20.2). Whereas 33.3% of patients (two cases) suffered a recurrence and/or died within an average of 16.5 ± 5.5 months after a negative second-look laparotomy, the rate is 22.2% (four cases) with an average lapse of 35 ± 12 months after negative laparoscopic second look (Table 20.1). The rate of remission after negative second-look laparotomy is 66.6% (four patients), with an average follow-up of 37.5 ± 4.9 months, which is not significantly different from the 77.8% (14 cases) found after negative

Table 20.1 Outcome for patients in cases of positive second look.

	Total cases (*n*)	Deceased		Living	
		n	%	*n*	%
Laparotomy					
Time		15.4 ± 3 months		52 ± 9.6 months	
All stages	14	10	71.4	4	28.6
Stages I–II	0	0		0	
Stages III–IV	14	10	71.4	4	28.6
Laparoscopy					
Time		26 ± 25 months		42 ± 40 months	
All stages	9	6	66.6	3	33.3
Stages I–II	2	1	50	1	50
Stages III–IV	7	5	71.4	2	28.6

Table 20.2 Outcome for patients in cases of negative second look.

	Total cases (*n*)	Deceased		Living	
		n	%	*n*	%
Laparotomy					
Time		16 ± 5.5 months		37.7 ± 4.9 months	
All stages	6	2	33.3	4	66.6
Stages I–II	1	0	0	1	100
Stages III–IV	5	2	40	3	60
Laparoscopy					
Time		35 ± 12 months		42 ± 35 months	
All stages	18	4	22.2	14	77.8
Stages I–II	9	1	11.1	8	88.9
Stages III–IV	9	3	33.3	6	66.7

Table 20.3 Recurrences after negative second look by laparotomy (SLL).

Authors	Year	Total cases of SLL (*n*)	Negative SLL		Recurrences after negative SLL	
			n	%	*n*	%
Phillips *et al.* [65]	1979	—	21	—	1	5
Schwartz & Smith [32]	1980	—	58	—	7	12
Curry *et al.* [70]	1981	—	17	—	3	18
Greco *et al.* [71]	1981	—	17	—	1	6
Roberts *et al.* [72]	1982	—	61	—	6	10
Stuart *et al.* [34]	1982	37	15	40	2	13
Mead *et al.* [35]	1984	20	4	20	2	50
Smirz *et al.* [73]	1985	88	35	40	8	27
Cain *et al.* [74]	1986	177	104	59	16	17
Dauplat *et al.* [62]	1986	51	24	47	4	17
Ho *et al.* [57]	1987	39	17	44	9	53
Carmichael *et al.* [75]	1987	173	55	31	30	57
Free & Webb [37]	1987	89	55	62	6	11
Chambers *et al.* [48]	1988	67	38	57	7	18
Potter *et al.* [15]	1992	212	128	60.4	24	19
Total			649		127	19.6

laparoscopic second look with an average follow-up of 42 ± 35 months (Table 20.1). More importantly, the results are similar, after a negative and after a positive second look, when comparing only patients with stage III and IV disease (Tables 20.1 & 20.2).

Our results are different from those already published. When reviewing the literature, the recurrence rate after negative second-look laparotomy was 19.6% (127 cases) in 649 patients, which is significantly lower than the 30% (51 cases) recurrence after negative laparoscopic second look (170 patients) (χ^2 = 8.44; P < 0.01) (Tables 20.3 & 20.4). However, these data need to be interpreted cautiously.

Because of the progress of laparoscopic surgery, the quality of laparoscopic second look carried out 10 years ago or more [11,33,34], at a time when laparoscopy was purely diagnostic, is not at all like that carried out today. In 1981 Ozols *et al.* [9], for example, whose rate of false-negative laparoscopic second look was 55%, reported that it was impossible to explore the pelvis properly in 50% of cases. The technique for laparoscopic second look was not the same in all series. For example, in the series reported by Rosenoff *et al.* [11], for whom the rate of false-negative laparoscopic second look is 50%, no peritoneal washing and sampling for cytology was carried out, probably increasing the false-negative rate; in other series 18–32% of cases had a positive cytology whereas the biopsies were negative [10,35]. Similarly, as microscopic recurrence may be the only sign of cancer at the time of the second look [18,34,36,37], multiple peritoneal biopsies should be made systematically [38–40]. Copeland *et al.* [36] reported that 43 of the 50 patients presenting microscopic recurrences had a negative peritoneal cytology.

To illustrate these comments, in the most recent series performed with an adequate technique (176 cases), the rate of false-negative laparoscopic second look obtained is 24.9% (25 cases) (Table 20.5). Although this result is slightly higher than the 19.6% (127 cases) of recurrences observed after negative second-look laparotomy (Table 20.3), the difference is not statistically significant. These results, and our experience, strongly suggest that, provided the technique is adequate, and the procedure satisfactory, laparoscopic second look seems as reliable as second-look laparotomy. However, this conclusion should be reserved for patients who undergo a complete staging before the medical treatment.

The adequacy of second-look laparoscopy when compared with laparotomy has recently been confirmed by two studies from the USA.

Childers *et al.* reported 44 second-look procedures performed on women who had previously undergone 'optimal' surgical cytoreduction and were treated with platin-based chemotherapy [41]. All were clinically without evidence of disease. Twenty-four (56%) women were positive for persistent disease; five of these 24 patients (20%) had microscopic disease only. The microscopic disease was discoved in the omentum, washings, pelvic peritoneum and para-aortic nodes. Casey *et al.* reported similar results when they compared 57 second-look laparoscopies to 69 second-look laparotomies [42]. The groups were evenly matched for age, tumour histology and grade, stage and degree of primary cytoreduction. There was no difference in the ability of laparoscopy to detect persistent disease compared with laparotomy (52.6% vs 53.6%). Furthermore, there were significant advantages of laparoscopy over laparotomy: estimated blood loss (34 ml vs 165 ml, $P = 0.0002$), operative time (81 minutes vs 130 minutes, $P = 0.0001$), hospital stay (0.3 days vs 6.8 days, $P = 0.0001$) and direct cost per case ($2765 vs $5420, $P = 0.0001$).

Is there a place for laparoscopic second look in the treatment of ovarian cancer?

Second look theoretically has a number of advantages.
1 It avoids chemotherapy being stopped prematurely when microscopic lesions are seen to persist at second look, despite complete clinical remission [15].
2 It avoids unnecessary prolongation of chemotherapy in cases of negative second look [15] decreasing the risk of secondary effects, notably that of induced cancer [43,44].

Table 20.4 Recurrences after negative second look by laparoscopy [38].

Authors	Year	Negative LSL (n)	Recurrences after negative LSL	
			n	%
Rosenoff *et al.* [11]	1975	4	2	50
Smith *et al.* [12]	1977	24	6	25
Mangioni *et al.* [8]	1979	18	6	33
Piver *et al.* [10]	1980	10	2	20
Queen *et al.* [76]	1980	20	3	15
Ozols *et al.* [9]	1981	22	12	55
Berek *et al.* [3]	1981	37	11	29.7
Lele & Piver [23]	1986	17	5	29.5
Authors' series		18	4	22.2
Total		170	51	30.0

LSL, laparoscopic second look.

Table 20.5 Recurrences after negative second look by laparoscopy [69].

Authors	Year	LSL (n)	Negative LSL		Recurrences after negative LSL	
			n	%	n	%
Piver *et al.* [10]	1980	10	10	100	2	20
Queen *et al.* [76]	1980	43	20	46.5	3	15
Berek *et al.* [3]	1981	57	37	65	11	29.7
Lele & Piver [23]	1986	39	17	43.6	5	29.5
Authors' series		27	18	61.5	4	22.2
Total		176	102		25	24.9

LSL, laparoscopic second look.

3 Exeresis of tumour lesions which has been rendered possible by chemotherapy [45].

4 It establishes the indication of complementary treatment. Various treatments are proposed, although their efficacy has not been demonstrated: radiotherapy [46, 47], second-intention chemotherapy [27,40,44,48–51], intraperitoneal chemotherapy [37,52,53] and intensive chemotherapy with autologous bone marrow infusion [20,54,55].

5 It provides a check on the results of new chemotherapy protocols in controlled trials.

Despite all these potential advantages, the therapeutic value of this operation is questionable because several studies [7,48,56–59] have demonstrated that a second look did not confer any survival benefit, particularly in patients who have been optimally treated with full surgical staging and adequate postoperative chemotherapy. The best management, according to the results of the second look, has not been established. This may explain the limited survival benefits of second-look procedures.

In patients with persistent disease, the value of secondary cytoreduction at second look is controversial [32,35,45,53,60–67]. Recently, Creasman [16] suggested classifying these patients into different groups.

1 Patients with clinical residual disease, for whom secondary optimal debulking did not have a significant effect on survival.

2 Complete clinical responders, among whom about 50% will have macroscopic disease at second-look laparotomy; despite some enthusiastic reports about the role of secondary debulking, it appears that it may be of benefit in only 10% of the patients who underwent a second-look laparotomy. Whatever the answer to this essential question, laparoscopy may be proposed as a very interesting tool in such patients. Indeed, if the survival rate is not significantly improved by secondary surgical reduction, carrying out the second look by laparoscopy avoids unnecessary laparotomy for all those patients who have a recurrence and/or persistence of tumour lesions. This concurs with Smart and Farquharson's opinion [68], who consider that when beginning second look by laparoscopy, 15–48% of laparotomies could be avoided. On the other hand, if secondary cytoreduction is decided, laparoscopy may be used to know whether or not a secondary debulking is necessary — if large tumour residuum (≥5 mm) are present, or if it is possible.

After a negative second look, 20–50% of patients will manifest recurrent disease. This was a major argument against a second-look procedure in patients who achieved a complete clinical response. Because of this very high recurrence rate, authors such as Dauplat *et al.* [62], Webb *et al.* [20] and Raju *et al.* [66] propose that chemotherapy should be continued in order to treat microscopic lesions

inevitably overlooked at second look, even by multiplying the biopsies. Patients found to be complete pathological responders are ideal candidates for consolidation treatments, as their tumours are probably sensitive to chemotherapy and may have a favourable tumour biology [10]. Several consolidation treatments have been proposed and require further evaluation in prospective randomized clinical trials. Second-look procedures are the gold standard in research protocols designed to compare new therapeutic regimens [14,33,35,57,69]. Laparoscopy again appears to be a very attractive alternative to laparotomy in patients who are complete pathological responders for whom a second look includes meticulous inspection of the peritoneal cavity, peritoneal washing and multiple biopsies.

As it has now been demonstrated that a second look can be safely achieved by laparoscopy and the results of this laparoscopic evaluation seem as reliable as the evaluation performed previously at laparotomy, we are convinced that all the arguments against a second-look operation should be used as arguments in favour of a laparoscopic approach. The advantages of the laparoscopic approach have not been exploited enough. Indeed, this approach allows the chemotherapy to begin 2–4 days after the surgical procedure, thus avoiding the delay required by abdominal wall healing. Using this approach, a surgical evaluation of the peritoneal cavity may be proposed more often, to assess the efficacy of new treatment, to check the situation of an intraperitoneal catheter or to look for adhesions which may decrease the efficacy of intraperitoneal treatments. The concept of an 'interval' laparoscopy, as proposed by Lele and Piver many years ago, now becomes more realistic and can be used as often as required by new therapeutic protocols.

References

1 Wangensteen OH, Lewis FJ, Tongen IA (1951). The 'second-look' in cancer surgery. *Lancet* **71**:303–307.

2 Rutledge F, Burns B (1966). Chemotherapy for advanced ovarian cancer. *Am J Obstet Gynecol* **96**:761–770.

3 Berek JS, Griffiths CT, Leventhal JM (1981). Laparoscopy for second-look evaluation in ovarian cancer. *Obstet Gynecol* **58**:192–198.

4 Canis M, Chapron C, Mage G *et al* (1992). Technique et résultats préliminaires du second-look percoelioscopique dans les tumeurs épithéliales malignes de l'ovaire. *J Gynecol Obstet Biol Reprod* **21**:655–663.

5 Childers JM, Brzechffa PR, Surwit EA (1993). Laparoscopy using the left upper quadrant as the primary trocar site. *Gynecol Oncol* **50**:221–225.

6 Lacey CG, Morrow CP, Disaia PJ, Lucases WE (1978). Laparoscopy in the evaluation of gynecologic cancer. *Obstet Gynecol* **52**:708–712.

7 Luesley D, Blackledge G, Kelly K *et al* (1988). (West Midlands

ovarian cancer group.) Failure of second-look laparotomy to influence survival in epithelial ovarian cancer. *Lancet* **ii**:599–603.

8 Mangioni C, Bolis G, Molteni P, Belloni C (1979). Indications. Advantages and limitations of laparoscopy in ovarian cancer. *Gynecol Oncol* **7**:47–55.

9 Ozols RF, Fischer F, Anderson T, Makuch R, Young RC (1981). Peritoneoscopy in the management of ovarian cancer. *Am J Obstet Gynecol* **140**:611–618.

10 Piver MS, Lele SB, Barlow JJ, Gamarra M (1980). Second-look laparoscopy prior to proposed second-look laparotomy. *Obstet Gynecol* **55**:571–573.

11 Rosenoff SH, Devita VT, Hubbard S, Young RC (1975). Peritoneoscopy in the staging and follow-up of ovarian cancer. *Semin Oncol* **2**:223–228.

12 Smith WG, Day TG, Smith JP (1977). The use of laparoscopy to determine the results of chemotherapy for ovarian cancer. *J Reprod Med* **18**:257–260.

13 Xygakis AM, Politis GS, Michalas JP (1984). Second look laparoscopy in ovarian cancer. *J Reprod Med* **29**:583–585.

14 Berek JS (1992). Second-look versus second nature. *Gynecol Oncol* **44**:1–2.

15 Potter ME, Hatch KD, Soong SJ, Partridge EE, Austin JM, Shingleton HM (1992). Second-look laparotomy and salvage therapy: a research modality only. *Gynecol Oncol* **44**:3–9.

16 Creasman WT (1994). Second-look laparotomy in ovarian cancer. *Gynecol Oncol* **55**:s122–s127.

17 Hunter JG (1991). Avoidance of bile duct injury during laparoscopic cholecystectomy. *Am J Surg* **162**:71–76.

18 Cook WA (1976). Needle laparoscopy in patients with suspected bowel adhesions. *Obstet Gynecol* **49**:105.

19 Tobias JS, Griffiths CT (1976). Management of ovarian carcinoma: current concepts and future prospects. *N Engl J Med* **294**:818–822.

20 Webb MJ, Snyder JJA, Williams TJ, Decker DG (1982). Second-look laparotomy in ovarian cancer. *Gynecol Oncol* **14**:285–293.

21 Williams PP (1976). The needlescope as a gynecologic endoscope. In: Sciarra JJ, ed. *Advances in Sterilization Techniques*. Hagerstown, MD: Harper & Row, 106.

22 Bruhat M-A, Mage G, Pouly J-L, Manhes H, Canis M, Wattiez A (1992). *Operative Laparoscopy*. New York: McGraw-Hill.

23 Lele SB, Piver MS (1986). Interval laparoscopy as predictor of response to chemotherapy in ovarian carcinoma. *Obstet Gynecol* **68**:345–347.

24 Menscer J, Modan M, Brenner J, Ben-Baruk G, Brenner H (1986). Completion of cisplatinium based combination chemotherapy. *Gynecol Oncol* **24**:149–154.

25 Siegel B, Golub RM, Lioacono IA *et al* (1991). Technique of ultrasonic detection and mapping of abdominal wall adhesions. *Surg Endosc* **5**:161–165.

26 Howell SB, Zimm S, Markman M *et al* (1987). Long-term survival of advanced refractory ovarian carcinoma patients with small-volume disease treated with intraperitoneal chemotherapy. *J Clin Oncol* **5**:1607–1612.

27 George M, Heron JF, Kerbrat P *et al.* (Féderation Nationale des Centres de Lutte Contre le Cancer) (1988). Phase II study of navelbine (nvb) in advanced ovarian cancer (adovca). A cooperative study of French oncology centers. *ASCO Proc* **7**(143): abstract 553.

28 Perone N (1983). Conventional vs. open laparoscopy. *Am Fam Physician* **27**:147–149.

29 Penfield AJ (1985). How to prevent complications of open laparoscopy. *J Reprod Med* **30**:660–663.

30 Lansac J, Fignon A, Body G, Chauvet B (1988). Traitements des tumeurs épithéliales après laparotomie de deuxième regard. In: Querleu D, Cappelare P, eds. *Tumeurs de l'Ovaire*. Paris: Doin editeurs, 203–212.

31 Piccart LJ, Abrams J, Dodion PF *et al* (1988). Intraperitoneal chemotherapy with cisplatin and melphalan. *J Natl Cancer Inst* **80**:1118–1124.

32 Schwartz PE, Smith JP (1980). Second-look operation in ovarian cancer. *Am J Obstet Gynecol* **138**:1124–1130.

33 Morgan MA, Noumoff JS, King S, Mikuta JJ (1992). A formula for predicting the risk of a positive second-look laparotomy in epithelial ovarian cancer: implications for a randomized trial. *Obstet Gynecol* **80**:944–948.

34 Stuart GCE, Jeffries M, Stuart JL, Anderson RJ (1982). The changing role of 'second-look' laparotomy in the management of epithelial carcinoma of the ovary. *Am J Obstet Gynecol* **142**:612–616.

35 Mead GM, Williams CJ, Macbeth FR, Boyd IE, Whitehouse JM (1984). Second look laparotomy in the management of epithelial cell carcinoma of the ovary. *Br J Cancer* **50**:185–191.

36 Copeland IJ, Wharton JT, Rutledge FN, Gershenson DM, Seski JC, Herson J (1983). Role of 'third-look' laparotomy in the guidance of ovarian cancer treatment. *Gynecol Oncol* **15**:145–153.

37 Free KE, Webb MJ (1987) Second-look laparotomy—clinical correlations. *Gynecol Oncol* **26**:290–297.

38 Ballon SC, Portnuff JC, Sikic BL *et al* (1984). Second-look laparotomy in epithelial ovarian carcinoma: precise definition, sensitivity and specificity of the procedure. *Gynecol Oncol* **17**:154–160.

39 Miller DS, Ballon SC, Teng N, Seifer DB, Soriero O (1986). A critical reassessment of second-look laparotomy in epithelial ovarian carcinoma. *Cancer* **57**:530–535.

40 Phibbs GD, Smith JP, Stanhope CR (1983). Analysis of sites of persistent cancer at 'second-look' laparotomy in patients with ovarian cancer. *Am J Obstet Gynecol* **147**:611–617.

41 Childers J, Lang J, Surwit E, Hatch K (1995). Laparoscopic surgical staging of ovarian cancer. *Gynecol Oncol* **59**:25–33.

42 Casey AC, Farias-Eisner R, Pisani A *et al* (1996). What is the role of reassessment laparoscopy in the management of gynecologic cancers in 1995? *Gynecol Oncol* **60**:454–461.

43 Green MH, Boice JD, Greer BE, Blessing JA, Dembo AT (1982). Acute non lymphocytic leukaemia after therapy with alkylating agents for ovarian cancer: a study of five randomised trials. *N Engl J Med* **307**:1416.

44 Rosen GF, Lurain JR, Newton M (1987). Hexamethylmelamine in ovarian cancer after failure of cisplatin-based multiple-agent chemotherapy. *Gynecol Oncol* **27**:173–179.

45 Wils J, Blijham G, Naus A (1986). Primary or delayed debulking surgery and chemotherapy consisting of cisplatin doxorubicin and cyclophosphamide in stage III–IV epithelial ovarian carcinoma. *J Clin Oncol* **4**:1068–1073.

46 Goldhirsh A, Greiner R, Dreher E *et al* (1988). Treatment of advanced ovarian cancer with surgery. Chemotherapy and consolidation of response by whole-abdominal radiotherapy. *Cancer* **62**:40–47.

47 Hacker NF, Berek JS, Burnison CM, Heintz APM, Juillard GJF, Lagasse ID (1985). Whole abdominal radiation as salvage therapy for epithelial ovarian cancer. *Obstet Gynecol* **65**:60–66.

48 Chambers SK, Chambers JT, Kohorn EI, Lawrence R, Schwartz PE (1988). Evaluation of the role of second-look surgery in ovarian cancer. *Obstet Gynecol* **72**:404–408.

49 Kuhnle H, Meerpohl HG, Lenaz I *et al* (1988). Etoposide in cisplatin-refractory ovarian cancer. *ASCO Proc* **7**(137): abstract 527.

50 Ozols RF, Behrens BC, Ostchega Y, Young RC (1985). High dose cisplatin and high dose carboplatin in refractory ovarian cancer. *Cancer Treat Rev* **12**(suppl a):59–65.

51 Surwit EA, Alberts DS, O'Toole RV *et al* (1987). Phase II trial of vinblastine in previously treated patients with ovarian cancer: a Southwest Oncology Group Study. *Gynecol Oncol* **27**:214–219.

52 Janisch H, Shieder K, Keebl H (1989). Diagnostic versus therapeutic second-look surgery in patients with ovarian cancer. *Surg Obstet Gynecol* **3**:197–200.

53 Podartz KC, Malkasian GD, Hilton JF, Harris EA, Gaffey TA (1985). Second-look laparotomy in ovarian cancer: evaluation of pathological variables. *Am J Obstet Gynecol* **152**:230–238.

54 Fitzgibbons RJ, Salerno GM, Filipi CJ (1991). Open laparoscopy. In: Zucker KA, ed. *Surgical Laparoscopy*. St Louis, Missouri: Quality Medical Publishing, 87–97.

55 Nores JM, Dalayeun J, Otmezguine Y, Le Douarin LA, Folgoas C, Nenna A (1987). Le traitement du cancer évolué par chimiothérapie intensive avec autogreffe de moelle osseuse. A partir d'un cas. Discussion et revue de la littérature. *Rev Fr Gynecol Obstet* **82**:355–359.

56 Cohen CJ, Golberg JD, Holland JF *et al* (1983). Improved therapy with cisplatin regimens for patients with ovarian carcinoma (FIGO stages III and IV) as surgical and staging (second-look operation). *Am J Obstet Gynecol* **145**:955–967.

57 Ho AG, Beller U, Speyer JL, Colombo N, Werns J, Beckman EM (1987). A reassessment of the role of second-look laparotomy in advanced ovarian cancer. *J Clin Oncol* **5**:1316–1321.

58 Luesley DM, Chan KK (1986). Second look laparotomy in ovarian cancer. In: Blackledge G, Chan KK, eds. *Management of Ovarian Cancer*. London: Butterworths, 83–96.

59 Wiltshaw E, Raju KS, Dawson I (1985). The role of cytoreductive surgery in advanced carcinoma of the ovary: an analysis of primary and second surgery. *Br J Obstet Gynaecol* **92**:522–527.

60 Berek JS, Hacker NF, Lagasse LD, Nieberg RK, Elashoff RM (1983). Survival of patients following secondary cytoreductive surgery in ovarian cancer. *Obstet Gynecol* **61**:189–193.

61 Bertelsen K, Hansen MK, Pedersen PH *et al* (1988). The prognostic and therapeutic value of second-look laparotomy in advanced ovarian cancer. *Br J Obstet Gynaecol* **95**:1231–1266.

62 Dauplat J, Ferriere JP, Gorbinet M *et al* (1986). Second-look laparotomy in the management of epithelial ovarian carcinoma. *Cancer* **57**:1627–1631.

63 Lipmann SM, Alberts DS, Slymen DJ *et al* (1988). Second-look laparotomy in epithelial ovarian carcinoma. Prognostic factors associated with survival duration. *Cancer* **61**:2571–2577.

64 Luesley DM, Chan KK, Fielding JWL, Hurlow R, Blackledge GR, Jordon JA (1984). Second-look laparotomy in the management of epithelial ovarian carcinoma: an evaluation of fifty cases. *Obstet Gynecol* **64**:421–426.

65 Phillips BD, Buchsbaum HJ, Lifshiitz S (1979). Re-exploration after treatment for ovarian carcinoma. *Gynecol Oncol* **8**:339–345.

66 Raju KS, Mckinna JA, Barker GH, Wittshaw E, Jones JM (1982). Second-look operations in the planned management of advanced ovarian carcinoma. *Am J Obstet Gynecol* **144**:650–654.

67 Vogl SE, Seltler V, Calanog A *et al* (1984). 'Second effort' surgical resection for bulky ovarian cancer. *Cancer* **54**:2220–2225.

68 Smart GE, Farquharson DI (1985). Second look surgery: a review. In: Hudson CD, ed. *Ovarian Cancer*. Oxford: Oxford University Press, 12–322.

69 Barnhill DR, Hoskins WJ, Heller PB *et al* (1984). The second-look surgical reassessment for epithelial ovarian carcinoma. *Gynecol Oncol* **19**:148.

70 Curry SL, Zembo MM, Nahhas WA, Jahsan AE, Whitney CW, Mortel R (1981). Second look laparotomy for ovarian cancer. *Gynecol Oncol* **11**:114–118.

71 Greco FA, Julian CG, Richardson RL *et al* (1981). Advanced ovarian cancer: brief intensive combination chemotherapy and second-look operation. *Obstet Gynecol* **58**:199–205.

72 Roberts WS, Hodel K, Rich WM, Disaia PJ (1982). Second-look laparotomy in the management of gynecologic malignancy. *Gynecol Oncol* **13**:345–355.

73 Smirz IR, Stehman FB, Ulbright TM, Sutton GP, Ehrlich CE (1985). Second-look laparotomy after chemotherapy in the management of ovarian malignancy. *Am J Obstet Gynecol* **152**:661–668.

74 Cain JM, Saigo PE, Pierce VK *et al* (1986). A review of second-look laparotomy for ovarian cancer. *Gynecol Oncol* **23**:14–25.

75 Carmichael JA, Shelley WE, Brown IB *et al* (1987). A predictive index of cure versus no cure in advanced ovarian carcinoma patients—replacement of second-look laparotomy as a diagnostic test. *Gynecol Oncol* **27**:269–278.

76 Queen MA, Bishop GJ, Campbell JJ *et al* (1980). Laparoscopic follow-up of patients with ovarian cancer. *Br J Obstet Gynaecol* **87**:1132.

21   **Vulvar and vaginal cancer**

Patrice Mathevet

Vulvar cancer

Introduction

Surgery in cancer therapy presently attempts to decrease the aggressiveness and the morbidity of surgical treatments without reducing the chances of survival. The application of laparoscopy in gynaecological oncology is a way of achieving these goals, but it also improves the surgical staging of gynaecological malignancies.

En bloc radical vulvectomy and bilateral groin dissection had been the standard treatment for a considerable time, whatever the stage and the size of the tumour. This operation, which was associated with a high incidence of postoperative complications, has been abandoned in favour of radical vulvectomy and inguinofemoral lymphnode dissections through separate incisions.

The increased medical education of the population, the development of preventive measures, and also the occurrence of vulvar cancer related to the human papillomavirus, have led to an increase in the reported incidence of small vulvar cancer, in particular in young patients who do not want any extensive damage to their body image and sexual function. Therefore vulvar surgery has evolved towards minimizing the morbidity of the surgical treatment in the cases of small vulvar cancer (associated with good prognosis), and individualizing oncological treatments and endoscopic techniques. Also better staging and management of advanced vulvar cancer can be achieved with the help of laparoscopic procedures for lymph-node evaluation.

Currently we have to answer the question: how can endoscopy improve the surgical management of vulvar cancer? Endoscopy cannot improve the efficacy of surgical treatments, but it can decrease the morbidity of these treatments. There are two different uses of endoscopy in vulvar cancer therapy: (i) inguinal lymph-node dissection through the endoscopic approach; and (ii) retroperitoneal (pelvic and para-aortic) laparoscopic lymph-node dissections during the staging of advanced vulvar malignancies.

Endoscopic inguinal lymph-node dissection

The surgical management of stage I and II vulvar cancers has to be defined, and in particular in which cases an inguinal lymphadenectomy should be performed.

When the depth of invasion is less than 1 mm, the risk of lymph-node metastases is nearly nil (less than 1%). If the invasion is deeper than this, the risk of lymph-node involvment increases with the size, grade and depth of invasion of the tumour [1]. Therefore, vulvar cancers less than 1 mm deep should be treated by wide local resection without groin dissections. The therapeutic efficacy of this procedure is nearly 100%.

For stage I lesions, two different types of conservative (less aggressive) surgery has been used recently [2]:
1 Reduction of the extension of the vulvar resection by performing radical resection adapted to the extension of the lesion, in order to decrease alterations of body image and sexual function.
2 Reduction of the fields of lymph-node dissections, in order to decrease the postoperative complications related to the lymphadenectomy (wound breakdown and infection, leg lymphoedema).

These major complications are frequent (more than 60% of cases) with the *en bloc* radical vulvectomy. Even if they are reduced when performing radical vulvectomy with separate incisions, their rate is about 15–20% of cases [3–6]. In order to lessen these complications, different authors have shown that ipsilateral groin lymphnode dissection is sufficient for small lateral vulvar cancer [7].

Recently, Di Saia [8] discussed femoral lymph-node dissection in those cases, and recommended performing only ipsilateral inguinal superficial lymph-node dissection (femoral lymphadenectomy and pelvic lymphadenectomy are performed only if extemporaneous assessment of the superficial nodes is positive). All these results are supported by studies of the natural history of vulvar cancer. It has been reported that vulvar carcinoma invades locally and spreads by embolization to regional lymph nodes, without significant involvment of the intervening

170

tissues [9]. The superficial inguinal lymph nodes are primarily involved [10].

The final evolution of this approach to less aggressive surgery is described in a recent feasibility study concerning the evaluation of the regional lymph nodes. The M.D. Anderson team [11] proposes to perform vulvar mapping, in order to carry out resection of only the sentinel lymph node of the vulvar cancer. This use of elective lymph-node dissection has been criticized by different authors, who argue that inguinal lymphadenectomy has therapeutic value. Monaghan evaluated the improvement of the 5-year survival rate of about 14% when performing inguinal lymphadenectomy compared with no lymph-node dissection. He stated that groin-node dissection improves the survival, by effectively removing micrometastases which are not detectable [1].

To benefit from the therapeutic value of groin dissection, we propose a different approach to less aggressive surgery, using inguinal lymph-node dissection through endoscopy. This technique aims to significantly reduce the rate of groin dissection complications (in particular lymphoedema and wound breakdown) without reducing the chances of survival. The principles of this technique, and our initial results, are given below.

The main advantages of endoscopic inguinal lymphadenectomy are:

1 Preservation of the great saphenous vein, reducing the risk of lymphoedema.
2 Reducing the cutaneous incisions, decreasing the risk of wound breakdown and infection.
3 Probably reducing the risk of postoperative lymphocystitis due to the small cutaneous incisions.

The disadvantages of this technique are:

1 Requirement of the surgical team to be trained in endoscopic techniques and the use of specific surgical instruments.
2 The therapeutic value of this technique still has to be proved. Currently, we are performing vulvar mapping during endoscopic lymph-node dissection, to localize the sentinel lymph node and to be sure this node is extracted.

For stage II vulvar cancers, recent reports have demonstrated that the same conservative procedures used for stage I (i.e. hemivulvectomy with selective ipsilateral inguinal lymphadenectomy) are as effective as radical vulvectomy with decreased morbidity. Therefore, stage II should be treated as stage I, with a wide radical local excision (including a margin of 1 cm of normal skin) and an ipsilateral endoscopic inguinal lymphadenectomy.

Vulvar cancer reaching the midline should be treated with bilateral endoscopic inguinal lymphadenectomy.

Laparoscopic pelvic lymph-node dissection

For more advanced lesions (stage III and IV and vulvar cancer with urethral or vaginal extension), our strategy is to begin with a laparoscopic retroperitoneal pelvic lymph-node dissection. This procedure is easy to perform, its morbidity is reduced and it does not impair radiotherapy by the formation of pelvic adhesions. If the pelvic lymph nodes are involved, radiotherapy is carried out first (plus chemotherapy if the patient is young), followed eventually by surgery. If there is no pelvic lymph-node metastases, traditional radical surgery is performed, including exenterative procedures for selected stage IV cases.

For tumour with clinically evident positive inguinal node, there is controversy about the adequate treatment. Retroperitoneal laparoscopic pelvic lymph-node dissection, as for advanced carcinoma, is carried out. Then, in the case of negative pelvic lymph nodes, an inguinal 'debulking' excision following the standard technique of groin dissection, associated with a radical vulvar resection and a contralateral endoscopic groin dissection, is performed.

Cancers of the clitoris and Bartholin's gland have been shown to spread directly to the interiliac lymph nodes. The occurrence of positive pelvic nodes without metastases to the inguinal nodes is very rare, and the majority of authors recommend performing pelvic lymph-node dissection only in cases with positive inguinal nodes [12,13].

Vaginal cancer

It is well known that cancers of the upper vagina spread to the pelvic nodes, whereas lower vaginal cancers spread to the inguinal lymphatics. However, because of extensive anastomotic connections of the vaginal lymphatics, there are numerous exceptions to this general rule.

Most oncological teams have a policy of treating by surgery only stage I vaginal carcinomas; more advance-stage carcinomas of the vagina are treated by a combination of external and internal radiotherapy [14].

Microinvasive carcinoma of the vagina can be defined as an early invasive lesion in which the risk of lymph-node involvment is low enough to allow treatment with local excision without specific therapy directed toward the regional lymph nodes. Even if the limits for this type of tumour are not well defined, it seems that the risk of lymph-node metastases is nearly nil when the depth of invasion is less than 3 mm and when where is no lymph-vascular invasion [15].

Stage I vaginal cancer can be treated with wide local resection by the vaginal approach and with laparoscopic retroperitoneal pelvic lymph-node dissection (or endoscopic inguinal lymphadenectomy for lesions of the lower third of the vagina).

Stage II vaginal cancer, in our opinion, can also be treated by surgery. The combination of laparoscopy and the vaginal approach allows vaginectomy with paracolpectomy and parametrectomy, in association with laparoscopic retroperitoneal pelvic lymph-node dissection (and endoscopic inguinal lymphadenectomy for lesions of the lower third of the vagina), to be carried out. Also it is possible, in association with a transperitoneal or a retroperitoneal laparoscopic lymph-node dissection, to perform a division of the parametrium under laparoscopic magnification. Then a laparoscopically assisted vaginal radical colpohysterectomy can be carried out [16]. This gives a good control rate with a decreased morbidity.

For more advanced lesions, there is still a place for laparoscopy. It is well known that the lymph-node status is the most important predictive factor of tumour relapse. This factor is assessed accurately only by surgical lymphadenectomy (clinical and imaging assessment of the lymph nodes is not accurate). Until recently, surgical staging of these advanced carcinomas did not include lymphadenectomy, as this procedure was associated with a high morbidity and increased radiotherapy complications (due to pelvic adhesions).

The development of laparoscopic retroperitoneal pelvic and aortic lymph-node dissections has greatly reduced the complication rate of these procedures, so, currently, these laparoscopic lymph-node dissections should be included in the surgical staging of advanced vaginal carcinomas. Oncological treatments should then be performed following results of lymph-node status: extension of radiotherapy fields, association with systemic therapy or exenterative surgery (in central stage IV lesions).

Operative technique of video endoscopic inguinal lymphadenectomy

The technique described here is designed to completely eliminate wound breakdown and may prevent secondary lymphoedema. The inspiration for this technique came from two innovations introduced by plastic surgeons, liposuction and subcutaneous video endoscopy [17,18]. Both innovations have been used successfully by F. Suzanne and A. Wattiez for axillary lymphadenectomy [19].

Technique

The patient is placed in a dorsal decubitus position and the lower extremities are abducted without flexure. The reference points of the femoral triangle are identified and

the triangle marked with a marker. Beginning at the lower corner, the space inside the triangle is infiltrated with a mixture of normal saline (100 ml), distilled water (100 ml) and Lidocaine (20 ml) with adrenaline (1%), using a 20-gauge 3.5 lumbar puncture needle. The needle is moved in a fan-like manner between the undersurface of the superficial fascia, about 5–10 mm from the skin, and the upper surface of the fascia lata, about 2–4 mm deeper, until the entire layer of subcutaneous fat is infiltrated.

Liposuction of the subcutaneous fat is the next step (Fig. 21.1). Two centimetres below the tip of the femoral triangle, a vertical microincision is made and a 7-mm-diameter curved Karmann cannula (CCD) is inserted. The cannula is connected to an aspirator and suction of 800 mmHg is applied. A canal is carved in the fat along the axis of the triangle to its base. The cannula is then moved back and forth within the space between the superficial fascia and the fascia lata, rotating the tip up and down, until the fat that is aspirated is tinged red. A second canal is made at a slightly different angle than the first and the process is repeated. The liposuction takes about 10 minutes. The aspirated tissue is sent to the laboratory.

When the liposuction is completed, the femoral incision is enlarged and a blunt-tip trocar (Origin) is inserted. The balloon is filled with 18 ml of normal saline, the shield is co-opted, and the space filled with carbon dioxide. The laparoscope is then inserted and two incisions are made on each side, 2 cm from the edges of the triangle. The incisions allow insertion of two 5-mm trocars, through which a grasping laparoscopic forceps and an atraumatic laparoscopic forceps are introduced into the operating field. The instruments are used to tear the conjunctival tracts connecting the deep layer of the superficial fascia and the superficial layer of the fascia lata (Fig. 21.2). Surgical dissection then begins.

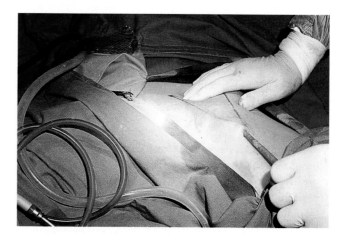

Fig. 21.1 Liposuction of the subcutaneous fat of the right femoral triangle.

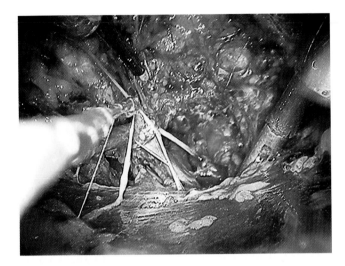

Fig. 21.2 Endoscopic view of the opening of the fascia lata.

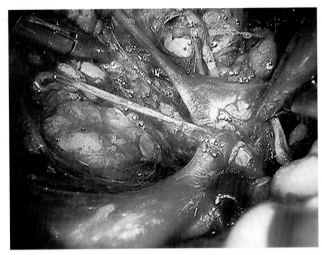

Fig. 21.4 Dissection of the arch of the saphenous vein.

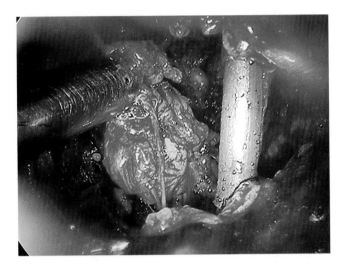

Fig. 21.3 Extraction of the lymph nodes using the coelio-extractor.

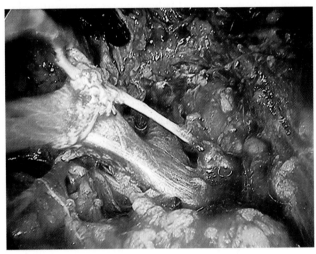

Fig. 21.5 Identification of the arch of the saphenous vein and femoral vessels.

Objective

The primary objective of surgical dissection is to locate and free the lymph nodes situated under and within the arch of the great saphenous vein, as well as those above the arch along the same vertical axis. The great saphenous vein or an accessory saphenous vein is usually found first. Dissection of the lymph nodes follows the path of the saphenous vein, starting at the bottom and moving up past the arch to the area where the lymph nodes are situated around the external pudendal veins, the superficial epigastric vein and the superficial circumflex vein. Note that all blood vessels effluent to the convex side of the arch can be preserved.

After freeing the superficial lymph nodes, one of the lateral incisions is enlarged. A 10-mm trocar is inserted in order to place the coelio-extractor in the operative field. The lymph nodes are then removed (Fig. 21.3). The dissection continues by dilacerating the fascia lata surrounding the arch of the great saphenous vein (Fig. 21.4) and identifying the femoral artery and vein (Fig. 21.5), in order to locate, free and resect the deep inguinal lymph nodes. These nodes are found on the medial aspect of the femoral vein, above and below its junction with the great saphenous vein. The highest of the deep femoral nodes is Cloquet's node. Upon completion of the lymphadenectomy, the operative field is washed with saline and a drain put in place.

Experience

Between July 1994 and May 1996, we performed inguinal lymphadenectomies in 13 patients using video laparoscopy. Cancer of the vulva was present in 11 cases and cancer of the inferior vagina in two. Lesions were lateralized in 11 cases and centralized in two cases. The size of the lesion was 12–40 mm. Ipsilateral metastatic adenopathy, as confirmed by cytopuncture, was present in three of the lateralized cases. In these cases, a routine lymphadenectomy was performed and video endoscopy was used for the contralateral lymphadenectomy. In the eight other cases, the nodes were palpably negative and ipsilateral lymphadenectomy was performed using video endoscopy. For the two patients with centralized disease, bilateral lymphadenectomy was performed. Ten years earlier, one of these patients had undergone treatment for thrombosis of the left femoral vein. The same inguinal incision was re-used for the lymphadenectomy on the left side. Video endoscopy was used for the right side only. The other patient with centralized disease underwent bilateral video laparoscopy.

Inguinal lymphadenectomy was performed concurrently with primary treatment in eight cases and subsequent to treatment in five other cases.

Results

Operations took 75 minutes on average, with a range of 50–120 minutes. Only one complication occurred: a transverse injury of the femoral vein under the junction point of the femoral and the great saphenous veins. A small transverse inguinal incision permitted repair. The irruption of carbon dioxide that occurred in this incident had no perceptible side effects on the patient.

Local complications of these procedures included the presence of a lymphocyst in three cases; two were drained and the third was treated by puncture. No wound breakdown was observed. None of the patients had any lymphoedema at the control examination between the sixth and ninth weeks. One patient experienced a cerebrovascular accident 1 hour postoperatively. In the previous year, this same patient had had a similar cerebrovascular accident which was completely reversible. Although this occurred 2 hours after infiltration, the Lidocaine and adrenaline added to the infiltrating solution may have added to the risk.

The length of stay in hospital varied according to the degree of healing of the vulvectomy incision in the eight cases where the lymphadenectomy was concurrent with the primary lesion treatment. In the five other cases, where lymphadenectomy was an isolated procedure, lengths of stay were 30, 9, 5, 4 and 3 days. The 30-day

length of stay involved the patient who experienced the cerebrovascular accident. The 9-day length of stay resulted from the use of conventional contralateral inguinal lymphadenectomy.

The number of lymph nodes removed per case ranged from two to 15, with a mean of eight. Histopathological examination showed metastases in one case and negative results for the other 12 cases.

Addendum

Since the writing of this chapter, we have observed a large inguinal recurrence in a patient with positive inguinal nodes explored with the described surgical technique. This complication led us to modify our endoscopic technique. Currently, we use a gasless system (Origin®), which holds the inguinal skin and creates a space where the inguinal lymph-node dissection is performed without the use of liposuction. We hope that this new approach will reduce the risk of dissemination during dissection of positive lymph nodes.

References

1 Monagham JM (1992). Surgery for invasive carcinoma of vulva. In: Coppleson M, ed. *Gynecologic Oncology*, 2nd edn. Edinburgh: Churchill Livingstone, 1171–1183.

2 Burke TW, Stringer CA, Gershenson DM *et al* (1990). Radical wide excision and selective inguinal node dissection for squamous cell carcinoma of the vulva. *Gynecol Oncol* **38**:328–332.

3 Hacker NF (1992). Conservative surgery for stage I carcinoma of vulva. In: Coppleson M, ed. *Gynecologic Oncology*, 2nd edn. Edinburgh: Churchill Livingstone, 1185–1189.

4 Hopkins MP, Reid GC, Morley GW (1993). Radical vulvectomy. *Cancer* **72**:799–803.

5 Sutton GP, Miser MR, Stehman FB, Lock KY, Ehrlich CE (1991). Trends in the operative management of invasive squamous carcinoma of the vulva at Indiana University, 1974 to 1988. *Am J Obstet Gynecol* **164**:1472–1481.

6 Cavanagh D (1990). Invasive vulvar carcinoma. *Am J Obstet Gynecol* **163**:1007–1015.

7 Stehman FB, Bundy BN, Dvoretsky PM, Creasman WT (1992). Early stage I carcinoma of the vulva treated with ipsilateral superficial inguinal lymphadenectomy and modified radical hemivulvectomy: a prospective study of the Gynecologic Oncology Group. *Obstet Gynecol* **79**:490–497.

8 Di Saia PJ (1987). The case against the surgical concept of en bloc dissection for certain malignancies of the reproductive tract. *Cancer* **60**:2025–2028.

9 Hacker NF, Berek JS, Lagasse SD, Nieberg RK, Leuchter RS (1984). Individualization of treatment for stage I squamous cell vulvar carcinoma. *Obstet Gynecol* **63**:155–162.

10 Andrews SJ, Williams BT, DePriest PD, Gallion HH *et al* (1994). Therapeutic implications of lymph nodal spread in lateral T1 and T2 squamous cell carcinoma of the vulva. *Gynecol Oncol* **55**:41–46.

11 Levenback C, Burke TW, Gershenson DM *et al* (1994). Intraoperative lymphatic mapping for vulvar cancer. *Obstet Gynecol* **84**:163–167.

12 Piver MX, Xynos FP (1977). Pelvic lymphadenectomy in women with carcinoma of the clitoris. *Obstet Gynecol* **49**:592–595.

13 Copeland LJ, Nour Sneige, Gershenson DM, McGuffie VB, Abdul Karim F, Rutledge FN (1986). Bartholin gland carcinoma. *Obstet Gynecol* **67**:794–801.

14 Lee WR, McCollough WM, Mendenhall WM *et al* (1993). Elective inguinal lymph node irradiation for pelvic carcinomas. *Cancer* **72**:2058–2065.

15 Manetta A, Gutrecht EL, Berman ML, Di Saia PJ (1990). Primary invasive carcinoma of the vagina. *Obstet Gynecol* **76**:639–642.

16 Dargent D, Mathevet P (1992). L'hystérectomie élargie laparoscopico-vaginale. *J Gynecol Obstet Biol Reprod* **21**:709–710.

17 Illouz YG, DeVillers YT (1989). *Body Sculpturing by Lipoplasty.* Edinburgh: Churchill Livingstone.

18 Isse NG (1994). Endoscopic facial rejuvenation: endoforehead, the functional lift. *Aesth Plast Surg* **18**:21–29.

19 Suzanne F, Anton MC, Ducroz F, Wattiez A, Jacquetin B (1994). Le curage axillaire dans le cancer du sein par aspiration graisseuse et ganglionnaire: à propos de 57 cas. *Ref Gynecol Obstet* **2**:255–266.

22 Restaging operations and staging before exenteration

Denis Querleu, François Dubecq and Eric Leblanc

Introduction

Restaging patients referred with incomplete staging is not uncommon in gynaecological oncology. The rationale for restaging is that some patients may be understaged and, consequently, undertreated. This concept applies especially to apparent stage I invasive ovarian tumours, but it may be extended to other pelvic malignancies. The traditional approach for restaging is exploratory laparotomy. The development of laparoscopic surgery in gynaecology has raised the hope of sparing the patient the discomfort of laparotomy for the only purpose of staging. However, staging operations involve a number of specific steps, including, in most patients, para-aortic lymphadenectomy and omentectomy. Laparoscopy is thus acceptable only if all these steps can be safely and accurately performed. Although the assessment of intraperitoneal disease has been the first indication for laparoscopy in oncology, this was impossible until laparoscopic para-aortic lymphadenectomy [1,2] and omentectomy [3] had been described.

Only restaging operations for inadequately staged cervical, endometrial, fallopian tube or ovarian carcinomata will be addressed in this chapter. The scope of this chapter does not include the more controversial second-look operations for monitoring of therapy, or the investigational staging operations before chemotherapy in advanced cancers. However, insight into the potential role of laparoscopy before exenteration will be given.

Restaging of ovarian or fallopian tube cancers

Rationale

The case of the referral patient with incomplete staging of adnexal (ovary or fallopian tube) malignancies, whether treated by laparoscopy or by laparotomy, is not uncommon. Only approximately one out of two patients managed by gynaecologists and one out of three patients managed by general surgeons are adequately staged [4].

In the Netherlands, only 15% of ovarian cancers are adequately staged [5].

In a majority of cases, the available information is sufficient to establish the diagnosis of stage II or III ovarian cancer. Adjuvant chemotherapy is required in such cases, whatever the result of the additional staging procedure, making the role of a restaging operation limited.

In another group of patients, the question of operability remains open. Many patients who are deemed inoperable by a non-specialist surgeon eventually benefit from optimal debulking by gynaecological oncologists [6–8]. Laparoscopy may be proposed to check the location, amount and potential operability of residual disease. In obviously inoperable patients, laparoscopic examination provides a precise assessment of residual disease before starting chemotherapy. When residual disease is thought to be operable, optimal or complete cytoreduction is indicated. In the vast majority of such cases, laparotomy is proposed. However, laparoscopic surgery may be applied in selected cases to the removal of small or medium-sized tumour grafts; this indication is acceptable only if the laparoscopic procedure leads to the same results as a laparotomy, and if the disease can be removed without any contamination of the abdominal wall. The laparoscopic approach is applicable to every place in the abdominal cavity. The implants are excised by sharp dissection, then taken out of the abdomen through the ancillary trocars, with a liberal use of endoscopic bags. The abdominal wall of the trocar sites must be irrigated at the end of the procedure, to prevent the development of tumour grafts [1].

In a significant number of patients, the macroscopic diagnosis is apparent stage I. In such cases, positive peritoneal washings or samplings, and positive lymph nodes, may be found in as many as one-third of the patients [9,10]. A significant number of patients are thus upstaged after a comprehensive staging operation, including sampling of peritoneal fluid for cytological examination, multiple peritoneal biopsies, omentectomy and lymphadenectomy. All these goals can be fulfilled by an experienced laparoscopic surgeon with a minimum of surgical trauma. The first relevant paper on this topic was published in 1994 [3].

Operative technique

The technique for laparoscopic reassessment is quite similar to the technique for the same operation performed by laparotomy. A thorough examination of the peritoneal surface includes the pelvis, paracolic gutters, mesentery, bowel surface, abdominal wall, diaphragm, liver and omentum. Multiple random or oriented biopsies, peritoneal fluid samplings or washings for cytological examinations are taken in a standard way, using sharp dissection rather than punch biopsies. The technique for excision of a peritoneal area is standard. The peritoneum is grasped and slightly elevated. The elevation creates a fold that is incised, showing the deep surface of the peritoneal lining. A patch of peritoneum is then dissected and removed without any injury to the underlying structures.

Laparoscopy is superior to laparotomy for two reasons.
1 The magnified view of the peritoneum facilitates the search for a small papillary growth or whitish thick implants.
2 The visual and instrumental access to the surface of the diaphragm is much easier than by any midline laparotomy incision.

Care must be taken to examine both sides of the mesentery and to unroll in a row all the small bowel loops, starting from the ileocaecal junction and ending when the duodenojejunal junction is identified. This step, as well as the examination of the upper quadrants of the abdominal cavity, the omentectomy and the para-aortic lymph-node dissection, is made easier if the surgeon stands between the patient's legs.

Technically, para-aortic node sampling in the staging of invasive ovarian cancers must be extended to the level of the left renal vein, including the nodes related to the origin of the ovarian vessels. This is more difficult to complete by laparoscopy (see Chapter 4) than the sampling of the lower para-aortic nodes in the staging of advanced cervical carcinoma [2].

Omentectomy may be easily performed using monopolar and bipolar cautery and lassos. We use mainly monopolar scissors to desiccate and divide the omentum. Bipolar cautery is used to control small bleeders close to the transverse colon. A lasso (Endoloop) is the fastest way to apply preventive haemostasis to the left gastroepiploic pedicle, after the omentum has been detached from the transverse colon. Our present strategy for laparoscopic infracolic omentectomy follows. The omentum is grasped and lifted with two graspers. Its midline is divided from the edge up to the level of the transverse colon using monopolar scissors. The right hemiomentum is detached from the colon, mainly with the help of monopolar scissors, and stored. The left hemiomentum is then detached from the colon, up to the point where it holds only to the splenic flexure. A PDS loop is placed and tied around the remaining pedicle, containing the gastroepiploic vessels. Appendectomy may be included in the staging procedure, especially in mucinous tumours.

Incomplete staging may be associated with inadequate surgery. In young women, after an ovarian cystectomy in the presence of invasive ovarian cancer, unilateral salpingo-oophorectomy is completed. In parous or menopausal patients, completion of total hysterectomy and bilateral salpingo-oophorectomy is feasible using laparoscopic or laparoscopically assisted surgery techniques.

Operative strategy

The patient is informed that laparotomy may be performed if necessary, either for unsatisfactory sampling or for intraoperative complication. She is placed in a supine position, with the legs in 15° abduction. The surgeon stands on the left side of the patient at the beginning of laparoscopy and when working in the pelvic area. When working in the abdominal cavity, the surgeon has to shift and stand between the legs of the patient. For that reason, two screens are necessary, one placed at the feet, another placed at the head of the patient.

The pneumoperitoneum rather than direct trocar insertion is advisable, using the left upper quadrant, immediately below the ribs, to place the Veress needle. A syringe test is carried out to check the umbilical area. If the test shows gas bubbles, blind insertion of the umbilical trocar is acceptable. Otherwise, a Needlescope is placed in the Veress needle in order to examine the peritonal surface of the abdominal wall. When the Needlescope is not available, a 5-mm trocar is placed in the left upper quadrant to accommodate a 5-mm endoscope. The view of the undersurface of the abdominal wall then allows safe placement of the 10-mm trocar to accommodate the standard endoscope. The insertion site of this trocar may be chosen in any place free of adhesions in the umbilical area or, when necessary, in another area of the abdomen.

In general, the placement of ancillary ports is conditioned by the presence of abdominal wall adhesions in addition to operative requirements. In most patients, both the pelvis as well as the undersurface of the diaphragm may be reached using two 5-mm ports placed 10 cm lateral to the umbilicus on the left and right side, respectively. An additional 10-mm port is placed in the midline or slightly laterally halfway between the symphysis pubis and the umbilicus. This last trocar may accommodate clip appliers, endoscopic bags and other specific instruments, as well as standard instruments.

The standard placement of trocars, as described above, may have to be modified according to the anatomy of the patient. The pelvis, along with the para-aortic area and the omentum, can almost always be reached through the two trocars placed lateral to the umbilicus. In some cases, a trocar placed in the left upper quadrant, at the place of insertion of the Veress needle, may be of help in completing the biopsies of the diaphragmatic peritoneum and the omentectomy.

The standard operative strategy that we suggest may be summarized using the example of surgical restaging and management of an apparently early ovarian carcinoma after diagnostic unilateral salpingo-oophorectomy or cystectomy. Begin the operation, in all cases, by a thorough examination of the entire peritoneal cavity and by samplings for cytological examination. Peritoneal fluid or peritoneal washings are sampled for cytological examination before any surgical procedure, to avoid contamination by blood cells. At this step in the procedure, proceeding with the laparoscopic approach is contraindicated if: (i) an obviously diseased remaining ovary is grossly enlarged, or adherent, and cannot be removed unruptured vaginally; or (ii) large extraovarian tumour grafts are visible. A laparoscopic approach is acceptable in: (i) apparent stage Ia cases; and (ii) apparent stage Ib cases with a moderately enlarged (less than 6 cm) and non-adherent contralateral ovary. In such cases, perform the laparoscopic para-aortic dissection first either transperitoneally (see Chapter 4) or, preferably, extraperitoneally (see Chapter 5). If this procedure cannot be completed while meeting the oncological standards, the surgeon must shift to a conventional laparotomy.

When the laparoscopic para-aortic node dissection is complete, the infracolic omentum is divided and stored in a paracolic gutter. Staging biopsies are taken in the upper abdomen. However, biopsies of the subdiaphragmatic peritoneum will be taken only at the end of the procedure, as diaphragmatic biopsies performed at an early stage of a long operation may lead to pneumomediastinum and subcutaneous emphysema.

The laparoscope is then directed toward the pelvis. The surgeon shifts to the left side of the patient, looks at the screen placed at the feet of the patient, and the operation continues in the pelvis. A bilateral pelvic lymphadenectomy and staging biopsies of the pelvic peritoneum are performed. Both infundibulopelvic (or the only remaining one) and round ligaments are cauterized or tied and divided. The anterior and posterior leaves of the broad ligament are incised. If an ovarian remnant, or the contralateral remaining ovary, are diseased, an endoscopic bag is placed around the adnexa and tied to avoid contamina-

tion of the vaginal cuff during vaginal removal of the specimen. The uterus and adnexae are thus ready for vaginal removal. The omentum is placed in the pouch of Douglas. The patient is then placed in the lithotomy position, and the operation is completed vaginally.

A modified version, without hysterectomy, is indicated in restaging operations after a previous hysterectomy and bilateral oophorectomy. In such cases, the omentum is placed in a bag and removed through an abdominal port or through an incision of the vaginal cuff.

When conservative surgery is planned after a previous unilateral oophorectomy or adnexectomy, a careful laparoscopic examination of the remaining ovary is performed. Biopsy of any suspicious area of the ovarian surface is obviously required, but random biopsies are not advised. When necessary, an ipsilateral salpingectomy or adnexectomy are performed.

In tumours of low malignant potential, peritoneal staging is performed in the same way as in invasive tumours. However, the significance of node involvement is unclear. Excellent survival is obtained after surgical therapy without node dissection [11]. For these reasons, laparoscopic lymph-node sampling has been abandoned in our department.

Results

Childers *et al.* mentioned five cases of restaging of ovarian carcinoma patients in their 1993 series of 61 para-aortic lymphadenectomies [12]. There was one major complication in the entire series — an injury to the inferior vena cava was controlled laparoscopically with clips. The mean operating time was 154 minutes and the mean postoperative stay was 1.3 days in cases with no concurrent hysterectomy. These authors concluded that laparoscopic restaging is worthy of further investigation.

The same authors extended their series in 1995, adding cases of patients staged laparoscopically during primary surgery [13]. Fourteen cases of apparent stage I invasive adenocarcinoma were recorded. Metastatic disease was discovered in eight patients: two patients were upstaged to stage IC, three patients to stage II and three patients to stage IIIc. The operating time ranged from 120 to 240 minutes, with an average of 149 minutes in the patients in whom hysterectomy was not performed during the same operative session. Two significant complications occurred, including the injury to the vena cava mentioned above. The second patient developed a large ecchymotic area on the abdominal wall. Hospital stays ranged from 0 to 3 days. The average hospital stay for patients in whom hysterectomy was not performed was 1.2 days.

In 1994, Querleu *et al.* reported 10 patients (nine with ovarian and one with tubal carcinoma) in whom initial surgical staging was judged unsatisfactory [3]. This series was updated in October 1998. Follow-up of the 10 patients has not revealed unexpected sites of recurrence. One patient, in whom laparoscopic biopsies showed persistent disease in the right diaphragmatic area, was prescribed second-line chemotherapy and is still alive with documented persistent disease. All eight stage I patients and one stage III patient are clinically free of disease. However, this series included patients with borderline tumours, and this favourable result may be a result of the general prognosis of the disease.

Additional cases have been included in this personal series (author's unpublished data). Overall, 32 attempts at laparoscopic restaging are included here. The pathological diagnosis was invasive epithelial ovarian cancer in nine patients, invasive adenocarcinoma of the fallopian tube in two patients, dysgerminoma in four patients and borderline epithelial or granulosa cell tumour in the remaining patients.

In two patients, the extent of pelvic adhesions precluded the use of laparoscopy for an additional hysterectomy, and a laparotomy was performed. Laparoscopic reassessment was successfully performed in 30 (94%) patients. The surgeon judged that the standards of oncological radical surgery and/or comprehensive staging were met in all 30 cases. The feasibility of laparoscopic restaging is thus 94%.

Data concerning 14 patients with invasive adnexal disease, including dysgerminoma, who were restaged laparoscopically, have been reviewed in detail. Ten had their first operation by laparotomy, four by laparoscopy. The average interval between primary and restaging surgery was 8.3 weeks (range 2–26 weeks). Staging biopsies and peritoneal cytology were taken in all cases, omentectomy was done in 11 cases, appendectomy in three, trocar site excision in three and additional hysterectomy in six. Right pelvic, left pelvic, right para-aortic, left para-aortic and full para-aortic lymphadenectomies were performed in 12, 11, four, one and nine cases, respectively. An average of 19.9 macroscopic nodes—excluding from the count microscopic nodes—were retrieved at bilateral para-aortic dissection. The total duration of the operations, including comprehensive staging and additional surgery of the genital tract, averaged 230 minutes (standard deviation 67.9). The average operating time for bilateral para-aortic dissection was 106.6 minutes.

Positive pelvic and para-aortic nodes were found in one patient, positive para-aortic nodes in two patients. Two of these patients had been initially staged IIIA, and had six cycles of platinum-based chemotherapy before node dissection. In one of these patients presenting with dysgerminoma, macroscopic (more than 1 cm in diameter) para-aortic nodal metastases were found. This patient had her only site of disease in the para-aortic nodes and was upstaged from IA to IIIC. Microscopic involvement was found in the omentum in two patients, in the appendix in one and at trocar site excision in one. Overall, four patients (28.6%) were upstaged. Two of these patients were proposed chemotherapy after restaging, and positive para-aortic nodes resistant to chemotherapy were removed in the other two.

The postoperative recovery was short in every case, and the average postoperative stay was 3.4 days (range 1–6 days). Bleeding from the para-aortic area was insignificant in all cases, although some small vessels had to be clipped or coagulated. Bleeding from the origin of the ovarian artery had to be managed by bipolar cautery in two cases, and bleeding from a vein of the left infrarenal area had to be managed by compression. The intraoperative blood loss was less than 300 ml in all patients. No major postoperative complication occurred. An ecchymosis of the right flank was noted in one patient. An ultrasound examination revealed no deep haematoma or significant intraperitoneal bleeding, and the patient recovered after posterior colpotomy and drainage. In four cases, peritoneal incision of the laparoscopic para-aortic lymphadenectomy was checked laparoscopically 8–24 months later. No adhesion was found. Instead, a fine linear scar was observed in all four cases.

The accuracy of laparoscopic staging seems to be excellent. A follow-up of more than 2 years did not show any unexpected site of abdominal recurrence. Specifically, all stage IA patients are presently free of disease. One patient with positive staging recurred after 2 years.

Pomel *et al*. [14] came to the same conclusion in a series of eight patients with a shorter follow-up.

Restaging of cervical cancers

Occasionally, pathological examination of a uterus removed for a benign indication reveals the presence of invasive cancer of the cervix. In such cases, the presence of residual gross disease, retrospectively determined tumour stage and lymphangiogram status are prognostic factors [15]. A radical parametrectomy, with lymph-node dissection or radiation therapy, may be proposed for these patients. Our method for laparoscopic paracervical lymphadenectomy (see Chapter 3) may also be applied in such cases. Before the initiation of therapy, examination of the peritoneal cavity, sampling of enlarged pelvic or para-aortic nodes or elective lymph-node dissection [2,16] may be performed laparoscopically.

Restaging of endometrial cancers

The question of restaging incompletely surgically staged

adenocarcinomata of the endometrium is more controversial, because the therapeutic value of lymph-node dissection is not generally recognized [17]. However, many gynaecological oncologists feel that knowing lymph nodes have a negative or positive diagnosis has an effect on adjuvant therapy recommendations. In addition, laparoscopic staging may be used to identify those patients with peritoneal disease, to remove remaining ovaries and to perform pelvic and/or aortic dissection in high-risk cases.

The potential yield of restaging apparent stage I endometrial cancer has been determined. In an Italian series of 1055 cases [18], metastases to the ovaries and/or fallopian tubes were found in 26 patients, to the pelvic peritoneum in eight patients, to the retroperitoneal nodes in 29 patients and in the abdominal cavity in three additional patients. Consequently, approximately 6% of endometrial cancer patients may be upstaged after surgical restaging.

The yield of surgical staging in high-risk cases has been assessed in the M.D. Anderson series [19], in which 295 patients with 'significant' myometrial invasion, or grade 2 or 3 adenocarcinomata or variant histology (papillary serous and/or clear cell), were assessed. Two hundred and twenty-four of these patients had at least an omental biopsy and peritoneal cytology; 22 patients (7.5%) showed gross evidence of peritoneal disease and an additional 28 patients had occult peritoneal involvement. Five peritoneal failures (false-negative cases) were observed between 12 and 37 months postoperatively.

The surgical technique is similar to that used for staging of ovarian cancers, including careful inspection of the entire abdominal cavity, washings and biopsies, lymph-node dissection as required, omentectomy (only for sero-papillary tumours) and, finally, oophorectomy.

Childers *et al.* [13] reported a series of 13 laparoscopic stagings in patients with incompletely staged adenocarcinoma of the endometrium. Extrauterine disease was found in three of these patients. Two patients had lymph-node metastasis and one had positive peritoneal washings. There were no intra- or postoperative complications. Three patients had their adjuvant therapy recommendations changed as a result of staging information.

Staging before exenteration

Medical and psychological preparation for pelvic exenteration is a traumatic experience for the patient. The operating room and the surgical team are scheduled for a long operation. The operation begins with an exploratory laparotomy. When contraindications to a curative removal of the pelvic content are found, the procedure is aborted. Having undergone an exploratory laparotomy without

any chance for cure adds to the disappointment of the patient. The long psychological preparation of the patient to the modification of her body image is then useless. Even though careful preoperative evaluation was carried out in all patients, 111 out of 394 planned exenterations were aborted in the M.D. Anderson series [20]. In these patients, the reasons for aborting the procedure were peritoneal disease in 46, nodal disease in 45 and involvement of the bowel or liver in five. A total of 96 contraindications to exenteration could, potentially, have been detected by a preliminary laparoscopy. However, significant intra-peritoneal adhesions were observed in 28 patients, potentially making laparoscopy longer and more hazardous. None the less, a minimum of 68 and a maximum of 96 abortive procedures would have been avoided in these series with the help of a minimally invasive procedure.

A staging laparoscopy can thus be proposed to all candidates for a pelvic exenteration. A pelvic examination under general anaesthesia gives further clinical information about involvement of the pelvic wall. Precautions specific to patients with a high risk of abdominal adhesions must be taken in all cases. The surgeon may choose between open laparoscopy, use of the Needlescope, or simple testing of the space under the umbilicus by means of the syringe test. In the majority of cases it remains possible to establish the pneumoperitoneum by inserting the Veress needle in the left upper quadrant. If the gas flows easily, the probability of adhesions in this area is quite low. It is then possible to introduce a 3-mm or 5-mm endoscope through the same upper quadrant site. The area under the umbilicus may be inspected, making the insertion of the umbilical trocar contraindicated or safe. If the extent of the adhesive process permits, the 10-mm trocar may also be introduced lateral or superior to the umbilicus. Examination of the liver and bowel, sampling of peritoneal fluid, examination of the entire peritoneal lining and biopsy of suspicious areas, palpation of the parametrial and nodal areas with a probe, and multiple blind peritoneal biopsies are performed.

Exenteration is contraindicated when one of the following criteria is met: (i) frozen examination of suspicious peritoneal areas confirming the presence of disease; (ii) fixation of the tumour to the pelvic wall; (iii) fixed pelvic nodes; and (iv) obviously diseased para-aortic nodes. In such cases, the procedure is aborted with a minimum of operative time, risks and cost. To proceed with para-aortic node dissection or node sampling, three criteria must be met: (i) the peritoneal lining, the bowel and the liver are macroscopically free of disease; (ii) the pelvic tumour is supposed to be resectable; and (iii) no evidence of para-aortic involvement is found. The posterior parietal peritoneum is opened. Suspicious nodes are sampled and sent for frozen section, in the same way as the surgeon would do for the open procedure. If no suspicious node is found, elective para-aortic dissection is performed. The indications for, counselling and information about stoma are deferred until definitive histology of all the peritoneal and lymph-node samplings has been made. This strategy may spare the patient the emotional burden of abortive exenteration, and may lead to better management of the operating room time for the nurses and surgical team.

This concept has been applied in three patients with recurrent stage IIIB cervical cancer by Plante and Roy [21], and in one patient with a previously untreated stage IVA cervical carcinoma in our department. The procedure was successful in all four patients, as a result of suitable patients being selected as candidates for pelvic exenteration. There was no intraoperative complication, but one deep phlebitis occurred postoperatively.

Conclusion

Although firm conclusions about the risks, cost, benefits and limitations of the procedure cannot be given, the feasibility of a comprehensive restaging of gynaecological tumours is well established.

Examination of the entire peritoneum, diaphragmatic and hepatic surfaces, sampling of the peritoneal fluid and biopsies of the peritoneal lining, as well as pelvic lymphadenectomy, are ideally performed by laparoscopy. Para-aortic lymphadenectomy up to the level of the renal vein, omentectomy or removal of significant peritoneal implants are also possible, although these require much more skill and training. It is possible to use all these techniques in the same patient to provide satisfactory staging, along with surgical therapy as required, in referral patients presenting with a postoperative diagnosis of apparent stage I endometrial or ovarian carcinoma, or with inadequately staged cervical cancer incidentally found on hysterectomy specimens. Such patients may be spared a laparotomy by midline incision with its inherent cost, pain and scar.

Potential surgical complications must not be overlooked. The laparoscopic approach is more hazardous in previously operated patients. Laceration of the vena cava, haemorrhage, laceration of the inferior mesenteric artery and ure-teral injury may occur during para-aortic dissection by laparoscopy as well as by laparotomy. Bowel injury is possible at laparoscopic adhesiolysis or omentectomy. However, the complication rate was low in the first large series published in this field [12]. Nevertheless, patients must be made aware that an unintended laparotomy may have to be performed. By contrast, the risk of wound dehiscence or infection is obviously avoided, and it is generally accepted that the risk of *de novo* abdominal adhesion is much lower after laparoscopy than it is after laparotomy. Finally, the occurrence of lymphocysts and adhesions is quite rare after laparoscopic lymphadenectomy without peritoneal closure (see Chapter 6).

Patient selection is required. Morbidly obese patients, in whom para-aortic dissection is problematical even by laparotomy, patients with extensive intra-abdominal adhesions or those with severe respiratory or cardiovascular disease should be excluded. However, moderately obese patients can be ideally managed laparoscopically, as infrarenal para-aortic dissection is not necessary. The learning curve is another problem. These techniques require a high level of skill and very delicate dissection. Therefore beginners are strongly advised against undertaking such operations. Training in gynaecological oncology and operative laparoscopy, and experience in standard abdominal para-aortic lymphadenectomy, in laparoscopic pelvic lymphadenectomy and in operative procedures in the upper part of the abdomen are required.

References

1 Childers JM, Hatch K, Surwit EA (1993). Laparoscopic para-aortic lymphadenectomy in gynecologic malignancies. *Obstet Gynecol* **82**:741–747.
2 Querleu D (1993). Laparoscopic paraaortic lymphadenectomy. A preliminary experience. *Gynecol Oncol* **49**:24–29.
3 Querleu D, Leblanc E (1994). Laparoscopic infrarenal paraaortic node dissection for restaging of carcinoma of the ovary or fallopian tube. *Cancer* **73**:1467–1471.
4 McGowan L, Lesher LP, Norris HJ, Barnett M (1985). Misstaging of ovarian cancer. *Obstet Gynecol* **65**:568–572.
5 Trimbos JB, Schueler JA, Vanlent M, Hermans J, Fleurens GJ (1990). Reasons for incomplete surgical staging in early ovarian carcinoma. *Gynecol Oncol* **37**:374–377.
6 Chen SS, Bochner R (1985). Assessment of morbidity and mortality in primary cytoreductive surgery for advanced ovarian carcinoma. *Gynecol Oncol* **20**:190–195.
7 Hacker NF, Berek JS, Lagasse LD, Nieberg RK, Elashoff RM (1983). Primary cytoreductive surgery for epithelial ovarian cancer. *Obstet Gynecol* **61**:413–420.
8 Piver MS, Baker T (1986). The potential for optimal (<2 cm) cytoreductive surgery in advanced ovarian carcinoma at a tertiary medical center: a prospective study. *Gynecol Oncol* **24**:1–8.
9 Burghardt E, Girardi F, Lahousen M, Tamussino K, Stettner H (1991). Patterns of pelvic and paraaortic lymph node involvement in ovarian cancer. *Gynecol Oncol* **40**:103–106.
10 Young RC, Decker DG, Wharton JT, Piver S, Sindelar WF, Edward BK (1983). Staging laparotomy in early ovarian cancer. *JAMA* **250**:3072–3076.
11 Trope C, Kaern J, Vergote IB, Kristensen G, Abeler V (1993). Are borderline tumors of the ovary overtreated both surgically and systemically? A review of four prospective randomized trials including 253 patients with borderline tumors. *Gynecol Oncol* **51**:236–243.
12 Childers JM, Lang J, Surwit EA, Hatch KD (1995). Laparoscopic surgical staging of ovarian cancer. *Gynecol Oncol* **59**:25–33.
13 Childers JM, Spirtos NM, Brainard P, Surwit EA (1994).

Laparoscopic staging of the patient with incompletely staged early adenocarcinoma of the endometrium. *Obstet Gynecol* **83**:597–600.

14 Pomel C, Provencher D, Dauplat J *et al* (1995). Laparoscopic surgical staging of ovarian cancer. *Gynecol Oncol* **58**:301–306.

15 Roman LD, Morris M, Follen-Mitchell M, Eifel PJ, Burke TW, Atkinson EN (1993). Prognostic factors for patients undergoing simple hysterectomy in the presence of invasive cancer of the cervix. *Gynecol Oncol* **50**:179–184.

16 Querleu D, Leblanc E, Castelain B (1991). Laparoscopic pelvic lymphadenectomy. *Am J Obstet Gynecol* **64**:579–581.

17 Kilgore LC, Partridge EE, Alvarez RD *et al* (1995). Adenocarcinoma of the endometrium: survival comparisons of patients with and without pelvic node sampling. *Gynecol Oncol* **56**:29–33.

18 Mangioni C, De Palo G, Marubini E, Del Vecchio M (1993). Surgical pathologic staging in apparent stage I endometrial carcinoma. *Int J Gynecol Cancer* **3**:373–384.

19 Marino BD, Burke TW, Tornos C *et al* (1995). Staging laparotomy for endometrial carcinoma: assessment of peritoneal spread. *Gynecol Oncol* **56**:34–38.

20 Miller B, Morris M, Rutledge F *et al* (1993). Aborted exenteration procedures in recurrent cervical cancer. *Gynecol Oncol* **50**:94–99.

21 Plante M, Roy M (1995). The use of operative laparoscopy in determining eligibility for pelvic exenteration in patients with recurrent cervical cancer. *Gynecol Oncol* **59**:401–404.

23   Present and future role of laparoscopic surgery in gynaecological oncology

Nicholas Kadar

Introduction

Debate surrounding the laparoscopic management of gynaecological malignancies has raised both technical and oncological issues, and, as with most laparoscopic cancer operations, technical considerations have been at the forefront. There are a number of reasons for this.

First, the oncological aspects of cancer treatment remain the same, regardless of the route by which the operation is carried out. For example, questions about the indications for lymphadenectomy, the type of lymphadenectomy to perform and the place, if any, of adjuvant pelvic radiation, which have dogged the management of stage I endometrial and cervical cancer, are not altered in any way just because the lymphadenectomy is carried out laparoscopically.

Second, *prima facie* the limitations of laparoscopic surgery are likely to be technical, related to such factors as obesity, exposure, the inability to palpate tissues, rupture of cysts or lymph-node capsules and extraction of the resected tissue from the peritoneal cavity.

Third, the quality of a cancer operation has always been judged by well-accepted surgicoanatomical and pathological criteria, such as node counts, frequency of positive nodes, quality of surgical planes, tumour margins, tumour handling, tumour spill, etc. Not surprisingly, therefore, the same criteria have been used to assess laparoscopic cancer operations, and it has been tacitly assumed that if by these criteria a laparoscopic operation met the same standards as its open counterpart, then its effectiveness as cancer treatment should also be the same.

In other words, questions about laparoscopic cancer operations have been couched in technical terms not because their effectiveness in treating cancer was ignored but simply because it was assumed that any reduction in that efficacy would be most likely to have a technical basis. This assumption has recently been questioned by numerous reports of abdominal wall recurrences at trocar sites (port-site recurrences) following laparoscopic resection of colon and other cancers, as well as diagnostic laparoscopy in ovarian cancer [1]. However, before dis-cussing this important question, some of the technical aspects of the operations used to treat gynaecological malignancies laparoscopically will be discussed.

What are we trying to achieve with a laparoscopic approach?

Most abdominal operations are performed laparoscopically to reduce the pain and discomfort associated with a laparotomy incision, the duration of hospitalization and the time to full recovery. In other words, the laparoscopic approach is not used to obtain a better primary surgical result, although it is possible that by reducing adhesion formation the laparoscopic approach to gynaecological malignancies may reduce the complications associated with adjunctive therapy, such as whole pelvic radiation following radical hysterectomy. Usually, however, the justification for a laparoscopic approach is not to be found in traditional criteria of improved outcome, namely, better survival, or even in a reduction in serious complications, such as pulmonary embolus, pneumonia, fistulae, etc. There are important corollaries.

Indications for surgery

Because the surgical goals do not change with the method of visualisation used, the indications for each laparoscopic operation should be the same as for its open counterpart. However, many aspects of the surgical management of gynaecological malignancies are controversial, and laparoscopic operation cannot be expected to be free from the unresolved controversies that surround the open procedure. Such controversies are, therefore, not a legitimate argument against the use of the laparoscopic approach, and disagreement over the indications for aortic lymphadenectomy and the type of lymphadenectomy to perform, for example, is no argument against performing aortic lymphadenectomy laparoscopically.

The treatment of malignant disease is, however, usually accompanied by significant morbidity, and in some circumstances this may sway the surgeon to withhold treatment, especially if the therapeutic gain to be expected is small. However, if the side effects can be reduced by laparoscopic management, this may tilt the risk–benefit ratio sufficiently for an operation to be undertaken where otherwise it might have been withheld. What has changed here is not really the indication for surgery, but the conclusion about where the risk–benefit ratio from treatment lies. Surgical staging of cervical cancer provides a good example because surgical morbidity is reduced very significantly if aortic lymphadenectomy is carried out laparoscopically rather than via an extraperitoneal approach, and this may sway even the opponents of surgical staging to undertake the procedure in advanced stage disease [2,3].

Evaluation of treatment efficacy

Traditional measures of outcome, namely survival and serious complications, cannot be used to assess the usefulness of the laparoscopic approach because these are not the variables it is designed to affect, and even if it did affect them, the magnitude of the treatment effect would, in all likelihood, be too small to be detectable statistically. For example, if laparoscopic management reduced survival from endometrial cancer by 5%, it would require a randomized trial with about 700 patients in each treatment arm to detect this as statistically significant. The same is true of serious complications, which are fortunately too uncommon for any salutary or undesirable effects of laparoscopic surgery to be statistically discernible.

However, the variables that laparoscopic management is meant to alter—postoperative pain, hospital stay, return to normal function—are largely subjective. To eliminate bias when different surgical approaches are compared with respect to these variables would require that both the surgeon and the patient are 'blinded' to the treatment received, which is obviously impossible if the treatments being compared are laparoscopy and laparotomy. Predictably, therefore, if we accept current dogma that a randomized clinical trial is the only reliable way to establish the effectiveness of clinical therapy, then it will be difficult to 'prove' that the laparoscopic approach is either an effective or a safe way to treat gynaecological malignancies. Therefore, other methods besides clinical trials must be used to evaluate both the efficacy and the safety of laparoscopic surgery [4].

Candidates for laparoscopic surgery

Because the purpose of laparoscopic surgery is to reduce morbidity, little will be gained by a laparoscopic approach if the morbidity from conventional surgery is already very low. The corollary is that if laparoscopic surgery is to realise its full potential, it must be applicable to patients who are difficult surgical candidates, such as those who are obese and who have extensive adhesions from prior surgery or advanced pathology, and it should not be confined to selected individuals who have very low morbidity from an open approach. Moreover, the introduction of laparoscopic techniques makes tremendous demands on a medical community and, except where individual surgeons are willing to make the sacrifices required, it may be unrealistic to expect widespread use of demanding techniques if they are applicable to only, say, 5–10% of women with these malignancies. Unfortunately, much of the literature on laparoscopic radical surgical techniques still applies only to highly selected cases—young, thin women with minimal pathology [5,6]. If we are to treat endometrial carcinoma laparoscopically, we need to know whether the requisite operations can be carried out safely and effectively in obese and elderly women. If we are to treat cervical cancer effectively, we need to know if fixed and enlarged nodes can be resected, not only normal nodes, because resection of clinically enlarged nodes may have a survival advantage [7].

Present situation

Can the oncological goals of surgical therapy be achieved laparoscopically?

Evidence that the surgical management of endometrial and cervical cancer can be carried out laparoscopically with a significant reduction in morbidity is, in the author's opinion, now compelling, even though comparative trials to prove this have not been carried out. However, only four operations are required for the primary surgical management of these malignancies: simple hysterectomy, radical hysterectomy, pelvic and aortic lymphadenectomy. It is quite indisputable that simple hysterectomy can be carried out laparoscopically, and the objection that many cases amenable to a laparoscopic approach could have been managed by vaginal hysterectomy, even if it were valid, is not relevant to the treatment of malignant disease. Vaginal hysterectomy, although sometimes possible and, as in obese women with serious medical problems, even desirable, is not an adequate cancer operation, making the laparoscopic approach preferable even if a vaginal one were feasible.

Laparoscopic hysterectomy can be successfully carried out in women who, historically, have not been candidates for vaginal hysterectomy, such as very obese nulliparous women, and those with very large fibroid uteri [8,9]. The reduction in morbidity is perhaps best reflected in the fact that in a small series of elderly women (age >65 years) laparoscopic surgery for endometrial or cervical cancer was associated with a shorter hospital stay than in age-matched controls undergoing abdominal hysterectomy. This is despite the fact that the operations performed laparoscopically were more extensive and complex than those in the control group, and involved pelvic or aortic lymphadenectomy or radical rather than a simple hysterectomy in most cases [10].

Radical vaginal hysterectomy has a history at least as long as its abdominal counterpart, and it fell into disuse only because the pelvic lymph nodes could not be removed vaginally, not because it was an inadequate operation for the central disease [11]. This is another indication for laparoscopically assisted radical vaginal hysterectomy. In centres where the operation continues to be used, it has yielded results comparable to the Wertheim hysterectomy [12]. Outstanding questions remain about which steps of the operation should be performed vaginally and which ones laparoscopically, as discussed in previous chapters and elsewhere [13], and the operation will also need to be re-learned by most gynaecological oncologists. However, once the procedure has been mastered there are no plausible reasons to believe that the operation will become less effective than it has been in the past by the addition of a laparoscopic lymphadenectomy or by facilitating the vaginal operation by, for example, laparoscopic development of the retroperitoneal spaces or laparoscopic division of the adnexal pedicles. Although some surgeons have recently claimed that an entirely laparoscopic approach (i.e. a laparoscopic Wertheim) may be associated with fewer complications [6], it has yet to be demonstrated that a laparoscopic radical hysterectomy can be carried out in other than highly selected, thin, young women with small or invisible (stage IA2) lesions.

Be that as it may, the question of whether the oncological goals of surgical therapy can be achieved laparoscopically really hinges on how effectively a lymphadenectomy can be carried out laparoscopically. The evidence that an adequate aortic lymphadenectomy can be carried out laparoscopically with less morbidity is irrefutable, as discussed in detail in Chapters 4 and 5. Although obviously refinement of the technique increases with experience, even in our first cases we were able to recover the same average number of lymph nodes (12.8) laparoscopically as other teams have using a retroperitoneal approach; the proportion of positive lymph nodes were, if anything, higher, and the morbidity and hospital stay much lower [3].

Some series have reported significant complications even in a selected, surgically low risk group of patients [5], but this has not been the general experience [1,2]. Some centres also had difficulty at first in performing a left-sided dissection, carrying the dissection above the inferior mesenteric artery or performing the operation in women weighing over 180 pounds (82 kg) [2], but most of these problems have been resolved. Currently, we have performed aortic lymphadenectomy in five women weighing over 180 pounds (82 kg), in two weighing over 250 pounds (114 kg), in three aged over 70 years; other teams have had a similar experience (G. Boike & Graham, personal communications). More importantly, however, obesity (although undefined) and age over 70 years have been contraindications to open aortic lymphadenectomy [14,15], and there is no evidence that aortic lymphadenectomy can be carried out with acceptable morbidity in a greater proportion of obese women (however defined) via laparotomy than laparoscopically. Photographic records clearly show that by every accepted surgical-anatomical criterion as extensive an anterolateral aortocaval dissection can be carried out laparoscopically as with an open technique.

The same is true for a pelvic lymphadenectomy, although information about morbidity is not as clear cut because pelvic lymphadenectomy is almost always combined with a simple or a radical hysterectomy. None the less, it is found that, again, the same average number of lymph nodes can be recovered as at a laparotomy [16–18], the same frequency of positive nodes obtained, even in elderly and obese women [8,19], and an essentially identical operation carried out with complete mobilization and skeletonization of the iliac vessels [17]. Currently we have performed pelvic lymphadenectomy in three women weighing over 300 pounds (136 kg), and in five women aged over 80 years.

Some surgeons have questioned the adequacy of laparoscopic pelvic lymphadenectomy because, in the first comprehensive report on this procedure, Querleu *et al.* [20] reported having recovered an average of only 8.7 nodes. However, like other French investigators who believe these are sentinel nodes, Querleu *et al.* [20] performed an interiliac rather than a complete pelvic lymphadenectomy for the treatment of endometrial and cervical cancer, and it is this fact, rather than the route used for the lymphadenectomy, which explains the lower lymph-node harvest. In their current experience (see Chapter 3), Querleu *et al.* remove an average of 20 nodes from the interiliac area.

Complications

The complications associated with specific operations have already been discussed in previous chapters and only a few general points will be discussed here. Laparoscopic operations are held to quite different standards to those expected of conventional operations. The surgical protocols of the Gynecologic Oncology Group (GOG), for example, have never required node counts or operating times to be recorded for conventional operations, yet they now require these for all its laparoscopic surgical protocols. Costs or operating times have never been the basis for choosing between two operations. No one, for example, has compared operating times or costs of a sacrocolpopexy and sacrospinous ligament fixation, or a needle suspension of the bladder neck and colposuspension. Yet, equality between laparoscopic and conventional operations is now being demanded for these variables.

The use of such double standards can be explained, at least in part, by the fact that, unlike the case for truly new operations, for which no alternatives exist, it is never necessary to manage a patient with a gynaecological malignancy laparoscopically. This might justify a somewhat lower tolerance for surgical complications, especially as there are no offsetting gains in survival to be expected. Nevertheless, these double standards have been applied very rigidly by some critics. For example, the appalling complications initially reported from the M.D. Anderson Cancer Center for surgical staging and extended-field radiation in advanced cervical cancer (16% overall treatment-related mortality and 27% serious bowel toxicity [21]), for which there were no offsetting benefits, did not have such a high level of criticism as the far more modest urinary tract injuries associated with the first cases of laparovaginal radical hysterectomies. The complications associated with conventional therapy have been either completely ignored or significantly downplayed in the comparisons between laparoscopic surgery and its open counterpart. In a report from Duke University, the mortality associated with the surgical staging of endometrial carcinoma was 2%, and the serious complication rate (thromboembolism, bowel obstruction) was over 10% [22]. Boike has shown that, compared with traditional surgical management, the laparoscopic treatment of endometrial carcinoma is associated with a 50% reduction in morbidity and a much shorter stay in hospital [23].

Obviously all operations and therapies in the developmental stages will be associated with an increased complication rate, but this will decline as experience with the procedure or operation increases. Therefore it is pertinent to note that complications after laparoscopic surgery have occurred most commonly when the operation in question could not be carried out in the same way as its open counterpart (e.g. laparoscopic hysterectomy), the corresponding operation was no longer being performed (e.g. Schauta–Amreich radical vaginal hysterectomy) or the endoscopic procedure had no real open counterpart

(laparovaginal radical hysterectomy). The complication rates associated with operations that can be approached exactly as their open counterparts (e.g. pelvic and aortic lymphadenectomy) were much less than those for the conventional operations. Thus, there is every reason to expect that the urinary tract injuries associated with simple hysterectomy will decline once it is recognized that the operation cannot be approached in the same sequence as an abdominal hysterectomy, that the ureters must be identified and that dissection of the bladder off the cervix is illogical unless the entire operation is carried out laparoscopically [24]. Also those injuries associated with laparoscopically assisted vaginal radical hysterectomy will be reduced by further experience with, and development of, the technique.

Outstanding questions

Can ovarian cancer be managed laparoscopically?

The most important unresolved question about the laparoscopic treatment of gynaecological malignancies is its role in the management of ovarian cancer. Laparoscopic management in this disease has largely been restricted to second-look procedures [25,26], partly because of the implicit proscription placed on it even by proponents of laparoscopic surgery. Parker, for example, commenting on the laparoscopic management of adnexal masses, wrote, 'laparoscopy should not be performed in any patient with clinical or ultrasonographic characteristics suspected of being malignant, or in any postmenopausal woman with an elevated CA-125 level', and 4 years later he was still of the opinion that, 'given the currently available data operative laparoscopy is not appropriate if the evaluation of the patient (with a pelvic mass) is suspicious for malignancy' [27,28]. His position is particularly difficult to understand because, by citing the study reported by Dembo *et al.* [29], which showed no significant impairment of survival by cyst rupture in women with stage I ovarian cancer, Parker would presumably not base his proscription on the possibly adverse effects of cyst rupture in the presence of a malignancy.

Although the basis for this belief has never been articulated by either proponents or opponents of laparoscopic surgery, the only potentially legitimate basis for the proscription is that either ovarian cancers cannot be adequately debulked laparoscopically or localized malignancies would be ruptured and the cancer disseminated. These are, of course, mutually exclusive concerns that need to be considered separately, for they arise in entirely different clinical situations.

TUMOURS/TUMOURS CANNOT BE 'DEBULKED' LAPAROSCOPICALLY

There is no question that resection of huge, fixed pelvic masses requires extensive retroperitoneal dissection and often proctocolectomy and retrograde hysterectomy. These cannot be removed laparoscopically. However, many of these women cannot be debulked at laparotomy either, and there is considerable evidence that neoadjuvant chemotherapy is preferable to immediate surgery, even a conventional laparotomy. Jacob *et al.* [30], in a retrospectively matched study, found that a significantly higher proportion of women deemed to have unresectable disease at primary surgery could be optimally debulked if they were first given two to four cycles of chemotherapy rather than re-explored immediately. The survival of patients treated with 'neoadjuvant' chemotherapy and interval debulking was similar to that of women suboptimally debulked at primary surgery. Schwartz *et al.* [31] obtained similar survival rates in 11 women treated with neoadjuvant chemotherapy or chemotherapy alone as with suboptimal cytoreductive surgery followed by chemotherapy. Although experience is still limited, neoadjuvant therapy followed by definitive laparoscopic surgery has been successfully employed, even in patients who had unresectable tumours at laparotomy [32]. Even if the disease cannot be treated laparoscopically after the neoadjuvant chemotherapy has taken its effect, the laparoscope will still have spared the patient one laparotomy, and in these patients this respite should not be dismissed lightly.

Survival after neoadjuvant chemotherapy and interval surgery has not, however, been compared with survival after primary optimal cytoreductive surgery. The available evidence justifies offering neoadjuvant chemotherapy as a primary treatment option to select women with advanced ovarian cancer, who cannot be optimally debulked at laparotomy. However, if *laparoscopically* unresectable pelvic disease is associated with minimal or clearly resectable upper abdominal disease, laparotomy is preferable to neoadjuvant chemotherapy at this time because the pelvis can almost always be debulked at laparotomy (Fig. 23.1). If, however, neoadjuvant chemotherapy is found to yield survival rates comparable to what has historically been obtained with optimal primary cytoreductive surgery, this recommendation would obviously need to be revised.

At the other extreme are cases of advanced ovarian cancer with normal size ovaries and, frequently, no bulk disease in the abdomen or pelvis [33]. Debulking plays no part in the management of these tumours, and, although these women do usually undergo laparotomy, hysterectomy, oophorectomy and omentectomy, it is legitimate to question what is actually being achieved by this. It could be argued that surgery achieves nothing besides a diagnosis, and that these women are ideal candidates for laparoscopic management.

CYST RUPTURE DURING LAPAROSCOPY

A great deal of controversy has surrounded the laparoscopic management of adnexal masses (Fig. 23.2). The main concern is that laparoscopic management, by causing rupture of a malignant cyst and dissemination of the malignancy within the peritoneal cavity, may adversely affect the survival of women who have localised ovarian cancer. Some authors, unthinkingly, cite the rapid development of abdominal wall implants, after *diagnostic* laparoscopy for pelvic masses that subsequently prove to be malignant, as the cause of this problem [34–36]. However, in every case in which this has occurred, the ovarian cyst was ruptured during surgery or disseminated disease was already present, proper histological examination of the cyst was not carried out at the time of laparoscopy and definitive treatment was delayed, usually by several weeks. Other than documented gross mismanagement and accelerated tumour growth at trocar sites (see below), these studies provide no further evidence on the safety or efficacy of laparoscopic management of frank or suspected ovarian malignancies. Indeed, the studies have no evidence to show that laparoscopic management entraps gynaecologists into mismanaging adnexal masses that prove to be malignant, because none of the surveys examined the fate of patients with malignant ovarian cysts who were managed by general gynaecologists with a laparotomy.

The preponderance of evidence suggests that rupture of a malignant cyst does not affect survival adversely, provided patients are treated with chemotherapy after surgery [29,37,38] and, currently, all women except those who have stage IA grade 1, lesions receive adjuvant therapy after surgery [39]. Therefore, cyst rupture potentially alters only the management of women with stage IA grade 1 carcinoma of the ovary, which comprise at most 20% of cases of stage I ovarian cancer, or 2–4% of all women with ovarian cancer [40]. In approximately 30% of stage I cases, the ovarian cyst is ruptured during laparotomy [40]. Therefore, even if every adnexal mass subjected to laparoscopy was malignant and every ovarian cyst removed laparoscopically ruptured, laparoscopic management would still entail administering chemotherapy to, at the most, three women for every 100 spared a laparotomy ($0.7 \times 0.04 = 0.028$ or 2.8%) [32].

However, only about one per 1000 ovarian cysts in pre-

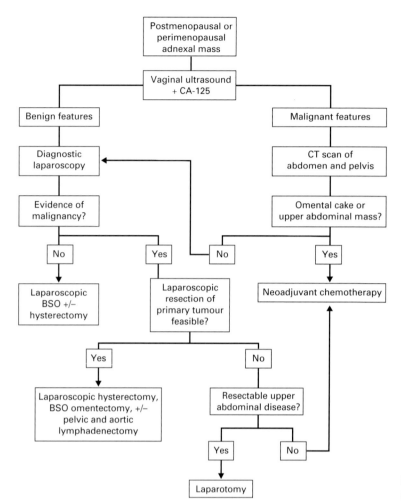

Fig. 23.1 Management of the postmenopausal adnexal mass.

menopausal women are caused by stage I ovarian cancer [41] and, if cases of obvious cancer are excluded (in which cyst rupture is not a concern), only about 30% of adnexal masses in women over the age of 50 prove to be malignant even on an oncology service [42]. Therefore, without belabouring the point further, it is easy to see that the risk associated with the laparoscopic management of adnexal masses is that a woman with stage I ovarian cancer who would not have required further treatment will need chemotherapy after surgery, but for every such case *at least* 110 laparotomies would have been avoided, which is, arguably, a bargain.

Limitations and possible solutions

Laparoscopic surgery is, by its very nature, limited in several ways: (i) it usually takes longer to perform than conventional surgery; (ii) pathology, such as large ovarian masses and extensive adhesions, can limit access; (iii) specimen removal from the abdominal cavity can be problematical; and (iv) obesity may make it impossible to carry

out some operations. The extent to which these factors limit laparoscopic management is, as yet, incompletely defined, and strategies to circumvent them are in their infancy.

PROLONGED OPERATING TIME

Usually, the prolongation in operating time that results from adopting a laparoscopic approach is inconsequential. As the pathology being treated increases, and more than one operation is required to treat the disease present, the effect on operating time quickly compounds. Therefore, a point is reached when the lengths to which one should go to avoid a laparotomy can be legitimately questioned. There are no clear answers to this question. Experience suggests that the primary surgical treatment of gynaecological malignancies can be carried out laparoscopically in most cases, without inordinate prolongations in operating time. Also, experience with the laparoscopic management of recurrent stage IV endometriosis, associated with cul-de-sac obliteration

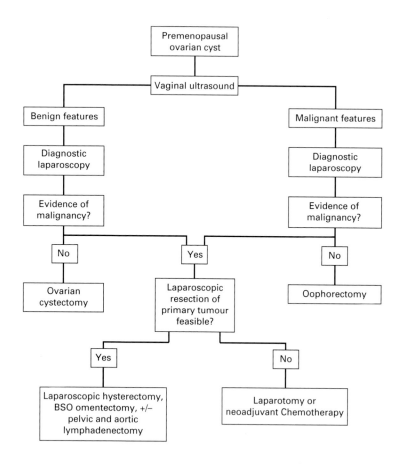

Fig. 23.2 Management of the premenopausal adnexal mass.

requiring rectal resection, suggests that very extended operations are remarkably well tolerated, albeit by relatively young women. There are situations in which a laparoscopic approach, although technically possible, may be unwise; for example, when many adverse features are present, such as obesity and multiple, dense adhesions, and/or when a complex operation has to be performed, such as resection of a pelvic mass, omentectomy and lymphadenectomy. However, in practice, contraindications to a laparoscopic approach are surprisingly few, and complex pathology can usually be successfully handled in this way.

LARGE PELVIC MASSES

Although we have successfully removed fibroid uteri weighing as much as 2.4 kg [43], very large pelvic masses that fill the pelvis and abdomen may simply not be amenable to laparoscopic management. The solutions to the laparospic treatment of what are presently irremovable masses are likely to be diverse. For example, large ovarian cancers may be first debulked with chemotherapy, as we have already discussed, and large cysts of uncertain character may be first drained by direct trocar puncture [44]. None the less, there will be the occasional patient whose abdominopelvic mass is so huge that it cannot be removed laparoscopically, although these cases are, again, relatively rare.

SPECIMEN REMOVAL

Specimen removal continues to be problematical. Current techniques for removing large masses have involved the use of either impermeable bags to facilitate removal of ovarian cysts without rupture or morcellators to fragment large fibroids. However, these techniques are not well suited to the removal of large ovarian cancers. A promising new approach, devised by McCartney, involves the use of transparent vaginal tubes [45]. These are inserted into the peritoneal cavity through the vagina and, because they have a pressure-reducing valve at their distal end, serve as a continuous conduit for tumour removal without loss of the pneumoperitoneum. The process of tissue extraction could be further facilitated by the development of a device that could homogenize tissue as it was fed down the tube (rather like a food processor).

OBESITY

Obesity hinders laparoscopic surgery in several ways. It is

more difficult to insert the auxiliary trocars and maintain them in place during extended procedures. The peritoneum can easily dissect away from the anterior abdominal wall, either during trocar insertion or during the dissection, if the trocar retracts past the peritoneum and gas escapes retroperitoneally. Exposure and access to the pelvis can then be significantly compromised. Higher insufflation pressures may also be required to obtain an adequate pneumoperitoneum, which can interfere with ventilation, and airways pressure can also increase significantly as the patient is placed in the Trendelenburg position. None the less, obesity has not significantly compromised our ability to perform simple hysterectomy or pelvic lymphadenectomy [8,19]. Although aortic lymphadenectomy is more problematical, the need to perform aortic lymphadenectomy in obese patients can be avoided in most patients by confining aortic lymphadenectomy to those who have pelvic lymph-node metastases [46].

Port-site recurrences

Many of the controversies about laparoscopic cancer operations have nothing to do with the route by which the operation is carried out. Port-site recurrences, on the other hand, are exclusively a laparoscopic problem. The many published cases of port-site recurrences after laparoscopic treatment of malignant disease, and recent animal studies showing that a pneumoperitoneum may facilitate intra-abdominal dissemination of tumour cell lines in experimental animals, have raised a disturbing concern. These laparoscopic operations may compromise the survival of patients with malignant disease, because the surgical environment created promotes tumour growth and dissemination; the traditional approach would allow satisfactory removal of malignant tumours [1].

Most port-site recurrences have occurred following laparoscopic colectomy for colon cancer or laparoscopic cholecystectomy for gallbladders that contained occult malignancies. The laparoscopic technique for both these operations entails dragging cancerous tissue through a small incision which, in the majority of cases, receives no further therapy (neither radiation nor chemotherapy) postoperatively. It is well known that tumour cells are frequently exfoliated from the surface of the colon, and that these cells can implant into healing wounds. There is also considerable evidence that healing wounds enhance the growth of tumour cells more than unwounded tissues, and that small wounds do so more than large wounds [1], although the reasons for this have not been elucidated.

Port-site recurrences associated with gynaecological malignancies have occurred almost exclusively following diagnostic laparoscopy for pelvic masses that subsequently proved to be malignant, and were always associated with disseminated intraperitoneal disease [34–36]. As noted above, in every case the ovarian cyst was ruptured during surgery or disseminated disease was already present, proper histological examination of the cyst was not carried out at the time of laparoscopy and definitive treatment was delayed, usually by several weeks.

By contrast, port-site recurrences following appropriate laparoscopic surgical therapy of gynaecological malignancies are uncommon. The one case reported by Childers *et al.* [47] represented a 1% incidence among women with metastatic (intraperitoneal or retroperitoneal) disease. Most of their patients, however, had ovarian cancer and received therapy after surgery. The patient with the port-site recurrence had a microscopically positive second-look laparoscopy and recurred before any further treatment was given. The author has treated four patients with endometrial or cervical cancer who had recurrences at seven trocar sites [48]. All had metastatic disease at the time of laparoscopy and all received postoperative radiation therapy, but the recurrences occurred at trocar sites that were outside the radiation fields in association with disseminated disease. There were no recurrences in women with metastatic ovarian cancer, all of whom received chemotherapy after surgery.

The following conclusions can be drawn from these observations [1,48]. The laparoscopic management of malignant disease in humans predisposes patients to port-site recurrences by creating small abdominal incisions which are conducive to tumour growth. Port-site recurrences result if the malignancy treated has a propensity to exfoliate cells into the peritoneal cavity and the trocar site remains untreated or the malignancy is refractory to adjuvant therapy. Whether a pneumoperitoneum enhances significantly the inoculation of exfoliated tumour cells into the trocar incisions is unknown and speculative. However, because gynaecological malignancies are sensitive to adjuvant therapy and women at increased risk of port-site recurrences can be reliably identified, these recurrences can be prevented by appropriate postoperative therapy. Nevertheless, it is important to be aware that the upper abdominal ports used for aortic lymphadenectomy are not within the standard radiation portals used for either pelvic or extended-field radiation, and that the lateral ports in the lower abdomen may also be outside the pelvic portals, and may need to be treated with radiation therapy.

The laparoscopic management of gynaecological malignancies can also potentially predispose patients to port-site recurrences by: (i) enhancing tumour cell exfoliation into the peritoneal cavity; (ii) causing rupture of ovarian cysts in patients with stage IA and IB ovarian cancer; (iii) rupture of the capsule of lymph nodes containing metastatic disease; and, possibly, (iv) manipulation of the uterus in patients with endometrial and cervical cancer. However, in most cases these problems can be potentially prevented, by modifying specimen extraction techniques (use of specimen bags and vaginal tubes) and, in those at risk, by appropriate postoperative therapy. Evidence that laparoscopic management of any malignancy impairs survival by promoting tumour dissemination within the peritoneal cavity or systemically is lacking.

Conclusion

Although the laparoscopic management of gynaecological malignancies is still in its infancy, progress has been so swift that the trend to use this technique is irreversible. Because this type of surgery has only been performed for a relatively short time, mature data and long-term follow-up series are not available. Over time, new concepts will emerge and some current strategies will be modified, but it is unlikely that this new approach will have to be abandoned. Rather, as the concerns raised by port-site recurrences illustrate, it is more likely that innovations in instrumentation and technology, coupled with new concepts in cancer treatment, will extend the scope of laparoscopic surgery. Therefore, the treatment of gynaecological malignancies will be much less of an ordeal for patients than it has been in the past.

References

1 Kadar N. The laparoscopic management of gynecological malignancies—time to quit? *Gynaecol Endosc.* (In press.)
2 Childers JM, Hatch KD, Tran A-N, Surwit EA (1993). Laparoscopic para-aortic lymphadenectomy in gynecologic malignancies. *Obstet Gynecol* **82**:741–747.
3 Kadar N, Pelosi MA (1994). Can cervix cancer be adequately staged by laparoscopic aortic lymphadenectomy? *Gynaecol Endosc* **3**:213–216.
4 Kadar N (1994). Radomized trials for laparoscopic surgery: valid research strategy or academic gimmick? [Editorial] *Gynaecol Endosc* **3**:69–74.
5 Spirtos NM, Schlaerth JB, Spirtos TW, Schlaerth AC, Indman PD, Kimball RE (1995). Laparoscopic bilateral pelvic and paraaortic lymph node sampling: an evolving technique. *Am J Obstet Gynecol* **173**:105–111.
6 Spirtos NM, Schlaerth JB, Spirtos TW, Schlaerth AC, Indman PD, Kimball RE (1996). Laparoscopic bilateral pelvic and paraaortic lymph node sampling: an evolving technique. *Am J Obstet Gynecol* **174**:1763–1768.
7 Downey GO, Potish RA, Adock LL, Prem KA, Twiggs LB (1989). Pre-treatment surgical staging in cervical carcinoma: therapeutic efficacy of pelvic lymph node resection. *Am J Obstet Gynecol* **160**:1056–1061.
8 Kadar N, Pelosi MA (1994). Laparoscopically assisted hysterectomy in women weighing 200 pounds or more. *Gynaecol Endosc* **3**:159–162.
9 Kadar N. Extraperitoneal hysterectomy for enlarged uteri. *Gynaecol Endosc.* (In press.)

10 Kadar N (1995). Laparoscopic surgery for gynaecologic malignancies in women aged 65 years or more. *Gynaecol Endosc* **4**:173–176.
11 Feroze R (1981). Radical vaginal operations. In: *Gynecologic Oncology*. Coppelson M, ed. Edinburgh: Churchill Livingstone, 840–853.
12 Massi G, Savino L, Susini T (1993). Schauta–Amreich vaginal hysterectomy and Wertheim–Meigs abdominal hysterectomy in the treatment of cervical cancer; a retrospective analysis. *Am J Obstet Gynecol* **168**:928–934.
13 Kadar N (1994). Laparoscopic radical vaginal hysterectomy: an operative technique and its evolution. *Gynaecol Endosc* **3**:109–122.
14 Winter R, Petru E, Haas J (1988). Pelvic and para-aortic lymphadenectomy in cervical cancer. In: Burghardt E, Monaghan JM, eds. *Operative Treatment of Cervical Cancer*. London: Ballière Tindall, 857–866.
15 Benedetti-Panici P, Scambia G, Baiocchi G, Greggi S, Mancuso S (1991). Technique and feasibility of radical para-aortic and pelvic lymphadenectomy for gynecologic malignancies. *Int J Gynecol Cancer* **1**:133–140.
16 Childers JM, Hatch K, Surwit EA (1992). The role of laparoscopic lymphadenectomy in the management of cervical carcinoma. *Gynecol Oncol* **47**:38–43.
17 Kadar N (1992). Laparoscopic pelvic lymphadenectomy for the treatment of gynecological malignancies: description of a technique. *Gynaecol Endosc* **1**:79–83.
18 Fowler JM, Carter JR, Carlson JW *et al* (1993). Lymph node yield from laparoscopic lymphadenectomy in cervical cancer: a comparative study. *Gynecol Oncol* **51**:187–192.
19 Kadar N (1995). Laparoscopic pelvic lymphadenectomy in obese women with gynecologic malignancies. *J Am Assoc Gynecol Laparoscopists* **2**:81–85.
20 Querleu D, Leblanc E, Castelain B (1991). Laparoscopic lymphadenectomy in the staging of early carcinoma of the cervix. *Am J Obstet Gynecol* **164**:579–581.
21 Wharton JT, Jones HW, Day TG, Rutledge FN, Fletcher GH (1977). Preirradiation celiotomy and extended field irradiation for invasive carcinoma of the cervix. *Obstet Gynecol* **49**:333–337.
22 Clarke-Pearson D, Cliby W, Soper J *et al* (1991). Morbidity and mortality of selective lymphadenectomy in early stage endometrial cancer. *Gynecol Oncol* **40**:168 (abstr).
23 Boike G, Lurain J, Burke J (1994). A comparison of laparoscopic management of endometrial cancer with traditional laparotomy. *Gynecol Oncol* **52**:105 (abstr).
24 Kadar N (1994). An operative technique for laparoscopic hysterectomy using a retroperitoneal approach. *J Am Assoc Gynecol Laparoscopists* **1**:365–377.
25 Casey AC, Farias-Eisner R, Pisani AL *et al* (1996). What is the role of reassessment laparoscopy in the management of gynecologic cancers in 1995? *Gynecol Oncol* **60**:454–461.
26 Childers JM, Lang J, Surwit EA, Hatch KD (1995). Laparoscopic staging of ovarian cancer. *Gynecol Oncol* **59**:25–33.
27 Parker WH (1992). Management of adnexal masses by operative laparoscopy: selection criteria. *J Reprod Med* **37**:603–606.
28 Parker WH (1995). The case for laparoscopic management of the adnexal mass. *Clin Obstet Gynecol* **38**:362–369.
29 Dembo AJ, Davy M, Stenwig AE, Berle EJ, Bush RS, Kjorstad AK (1990). Prognostic factors in patients with stage I epithelial ovarian cancer. *Obstet Gynecol* **75**:263–273.
30 Jacob JH, Gershenson DM, Morris M, Copeland LJ, Burke TW, Wharton JT (1991). Neoadjuvant chemotherapy and interval

debulking for advanced epithelial ovarian cancer. *Gynecol Oncol* **42**:146–150.

31 Schwartz PE, Chambers JT, Makuch R (1994). Neoadjuvant chemotherapy for advanced ovarian cancer. *Gynecol Oncol* **53**:33–37.

32 Kadar N (1998). The laparoscopic management of ovarian carcinoma: preliminary observations and suggested protocols. *Gynaecol Endosc* **7**:151–156.

33 Ben-Baruch G, Sivan E, Moran O *et al* (1996). Primary peritoneal serous papillary carcinoma: a study of 25 cases and comparison with stage III–IV ovarian papillary serous carcinoma. *Gynecol Oncol* **60**:393–396.

34 Maiman M, Seltzer V, Boyce J (1991). Laparoscopic excision of ovarian neoplasms subsequently found to be malignant. *Obstet Gynecol* **77**:563–565.

35 Gleeson NC, Nicosia SV, Mark JE, Hofman MS, Cavanagh D (1993). Abdominal wall metastases from ovarian cancer after laparoscopy. *Am J Obstet Gynecol* **169**:522–523.

36 Kindermann G, Massen V, Kuhn W (1995). Laparoskopisches 'Anoperieren' von ovariellen Malignomen. *Geburtshilfe Frauenheilk* **55**:687–694.

37 Sevelda P, Dittrich C, Salzer H (1989). Prognostic value of the rupture of the capsule in stage I epithelial ovarian carcinoma. *Gynecol Oncol* **35**:321–322.

38 Sjövall K, Nilson B, Einhorn N (1994). Different types of rupture of the tumor capsule and the impact on survival in early ovarian carcinoma. *Int J Gynecol Cancer* **4**:333–336.

39 Young RC, Walton LA, Ellenberg SS *et al* (1991). Adjuvant therapy in stage I and stage II epithelial ovarian cancer. Results of two prospective randomized trials. *N Engl J Med* **322**:1021–1027.

40 Einhorn N, Nilson B, Sjövall K (1985). Factors influencing survival in carcinoma of the ovary. *Cancer* **55**:2019–2025.

41 Nezhat F, Nezhat C, Welander CE, Benigno B (1992). Four ovarian cancers diagnosed during laparoscopic management of 1011 women with adnexal masses. *Am J Obstet Gynecol* **167**:790–796.

42 Vasilev SA, Schlaerth JB, Campeau J, Morrow CP (1988). Serum CA-125 levels in preoperative evaluation of pelvic masses. *Obstet Gynecol* **71**:751–756.

43 Kadar N (1995). Suprapubic microceliotomy: an aid to the morcellation of fibroid uteri weighing ≥2000 grams. *Gynaecol Endosc* **4**:63–65.

44 Pelosi MA, Pelosi MA (1996). Laparoscopic removal of a 103 pound tumor. *J Am Assoc Gynecol Laparoscopists* **3**:413–418.

45 McCartney AJ (1995). Using a vaginal tube to exteriorize lymph nodes during a laparoscopic pelvic lymphadenectomy. *Gynecol Oncol* **57**:304–306.

46 Kadar N, Homesley H, Malfetano J (1995). New perspectives on the indications for pelvic and para-aortic lymphadenectomy in the management of endometrial carcinoma: implications for laparoscopic management. *Gynaecol Endosc* **4**:109–118.

47 Childers JM, Aqua KA, Surwit EA, Hallum AV, Hatch KD (1994). Abdominal-wall tumor implantation after laparoscopy for malignant conditions. *Obstet Gynecol* **84**:765–769.

48 Kadar N (1997). Mechanism and prevention of port-site recurrences following laparoscopic treatment of gynecologic malignancies. *Br J Obstet Gynecol* **104**:1308–1313.

Index